T0132655

Chronic Rhinosinusitis

CLINICAL ALLERGY AND IMMUNOLOGY

Series Editors

MICHAEL A. KALINER, M.D.

Medical Director
Institute for Asthma and Allergy
Washington, D.C.

RICHARD F. LOCKEY, M.D.

Professor of Medicine, Pediatrics, and Public Health
Joy McCann Culverhouse Professor of Allergy and Immunology
Director, Division of Allergy and Immunology
University of South Florida College of Medicine
and James A. Haley Veterans Hospital
Tampa, Florida

Chronic Rhinosinusitis

Pathogenesis and Medical Management

Edited by

Daniel L. Hamilos

Massachusetts General Hospital
Harvard Medical School
Boston, Massachusetts, USA

Fuad M. Baroody

University of Chicago
Chicago, Illinois, USA

informa
healthcare

New York   London

Informa Healthcare USA, Inc.
52 Vanderbilt Avenue
New York, NY 10017

Library of Congress Cataloging-in-Publication Data

Chronic rhinosinusitis : pathogenesis and medical management / edited by
    Daniel L. Hamilos, Fuad M. Baroody.
      p. ; cm.–(Clinical allergy and immunology; 20)
    Includes bibliographical references and index
    ISBN-13: 978-0-8493-4052-9 (hb : alk. paper)
    ISBN-10: 0-8493-4052-7 (hb : alk. paper)
    1. Sinusitis. I. Hamilos, Daniel L. II. Baroody, M. Fuad III. Series.
    [DNLM: 1. Rhinitis. 2. Chronic Disease. 3. Sinusitis. W1 CL652 v.20 2007/WV
335 C557 2007]

    RF425.C47 2007
    616.2'1–dc22   2006103466

Visit the Informa web site at
www.informa.com

and the Informa Healthcare Web site at
www.informahealthcare.com

*This monograph is dedicated to our patients
who have inspired us, taught us, and given us purpose.*

Introduction

It was not too long ago when the treatment paradigm for chronic rhinosinusitis was a failure to respond to several courses of antibiotics, followed by surgery, which usually consisted of nasal-antral windows and/or a Caldwell-Luck procedure. Both procedures were developed many years ago and have been almost uniformly abandoned within the last 10 to 15 years. If physicians today are frustrated with the difficulty in managing chronic rhinosinusitis, they need only remember that the standards described above, although they seem to be ancient relative to our options today, were followed until very recently.

Yet even today the symptoms of chronic rhinosinusitis are not always well defined, it is still difficult to properly examine and assess the sinus cavities, and the treatments employed are often less than spectacular. Thus, it takes a specialist physician to diagnose and treat this chronic disorder. Rhinosinusitis is an exceptionally prevalent disease, and its frequency appears to be increasing. Not only is the disease disabling in its own right, it often complicates the ability to smell, taste, and hear, causes chronic cough and headache, and is a co-morbid condition for asthma. New understanding of rhinosinusitis has improved our knowledge of its pathophysiology, classification, symptoms, and signs, and has led to more effective medical and surgical treatments.

For these reasons, it is indeed a pleasure to welcome *Chronic Rhinosinusitis* as the 20th volume in the Clinical Allergy and Immunology Series. This work represents the combined talents of two outstanding leaders—one in the field of allergy/immunology and one in the field of otolaryngology—and their guidance has led to a wonderfully readable and important book. Thanks to Drs. Daniel Hamilos and Fuad Baroody for their creativity and hard work in bringing this fine book to publication. The authors are a "Who's Who" of leaders in this field, and the chapters included allow the reader to better understand the pathogenesis, diagnosis, and new and novel treatments for chronic rhinosinusitis.

The series of books that this volume joins is designed to translate basic science into clinical medicine. *Chronic Rhinosinusitis* continues this tradition. It should be of interest to both scientists and clinicians, and should be required reading for all physicians interested in rhinosinusitis, including those in family medicine, internal medicine, pediatrics, allergy, and otolaryngology. Each of the editors is pleased to welcome this new and worthwhile book.

Michael A. Kaliner, MD
Richard F. Lockey, MD

Preface

When Marcel Dekker, Inc., first contacted us about publishing a monograph on chronic rhinosinusitis, we were excited. It seemed that the timing was good for writing a book for clinicians focusing on medical management of this condition. In the interim, our publisher's name changed (it is now Informa Healthcare USA, Inc.) but our mission remained the same. A decision was made to invite experts across the globe and embrace the discipline broadly beginning with its clinical appearance, health care impacts, pathologic features, and emerging concepts regarding pathogenesis, and ending with its clinical management. A content list was prepared, authors were contacted, and we began working. Upon receiving all contributions, and after careful editing and some revisions, we have compiled a comprehensive review and state-of-the-art update on classification, pathophysiology, and management options for chronic rhinosinusitis. More than ever before, this exercise taught us how little we know, and how much still needs investigation. It also inspired us to search deeper for answers and novel insights into a condition that deserves more attention and better treatments.

To say chronic rhinosinusitis is complex is merely to acknowledge its heterogeneity and unknown causes. Research in this field has lagged behind other areas, such as asthma, owing in part to the fact that, although it is common, it rarely results in hospitalization or mortality. These facts are offset by the sheer magnitude of the problem. Allergists/immunologists devote 20% to 30% of their practice time caring for patients with rhinosinusitis (1), and this percentage is even higher for otolaryngologists.

At first glance, we seem to have advanced only modestly from the description of chronic rhinosinusitis offered by Noah Fabricant in 1942, or from Max Samter in 1961. Fabricant wrote:

> Repeated acute infections eventually lead to chronic infections of the nasal cavity and in the associated nasal sinuses. The changes in the individual layers of the mucous membranes vary considerably according to the severity and the duration of the infection. In chronic inflammatory processes the fundamental pathologic change is one of cellular proliferation. ... The epithelium is definitely thickened, and the degree of thickening is more pronounced in chronic nasal infection than in acute inflammatory processes or in allergy. The basement membrane is also markedly thickened. ... While the lymphocyte is the predominating cell, there are often large numbers of neutrophiles, monocytes, histiocytes, plasma cells, fibroblasts and a few eosinophils (2).

Max Samter described nasal polyp formation, discussing the involvement of polymorphonuclear cells, mast cells, and eosinophils in polyps, and the peculiar phenotype of "nasal polyps which form in middle-aged, nonallergic persons that experience acute exacerbation of hyperplastic changes of the nasal mucous membrane in response to small doses of acetylsalicylic acid" (3). He speculated that "a systematic search might uncover at least one enzyme system which might be inhibited in vitro by this drug."

Yet we are certainly making progress. And, in retrospect, the "gaps" in our knowledge base that may have once looked small now appear as vast expanses of information dealing with inflammatory pathways, cytokines, chemokines, growth factors, and enzymes that collectively orchestrate both acute and chronic inflammation and the tissue remodeling that accompanies or follows it.

This monograph highlights several concepts that have emerged or crystallized over the past decade. First is the greater appreciation for the role of eosinophilic (Th2-type) inflammation as a central feature not just in nasal polyps but more broadly in chronic rhinosinusitis. This observation, made by Harlin, Gleich, and colleagues (4) in 1988, continues to be a focal point for studies of chronic rhinosinusitis pathogenesis. The second is the observation that specific pathogens, such as colonizing fungi or, in the case of nasal polyposis, *Staphylococcus aureus*, may be a driving stimulus for chronic rhinosinusitis inflammation. The third is a growing appreciation for the importance of the innate host defense molecules in maintaining normal sinus health. Innate factors in nasal mucus were studied by Kaliner in the early 1990s (5). However, the science of host/microbial interactions expanded greatly over the past decade and is now poised to address critical questions about the role of defective innate immunity in human diseases such as chronic rhinosinusitis.

There has been an evolving consensus that the different phenotypes of chronic rhinosinusitis, namely chronic rhinosinusitis without nasal polyps, chronic rhinosinusitis with nasal polyps, and allergic fungal rhinosinusitis, represent distinct clinical syndromes and pathologic processes. Although this remains controversial, it provides an important framework for investigations and therapeutic interventions, and was adopted for use in this monograph. It is encouraging that interest in chronic rhinosinusitis is increasing. This is evidenced by several excellent consensus reports published over the past three years and increased funding for research from the National Institutes of Health over the past decade. The contributors to this monograph were carefully selected to showcase their involvement in these important initiatives.

The authors wish to thank the many contributors to this monograph whose unselfish contributions reflect their true passion for what they do. We thank our spouses and families for their forbearance during those many weekends when "the book" took priority over other duties. And we especially thank Ms. Sandra Beberman from Informa who first approached us with the idea for the monograph, and who patiently guided us through every step of the process. We reached this point in large part owing to her patience and encouragement.

We and our co-authors hope our goal of producing a monograph that improves the lives of patients with chronic rhinosinusitis will be realized. If that happens, even in some small way, our efforts will not have been in vain.

Daniel L. Hamilos
Fuad M. Baroody

REFERENCES

1. http://www.aaaai.org/patients/publicedmat/sinusitis/kindofdoctor.stm
2. Nasal Medication: A Practical Guide. ND Fabricant. The Williams & Wilkins Co., Baltimore, 1942.
3. Samter M. Nasal polyps: An inquiry into the mechanism of formation. Arch Otolaryngol 1961; 73:334–41.
4. Harlin SL, Ansel DG, Lane SR, Myers J, Kephart GM, Gleich GJ. A clinical and pathologic study of chronic sinusitis: the role of the eosinophil. J Allergy Clin Immunol. 1988; 81:867–75.
5. Kaliner MA. Human nasal host defense and sinusitis. J Allergy Clin Immunol. 1992 Sep; 90(3 Pt 2):424–30.

Contents

Contributors

Claus Bachert Upper Airway Research Laboratory, ENT-Department, University Hospital Ghent, Ghent, Belgium

James N. Baraniuk Georgetown University Proteomics Laboratory, Washington, D.C., U.S.A.

Fuad M. Baroody Section of Otolaryngology–Head and Neck Surgery, Departments of Surgery and Pediatrics, Pritzker School of Medicine, University of Chicago, Chicago, Illinois, U.S.A.

Itzhak Brook Georgetown University School of Medicine, Washington, D.C., U.S.A.

Begona Casado Georgetown University Proteomics Laboratory, Washington, D.C., U.S.A.

Marc G. Dubin Department of Otolaryngology–Head and Neck Surgery, Johns Hopkins University School of Medicine, Greater Baltimore Medical Center, Baltimore, Maryland, U.S.A.

Wytske Fokkens Department of Otorhinolaryngology, Academic Medical Centre, Amsterdam, The Netherlands

Susan Foley Meakins-Christie Laboratories, McGill University, Montreal, Quebec, Canada

Philippe Gevaert Upper Airway Research Laboratory, ENT-Department, University Hospital Ghent, Ghent, Belgium

Qutayba Hamid Meakins-Christie Laboratories, McGill University, Montreal, Quebec, Canada

Daniel L. Hamilos Division of Rheumatology, Allergy, and Immunology, Massachusetts General Hospital, Harvard Medical School, Boston, Massachusetts, U.S.A.

Michael A. Kaliner George Washington University Hospital, Chevy Chase, Maryland, U.S.A.

J. Kim Department of Otolaryngology–Head and Neck Surgery, Johns Hopkins University, Baltimore, Maryland, U.S.A.

Hirohito Kita Division of Allergic Diseases, Department of Internal Medicine, Mayo Clinic, Rochester, Minnesota, U.S.A.

Andrew P. Lane Department of Otolaryngology–Head and Neck Surgery, Johns Hopkins University, Baltimore, Maryland, U.S.A.

Kun Hee Lee Department of Otolaryngology, Nippon Medical School, Tokyo, Japan

Valerie J. Lund Professorial Unit, Institute of Laryngology and Otology, University College London, London, U.K.

Rodney Lusk Boys Town ENT Institute, Boys Town National Research Hospital, Omaha, Nebraska, U.S.A.

Mahmood F. Mafee Department of Radiology, University of California, San Diego, California, U.S.A.

Sonya Malekzadeh Department of Otolaryngology–Head and Neck Surgery, Georgetown University, Washington, D.C., U.S.A.

Christopher T. Melroy Georgia Nasal and Sinus Center, Savannah, Georgia, U.S.A.

Robert M. Naclerio Section of Otolaryngology–Head and Neck Surgery, Department of Surgery, University of Chicago, Chicago, Illinois, U.S.A.

Manabu Nonaka Department of Otolaryngology, Nippon Medical School, Tokyo, Japan

Joke Patou Upper Airway Research Laboratory, ENT-Department, University Hospital Ghent, Ghent, Belgium

Ruby Pawankar Department of Otolaryngology, Nippon Medical School, Tokyo, Japan

Jayant M. Pinto Section of Otolaryngology–Head and Neck Surgery, Department of Surgery, University of Chicago, Chicago, Illinois, U.S.A.

Jens U. Ponikau Department of Otorhinolaryngology, University at Buffalo, State University of New York, Buffalo, New York, U.S.A.

Mark D. Scarupa Institute for Asthma and Allergy, Johns Hopkins Asthma and Allergy Center, Chevy Chase, Maryland, U.S.A.

R. P. Schleimer Division of Allergy-Immunology, Northwestern University Feinberg School of Medicine, Chicago, Illinois, U.S.A.

Mark S. Schubert Department of Medicine, University of Arizona College of Medicine, and Allergy Asthma Clinic, Ltd., Phoenix, Arizona, U.S.A.

Brent A. Senior Department of Otolaryngology–Head and Neck Surgery, University of North Carolina Hospitals, Chapel Hill, North Carolina, U.S.A.

David A. Sherris Department of Otorhinolaryngology, University at Buffalo, State University of New York, Buffalo, New York, U.S.A.

Raymond G. Slavin Division of Allergy and Immunology, Department of Internal Medicine, St. Louis University School of Medicine, St. Louis, Missouri, U.S.A.

Ryuta Takizawa Department of Otolaryngology, Nippon Medical School, Tokyo, Japan

Paul van Cauwenberge Upper Airway Research Laboratory, ENT-Department, University Hospital Ghent, Ghent, Belgium

Thibaut van Zele Upper Airway Research Laboratory, ENT-Department, University Hospital Ghent, Ghent, Belgium

Nan Zhang Upper Airway Research Laboratory, ENT-Department, University Hospital Ghent, Ghent, Belgium, and ENT-Department, Zhongshan City Peoples Hospital, Zhongshan, Guangdong Province, China

1 Chronic Rhinosinusitis Patterns of Illness

Daniel L. Hamilos

Division of Rheumatology, Allergy, and Immunology, Massachusetts General Hospital, Harvard Medical School, Boston, Massachusetts, U.S.A.

INTRODUCTION

Clinicians experienced in treating chronic rhinosinusitis (CRS) recognize it as a syndrome rather than a single disease process. They also recognize that not everyone with complaints of "sinusitis" or a "sinus problem" actually has rhinosinusitis. There is considerable overlap of the symptoms of rhinosinusitis with other conditions, including allergic and nonallergic types of rhinitis, especially conditions associated with facial pain or headaches. Nonetheless, certain "patterns" of illness can be described within the syndrome of rhinosinusitis, and these provide some insight into the underlying causes of illness. This chapter describes these patterns based on clinical case series, including the results of an Outcomes Study performed at Washington University School of Medicine (WUSM) and the author's more recent experience at Massachusetts General Hospital (MGH). Understanding the pattern of illness can lead to more accurate diagnosis of causative and contributive factors in the disease and should ultimately translate to more effective therapies.

DEFINITION OF CRS

Chronic rhinosinusitis is defined as an inflammatory condition involving the paranasal sinuses as well as the lining of the nasal passages. The diagnosis of CRS with or without nasal polyposis requires that symptoms must be present for 12 weeks or longer despite attempts at medical therapy. There are four cardinal symptoms, namely: (i) anterior or posterior mucopurulent drainage or both; (ii) nasal congestion (or nasal blockage); (iii) facial pain/pressure/fullness; and (iv) decreased sense of smell. Generally, two or more of these symptoms must be present. In addition to compatible symptoms, objective documentation is required by direct visualization of the middle meatus through anterior rhinoscopy (after decongestion) or nasal endoscopy or by sinus radiographs to confirm the diagnosis of CRS. Bilateral nasal polyps (NP) present in the middle meatus are required to distinguish CRS with NP from CRS without NP. (Medical records documenting removal of bilateral NP during surgery would satisfy this requirement.) To satisfy the criteria for "allergic fungal rhinosinusitis" (AFRS), the patient must have CRS and evidence of sinus opacification with "allergic mucin" (inspissated mucus with degranulating eosinophils) also containing fungal hyphae as well as evidence of fungal specific IgE (by in vitro or skin testing). AFRS patients may also have sinus opacification that shows distinct hyperdensities on sinus computed tomography (CT) images and corresponding hypointensities on T2-weighted magnetic resonance images (MRI) (see Chapters 12 and 16).

PREVALENCE AND SPECIFICITY OF CRS SYMPTOMS
AND DIFFERENTIAL DIAGNOSIS
Cardinal Symptoms of CRS

The cardinal symptoms of CRS can also be seen in other diseases and should therefore be considered suggestive but not specific for CRS. The "differential diagnosis" of these symptoms will be discussed along with the prevalence of each in CRS patients.

Facial Pain, Facial Pressure, and Sinus Headache

The description of facial pain/pressure/headache ranges from vague and poorly localized to sharp and focal, with most patients describing vague discomfort (including "fullness" or "pressure") in the cheeks, above or below the eyes, or across the bridge of the nose. Many patients point to an area on the face that anatomically localizes to the ostiomeatal complex or unit (OMU) on one or both sides. Patients also frequently report "sinus headaches," but this symptom requires further refinement since it could signify anything from vague sinus pain/pressure to focal sharp pain or pulsatile vascular-type headaches. True sinus-related pain/ pressure or headaches may intensify as the patient bends forward, but even this symptom can have other causes. Less commonly, patients describe a more sharply localized pain in the right or left forehead, cheek, or temple, or pain in the upper teeth. Focal and sharp facial pain over one or more sinus areas may be rhinogenic in origin but is often unassociated with radiographic evidence of sinus disease and ultimately may be deemed a manifestation of "neurogenic" or "psychogenic" pain without more precise explanation for its cause despite further investigation. Pain in the upper teeth is suggestive of nerve irritation caused by an inflammatory process adjacent to tooth roots. This symptom is typically intermittent and associated with an increase in other symptoms, such as nasal purulence. Although it may be present in up to 5% of patients, an "odontogenic" cause for the pain is less commonly found. In the series reported by Bhattacharyya (1), facial pressure and headache were both reported by 83% of patients and dental pain was reported by 50% of patients (1).

Occasionally, symptoms suggesting "migraine" headaches may be attributed to a mucosal "contact point" between the nasal septum and the middle or superior turbinate or between the septum and the medial wall of the ethmoid sinus (2,3). Patients may have headaches in the absence of other symptoms of CRS and frequently have other symptoms suggestive of migraine headaches, such as pulsating headaches and photophobia (4). There is considerable debate over the prevalence of this condition and the means to establish it as a cause of headache. A contact point headache should be reproducibly relieved with local decongestion and anesthesia that relieves or anesthesizes the mucosal contact point on more than one occasion.

Facial pain/pressure have been shown to lack specificity with respect to predicting the presence of rhinosinusitis by other objective measures. In one study, headache and facial pain were much less predictive of the presence of sinusitis by nasal endoscopy or sinus CT scan than the symptoms of nasal obstruction or postnasal drip (5). In another study, patients' cumulative symptoms as recorded with the Sino-Nasal Outcome Test (SNOT-20) were found to lack correlation with sinus CT scoring by the Lund and Mackay method (6). Furthermore, endoscopy-negative, sinus CT-negative patients with facial pain were found to be unresponsive to medical treatment for sinusitis (7).

In the excellent case series report of West and Jones (7), out of 679 patients with sinonasal disease by rhinoscopy, endoscopy, or sinus CT, only 18% had facial pain. This prevalence, however, is an underestimate of facial pain in CRS because West and Jones' population also included patients with allergic or idiopathic rhinitis. In roughly one-third of the patients, the facial pain was felt to be incidental, and in these patients the facial pain failed to resolve despite either medical or surgical treatment of their sinonasal disease. The facial pain did respond to medical treatment directed at a neurologic cause, however. The breakdown of neurological causes of facial pain in patients with a normal sinus CT scan in this study ($N = 101$ patients) was: midfacial segment pain (35 patients), atypical facial pain (30 patients), tension headache (16 patients), migraine (10 patients), cluster headache (five patients), temporomandibular joint (TMJ) dysfunction (three patients), and trigeminal neuralgia (one patient). Interestingly, none of the patients in this series were felt to have contact point headaches, probably reflecting the fact that the authors dispute the existence of this condition. The distinguishing features of the other facial pain syndromes listed are summarized in Table 1.

Studies analyzing the relationship between headaches and rhinosinusitis have yielded widely disparate results suggesting that the studies themselves suffer from a certain degree of bias. Thus, in the study by Bhattacharyya, an otolaryngologist, 80% of patients diagnosed with CRS reported headaches, and the clinical impression was that this symptom was reflective of the underlying condition. In contrast, in the study of Schreiber et al. (11), which was conducted at multiple primary care sites, 2991 patients were enrolled if they had experienced at least six episodes of self-described or physician-diagnosed "sinus headaches" in the preceding 6 months. Patients were excluded if they had signs of nasal purulence or postnasal drainage with their self-described "sinus" headaches or if they had radiographic evidence of sinus infection in the previous 6 months. In this study, 80% of the patients were found to meet International Headache Society criteria for "migraine" headache and another 8% met criteria for "migrainous" headaches. Only a minority were felt to have rhinosinusitis. Whereas this study seems to highlight the common misdiagnosis of migraine headaches as "sinus" headaches, the results of the study should not be generalized to the population of CRS patients, since the study sought to exclude patients with obvious signs of CRS at entry and did not thoroughly exclude CRS in the study population by any objective diagnostic tests. In Tarabichi's study of 82 patients with CRS, 38% of patients with facial pain plus radiographic and endoscopic evidence of CRS had a persistence of facial pain 1 year following sinus surgery despite a lack of evidence for persistent sinus disease (12). The author concluded that roughly one-third of patients with facial pain underwent sinus sugery for a non-sinus indication. Perhaps it would be fairer to say that one-third of patients with facial pain and sinusitis failed to experience relief of facial pain despite surgical correction of their sinusitis.

The author's own experience lies somewhere in between these two extremes. In our Sinusitis Outcomes study, we found that patients with an initial complaint of facial pain/pressure had a poorer response to medical management compared to patients without this complaint (discussed on p. 7). Facial pain or pressure also correlated poorly with sinus CT scan findings. Of our 91 enrolled patients, 11 had a negative baseline sinus CT scan. Of these, 10 had either facial pain or facial pressure along with other CRS symptoms as part of their presenting symptom complex. Nonetheless, considering our entire patient population, a highly significant

TABLE 1 Most Common Causes of Non-rhinogenic Facial Pain and Their Distinguishing Clinical Features[a,b]

Syndrome	Typical clinical features	Ref.
Midfacial segment pain	Similar to tension headache but involves the middle of the face; symmetric; usually described as facial pressure. May involve the nose, cheeks or orbital regions in a symmetric fashion	Jones (8)
Atypical facial pain[c]	Throbbing pain situated deep in the eye and malar region, often radiating to the ear, neck, and shoulders. The pain generally is not confined to a dermatomal or anatomic boundary	Kanpolat et al. (9), ICHD (10)
	ICHD description: Persistent facial pain that does not have the characteristics of other cranial neuralgias. Present daily and usually present for all or most of the day. Confined at onset to a limited area on one side of the face, deep, and poorly localized. Not associated with sensory loss or other physical signs	
	Pain may be initiated by surgery or injury to the face, teeth, or gums but persists without any demonstrable local cause	
Tension headache	Infrequent, episodic or chronic headache lasting minutes to days. Typically bilateral, pressing or tightening in quality, of mild to moderate intensity, and it does not worsen with routine physical activity. There is no nausea but photophobia or phonophobia may be present	ICHD (10)
Migraine	Recurrent headache with attacks lasting 4–72 hr. Typically unilateral, pulsating, moderate or severe intensity, aggravation by routine physical activity, and association with nausea and/or photophobia and phonophobia.	ICHD (10)
Cluster headache	Severe, strictly unilateral pain which is orbital, supraorbital, temporal or in any combination of these sites, lasting 15–180 min and occurring from once every other day up to eight times a day. The attacks usually cause restlessness and agitation and are associated with one or more ipsilateral symptoms, including: conjunctival injection, lacrimation, nasal congestion, rhinorrhoea, forehead and facial sweating, miosis, ptosis, and eyelid edema	ICHD (10)
TMJ dysfunction	Recurrent facial pain in one or more regions of the head and/or face occurring in association with radiographic evidence of TMJ disease.	ICHD (10)
	Associated with at least one of the following:	
	Pain is precipitated by jaw movements and/or chewing of hard or tough food	
	Reduced range of or irregular jaw opening	
	Noise from one or both TMJs during jaw movements	
	Tenderness of the joint capsule(s) of one or both TMJs	
Trigeminal neuralgia	Unilateral and characterized by brief electric shock-like pains, abrupt in onset and termination, limited to the distribution of one or more divisions of the trigeminal nerve. Pain typically remits for variable periods	ICHD (10)

[a]In these conditions, nasal endoscopy and sinus CT scans are typically normal. Also, investigations including X-ray of the face and jaws do not demonstrate any relevant abnormalities (except in the case of TMJ dysfunction). However, these conditions can coexist with CRS, which leads to the difficulty in establishing an accurate diagnosis.

[b]The diagnosis of these conditions also requires that no other underlying disorder can be identified to cause the facial pain.

[c]The term atypical odontalgia has been applied to a continuous pain in the teeth or in a tooth socket after extraction in the absence of any identifiable dental cause (10).

Abbreviations: CT, computed tomography; ICHD, International Classification of Headache Disorders; TMJ, temporomandibular joint.

improvement in facial pain/pressure was reported by patients after medical treatment for their rhinosinusitis. Therefore, if other symptoms of CRS are present, it is worth considering that the patient's facial pain/pressure/headaches may have a rhinogenic component. If these symptoms fail to improve after treatment, other causes should certainly be sought.

The key point is that facial pain/pressure/headache may have multiple etiologies and are probably the least specific of the cardinal symptoms of CRS. Patients with facial pain/pressure/headache should be questioned further for diagnosing more precisely the underlying condition (see Table 1). Often, despite further questioning, the etiology of facial pain/pressure/headache remains difficult to establish. In such cases, improvement of the symptom complex in response to treatment of documented rhinosinusitis can be very helpful.

The disparity between the symptoms of facial pain/pressure and the extent of disease on sinus CT scan relates in part to the paucity of innervation in the sinus cavities and also to the causes for mucosal abnormalities. Some patients, particularly those with polypoid CRS, may have extensive sinus opacification in the absence of facial pain or facial pressure (13). This also underscores a limitation of CT scanning itself as well as the currently used radiologic scoring systems for CRS, insofar as they fail to differentiate "polypoid" mucosal thickening from "infectious" thickening or fluid accumulation in the sinuses, and they specifically fail to assess the significance of sinus ostial obstruction (with the exception of the OMU).

For the reasons outlined above, expert panels have recommended that the diagnosis of CRS not be made on the basis of a single major symptom of facial pain/pressure (14).

Anterior and/or Posterior Nasal Drainage

Other than CRS, anterior and/or posterior nasal drainage may be a symptom of seasonal or perennial allergic rhinitis, nonallergic idiopathic (orvasomotor) rhinitis, rhinitis medicamentosa and rhinitis associated with medication use. Other less common causes include cerebrospinal fluid (CSF) rhinorrhea, nasal and sinus secreting tumors, inverted papilloma, and nasal foreign bodies (typically unilateral, foul smelling drainage). The nature of the drainage is worth noting. Clear, watery rhinorrhea is most typically associated with allergic rhinitis, idiopathic rhinitis, rhinitis medicamentosa, rhinitis associated with medication use, or CSF rhinorrhea. Opaque white or colored drainage is more likely to represent "purulence" and is more likely to be associated with sinus pathology, including acute or chronic infection or chronic noninfectious inflammatory disease, including that seen in association with chronic rhinosinusitis without and with the nasal polyps (CRS without NP, CRS with NP), and AFRS. Thick, yellow, green, or brown mucus may be seen in recurrent acute rhinosinusitis or in refractory CRS cases, including cases of classic AFRS. Viral URIs may also cause discolored drainage, which may be difficult for the patient to differentiate from that caused by CRS. Some patients complain of greenish anterior or posterior drainage, particularly in the morning, despite a lack of endoscopic evidence of abnormal mucus or sinus pathology. Post-surgical patients may also have this complaint. In these cases, a negative endoscopic examination may be reassuring that the patient does not have a chronic infection.

Occasionally, the perception of mucus buildup in the throat may be a symptom of gastroesophageal reflux (GERD), particularly laryngopharyngeal reflux (LPR) (discussed in Chapter 17). In this case, other associated symptoms might include heartburn, chronic throat clearing and hoarseness (15).

Nasal Congestion (or Nasal Blockage)

Nasal congestion is often described by the patient as nasal blockage, stuffiness, or less commonly as nasal "fullness". The differential diagnosis of nasal congestion includes: allergic rhinitis, idiopathic rhinitis, rhinitis associated with medication use, CSF rhinorrhea, and "empty nose syndrome". Unilateral nasal congestion/blockage raises the question of a local anatomic problem or tumor, such as septal deviation or, less commonly, an antral choanal cyst.

Hyposmia, Anosmia, and Ageusia

Disturbance in the sense of smell may be perceived as a reduced or completely absent sense of smell (hyposmia or anosmia, respectively). Patients may also report a reduced ability to taste foods (ageusia). Less commonly, they may experience a reduced taste sensation with preservation in the sense of smell.

Minor CRS Criteria

Many published definitions for CRS have included "minor criteria" for the diagnosis, including headache, fever, halitosis, fatigue, dental pain, cough, and ear pain/pressure/fullness (16). In the consensus document of 1997, the presence of one major symptom and two or more minor symptoms satisfied the criteria for the diagnosis of CRS (16). However, facial pain alone could not be used as the sole major criterion to establish the diagnosis of CRS. A problem with the minor criteria is their lack of specificity for CRS, and recent consensus documents have not used them to define CRS (17). It is noteworthy that in the Bhattacharyya series fatigue was the most common minor symptom and was reported by 83% of CRS patients. Similarly, in our outcome study (see below), fatigue was the fourth most bothersome CRS symptom behind post-nasal discharge, thick nasal discharge and facial pain (18).

Importance of CRS Symptoms Based on SNOT-20 + 1 Survey

Another way to gauge the importance of CRS symptomatology is to ask patients to rate them on a severity scale from 0 (no bother) to 5 (as bad as can be) and to ask them to prioritize them from a list of symptoms. Both types of rating are included in the SNOT-20 instrument (see below). In our rhinosinusitis outcomes study, the SNOT-20+1, was completed at each patient's first visit to the clinic. The most frequent symptoms were: post-nasal drainage (96%), thick nasal discharge (93%), waking up tired (90%), and facial pain (86%). The most bothersome symptoms were: post-nasal discharge (42%), thick nasal discharge (41%), facial pain (40%), and fatigue (37%) (17).

CURRENT CRS CLASSIFICATION

A recent consensus conference classified CRS into three distinct subsets, including: CRS without NP, CRS with NP, and classic allergic fungal rhinosinusitis (AFRS) (17). Symptom criteria and minimal duration of illness (>12 weeks) are basically the same for each condition. An additional requirement for CRS with NP is the presence of bilateral NP visible in the middle meatus. There is an "intermediate" phenotype characterized by the presence of polypoid mucosa in one or more sinus areas or unilateral NP. We have used the term "polypoid CRS" to describe this subset (19). Although polypoid CRS is currently classified under CRS without NP, it may in fact represent an early stage of CRS with NP (20), and for this reason we feel it should be viewed differently. Nearly all patients with classic AFRS fall under the heading of CRS with NP but have additional distinguishing features of fungal involvement. These are reflected in the strict criteria for the diagnosis of classic AFRS, including documentation of the presence of "allergic mucin", fungal hyphae within the mucus, and fungal-specific IgE by skin testing or in vitro testing. Allergic mucin is defined as thick, inspissated mucus that contains sheets of eosinophils, often with signs of eosinophil degranulation. Classic AFRS is discussed in detail in Chapter 16. A more expansive view of fungal involvement in CRS is discussed in Chapter 11. The latter "fungal hypothesis" proposes a role for fungal hypersensitivity in CRS involving a modified Th2 response as central to the pathogenesis of CRS, regardless of subclassification.

The rationale for subcategorizing CRS into "without" and "with" NP was based primarily on studies showing different pathologic features in sinus tissue and middle turbinate biopsies from patients with the two conditions. These differences are discussed in Chapters 8 and 10.

CLINICAL FEATURES OF CRS IN THE WASHINGTON UNIVERSITY SCHOOL OF MEDICINE OUTCOMES STUDY

We conducted an outcomes study to evaluate the effects of medical management of CRS at WUSM in St. Louis, MO between November 1999 and June 2001. A total of 126 new patients referred to the ENT or Allergy/Immunology Clinic were enrolled, and 91 submitted sufficient data to assess outcomes over the one-year period. Patients with known humoral or cellular immune deficiency, cystic fibrosis, immotile cilia syndrome, or those who had undergone a Caldwell-Luc procedure were excluded from participation in this study. The patients received medical treatment determined by the judgment of the treating specialists and completed an extensive initial evaluation and monthly health status questionnaires assessing their symptoms and medication use. Patients were followed for 12 months. The SNOT-20 modified to include the symptom of "sense of smell" ("SNOT-20+1") was used as the primary outcome measure (18). A sinus CT scan was obtained at the beginning of the study and scored for extent of mucosal diseases (21).

In this study, the most frequent symptoms at presentation included postnasal drainage (96%), thick nasal discharge (93%), waking up tired (90%), and facial pain (86%). Although the symptom of nasal congestion was not captured, the related symptom of "need to blow nose" was reported with a prevalence of 68%. Hyposmia/anosmia was the least common of the cardinal CRS symptoms (22%); however, this symptom was often ranked as the most bothersome.

During the study, the most common treatments used were intranasal steroids (73%), intranasal saline (46%), and oral or intranasal antihistamines (35%). Oral antibiotics or systemic corticosteroids were prescribed based on the clinician's judgment after reviewing the clinical and endoscopic findings. Overall, the patients experienced a modest improvement in (SNOT-20+1) scores throughout the study ($\Delta = -0.60$) which, although significant ($P < 0.0001$), did not reach the predetermined level of a clinically meaningful effect (ΔSNOT-20+1 $= -0.80$). The most significant finding in the study was that the presence of baseline facial pain or pressure was negatively associated with outcome and did not correlate with the extent of disease by sinus CT scoring. The negative impact of facial pain or pressure in this study exemplifies a potential confounding effect of these symptoms on assessment of outcomes in CRS. As previously mentioned, facial pain or facial pressure lack specificity with respect to predicting the presence of rhinosinusitis by other objective measures. Other factors, including nasal discharge, hyposmia, cough, NP, and sinus CT stage, did not predict outcomes. Use of oral antibiotics or oral steroids was not associated with improved outcomes; however, given the limitations of the study, it was not possible to carefully assess each patient's response to these interventions.

CONTRASTING FEATURES OF CRS WITHOUT NP, POLYPOID CRS, AND CRS WITH NP

Each of the 126 patients enrolled in the WUSM Outcomes Study had a baseline sinus CT and underwent nasal endoscopy. Patients were classified as having CRS without NP, CRS with NP, or "polypoid CRS." Polypoid was defined as an area of raised edematous mucosa that appeared distinct from the adjacent normal mucosa. Polypoid changes were typically seen on the middle turbinate, in the post-operative ethmoid or maxillary sinus, or near the ostium of the sphenoid or posterior ethmoid sinus. The breakdown of patients in the three subgroups was: 67.5%, 16.7%, and 15.8%, respectively. The subgroups had overlapping but different symptom profiles (Fig. 1). Facial pain/pressure/headache was statistically more prevalent in CRS without NP than in CRS with NP. Nasal obstruction and hyposmia/anosmia were both more prevalent in CRS with NP. Polypoid CRS represented an intermediate phenotype. Furthermore, we found that polyp or polypoid changes were concordant (left and right side) in approximately 85% of patients, whereas, mucus/purulence was concordant in only about 50% of cases. This suggested that the "polyp/polypoid" phenotype was reflective of a diffuse rather than a localized inflammatory process.

A significant relationship was found between having undergone prior sinus surgery and the presence of either polyps or polypoid changes in both the middle meatus (MM)/OMU and superior meatus (SM) (P = 0.01 and 0.001, respectively). Both CRS with NP and polypoid CRS had a significantly higher rate of prior sinus

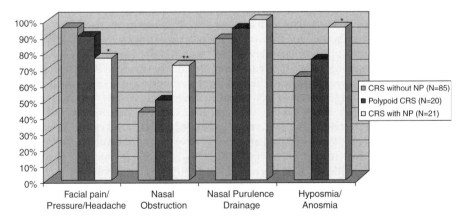

FIGURE 1 The breakdown of patients was 67.5%, 16.7%, and 15.8%, respectively. The subgroups had overlapping but different symptom profiles. *Source*: From Ref. 19.

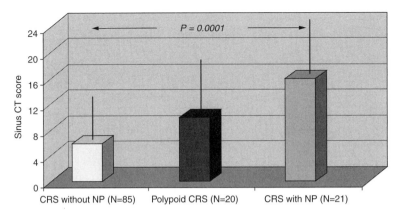

FIGURE 2 Sinus CT, comparison of CRS without NP, CRS with NP, and polypoid CRS. *Source*: From Ref. 19.

surgery and more severe disease on sinus CT compared to CRS without NP (Fig. 2). Positive allergy skin tests were found in 70% of patients tested (somewhat higher than in other published studies), with the most common positive tests being to perennial allergens including dust mite, molds, or animal danders. However, the prevalence of allergy was similar in each CRS category. By multivariate analysis, the factors most predictive of either polyp or polypoid phenotype were: prior sinus surgery (odds ratio = 28.3), high sinus CT scan score (OR = 1.16 for each unit of increase in CT score) and male gender (OR = 3.92). The combination of these three factors gave an 85% likelihood that the patient had either the polyp or polypoid phenotype.

PATTERNS OF ILLNESS IN CRS BASED ON MGH CASE SERIES

A total of 100 consecutive cases of CRS from the author's clinic at MGH in Boston, MA were reviewed for clinical features and underlying contributive factors to their illness. In this analysis, all patients with CRS were included to give a better appreciation of the frequency of conditions such as hypogammaglobulinemia, gram-negative infection, cystic fibrosis, and oral-antral fistula in a CRS referral population. Patients were classified according to the CRS classification system described above, and the results are summarized in Table 2.

In comparing CRS without NP and CRS with NP, several significant differences were noted. As in the WUSM Outcomes Study, male gender, previous sinus surgery, and hyposmia/anosmia were all more common in CRS with NP (although male gender failed to reach statistical significance). In addition, ongoing asthma, aspirin sensitivity, and suspected allergic AFRS were statistically more prevalent in CRS with NP. Again consistent with the WUSM Outcomes Study, facial pain and headache were more prevalent in CRS without NP.

In terms of medication use, four or more courses of antibiotics per year was more common in CRS without NP, whereas use of oral steroids more often than every four months was more frequent in CRS with NP. Furthermore, the pattern of chronic recurrent infection was found in 20% of the CRS without NP subgroup but was not found at all in the CRS with NP subgroup (P = 0.0017). Hypogammaglobulinemia was also more prevalent in CRS without NP, although this did not

TABLE 2 Demographic, Clinical, Allergic, Immunologic, and Microbial Differences Between CRS Without NP and CRS with NP Based on a Series of 100 Consecutive Patients Seen at MGH

	Characteristic	CRS without NP	CRS with NP	P-value for comparison of CRS without NP versus CRS with NP[e]
Demographics[a]	Percent of cases (N)	55	45	
	Sex (%female)	54.5	35.6	0.09
	Age	49.8	47.9	0.42
Clinical history	Duration of CRS symptoms	9.0	7.1	0.14
	Antecedent history of SAR	15/55	15/45	0.66
	Ongoing symptoms of SAR	13/55	13/45	0.71
	Previous surgery (%)	52.7	77.8	0.017
	Avg. no. surgeries/patient	0.89	1.27	0.09
	Ongoing asthma (%)	21.8	51.1	0.004
	Aspirin sensitivity (%)	1.8	17.8	0.015
	GERD (%)	14.5	13.3	0.91
% of cases with each symptom	Nasal congestion	72.7	80	0.54
	Anterior or posterior nasal drainage	85.4	73.3	0.21
	Facial pain	50.9	9.8	<0.0001
	Facial pressure	36.4	20.0	0.12
	Headache	29.1	11.1	0.05
	Localized headache	10.9	2.2	0.19
	Chronic cough	18.2	20.0	0.98
	Anosmia	29.1	82.2	<0.0001
	Ageusia	5.4	24.4	0.015
% with medication usage of each type[d]	Antibiotic use >4 times per year	52.7	24.4	0.008
	Use of oral steroids every >4 month	12.7	40.0	0.004
Pattern of illness	Chronic recurrent infection[b]	11 (20%)	0	0.0017[f]
Unusual bacterial infection	Gram-negative infection%	9.1	4.4	0.62[f]
	Staph aureus or MRSA (%)	0	4.4	0.40[f]
% of cases with positive allergy skin tests	Pollen allergy	32.7	33.3	0.88
	Dust mite allergy	21.8	46.7	0.016
	Mold allergy	21.8	40.0	0.079
Immune deficiency[c] (%)	IgA or IgM deficiency	5.4	0	0.32
	IgG or IgG subclass deficiency	10.9	2.2	0.19[f]
	Any hypogamm.	12.7	2.2	0.12[f]
Fungal disease (%)	Suspected allergic fungal rhinosinusitis	1.8	24.4	0.001[f]

[a]The ethnic breakdown of these patients was: Caucasian 91%, Hispanic/Latino/South American 4%, Asian 2%, African American 1%, Moroccan 1%, and Iranian 1%.
[b]Defined as having ≥ 4 episodes/year of acute rhinosinusitis exacerbations that respond to antibiotic treatment spaced between periods of wellness.
[c]Cystic fibrosis and ciliary dyskinesia syndrome were not represented in this CRS population. Two patients in the CRS without NP group experienced local complications, including one with an oral-antral fistula and one with osteomyelitis of the maxillary sinus. None of the patients had an underlying vasculitis (Wegener's, Churg-Strauss syndrome).
[d]Based on information obtained from patients at their initial visit to the clinic.
[e]Continuous variables were compared by Student's *t*-test. Dichotomous variables were compared using chi-square analysis unless otherwise indicated.
[f]By Fisher exact test.

reach statistical significance. These features suggest that defects in either systemic or local immune function play a greater role in CRS without NP than in CRS with NP. In contrast, the prevalence of infection with either a gram-negative bacteria or *Staphylococcus aureus* was not statistically different in these two subgroups.

The prevalence of pollen allergy was no different in CRS without NP and CRS with NP. However, allergy to house dust mite was more prevalent in patients with CRS with NP.

IMPACT OF CRS PHENOTYPE ON RESPONSE TO MEDICAL OR SURGICAL TREATMENT

Previous reports also suggested that patients with CRS without NP and CRS with NP respond differently to surgical and medical management. Specifically, Senior et al. found that patients with "advanced mucosal disease" were more likely to show persistence of mucosal disease following functional endoscopic sinus surgery, and these same patients were more likely to undergo revision surgery (22). Stankiewicz (23) and Deal and Kountakis (24) similarly showed that the presence of NP or polypoid rhinosinusitis had a negative impact on CRS surgical outcomes. In the latter study of 201 patients, CRS with NP patients had more severe symptoms, higher SNOT-20 scores prior to surgery, less improvement with sinus surgery, and a higher rate of repeat sinus surgery. Similarly, our group found that symptomatic relapses of CRS following intensive medical treatment occurred sooner in patients with current or past NP (25). In that study, patients were assessed for relapses after receiving a combination of oral antibiotics and oral corticosteroids designed to eradicate infection and control mucosal inflammation. Thus, there are important differences in the natural history of patients classified as CRS without NP and CRS with NP with the latter representing the more severe and refractory subclass.

CONCEPTUAL CLINICAL FRAMEWORK—FORMULATION OF THE "CRS MATRIX"

The results from the WUSM CRS Outcomes Study and the MGH case series are in general agreement and illustrate several important clinical differences between CRS without NP and CRS with NP. Conceptually, these can be summarized in terms of a "CRS matrix" illustrating the relative tendency of clinical factors to associate with either phenotype (Fig. 3).

SUMMARY

Chronic rhinosinusitis is a complex, multifactorial illness that has genetic, infectious, immune, anatomic, allergic, and inflammatory components. The syndrome is defined based on imprecise symptoms that lack specificity for the condition. Nonetheless, certain relatively characteristic patterns of illness can be identified within the syndrome, and these provide some insight into the underlying cause(s) of CRS. Furthermore, they form a basis for the clinical assessment and management of patients. In general, CRS without NP is a more heterogeneous subgroup of patients more likely to have facial pain, headache, chronic recurrent infection, defects in systemic or local immune function, and more likely to experience local infectious complications, such as facial osteomyelitis. In contrast, CRS with NP patients are more likely to have male gender, anosmia/hyposmia, a history of

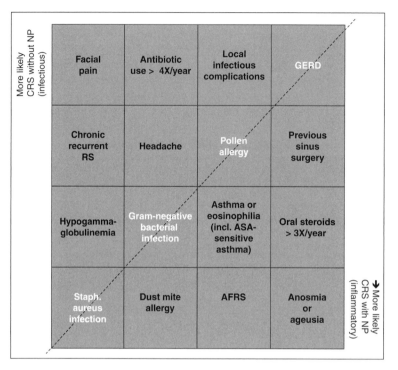

FIGURE 3 (*See color insert.*) Clinical/pathologic matrix of symptoms and clinical features associated with CRS without NP or CRS with NP. The symptoms and clinical features shown toward the upper left corner of the matrix are statistically more common in CRS without NP. In contrast, the symptoms and clinical features shown toward the lower right corner of the matrix are statistically more common in CRS with NP. Clinical features shown on the dotted line do not distinguish CRS without NP from CRS with NP. See text for details.

prior sinus surgery, asthma and aspirin sensitivity, allergy to house dust mite, and AFRS. In the next 17 chapters, an in-depth discussion of factors contributing to the pathophysiology of CRS will be presented that will provide further insight into the clinical patterns of illness described herein. Armed with this information plus the clinical framework outlined in this chapter, a stepwise medical evaluation and treatment strategy will be presented in Chapter 19.

REFERENCES

1. Bhattacharyya N. The economic burden and symptom manifestations of chronic rhinosinusitis. Am J Rhinol 2003; 17:27–32.
2. Behin F, Behin B, Behin D, Baredes S. Surgical management of contact point headaches. Headache 2005; 45:204–10.
3. Parsons DS, Batra PS. Functional endoscopic sinus surgical outcomes for contact point headaches. Laryngoscope 1998; 108:696–702.
4. Behin F, Behin B, Bigal ME, Lipton RB. Surgical treatment of patients with refractory migraine headaches and intranasal contact points. Cephalalgia 2005; 25:439–43.
5. Rosbe KW, Jones KR. Usefulness of patient symptoms and nasal endoscopy in the diagnosis of chronic sinusitis. Am J Rhinol 1998; 12:167–71.

6. Bhattacharyya T, Piccirillo J, Wippold FJ. Relationship between patient-based descriptions of sinusitis and paranasal sinus computed tomographic findings. Arch Otol Head Neck Surg 1997; 123:1189–92.
7. West B, Jones NS. Endoscopy-negative, computed tomography-negative facial pain in a nasal clinic. Laryngoscope 2001; 111:581–6.
8. Jones NS. Midfacial segment pain: implications for rhinitis and sinusitis. Curr Allergy Asthma Rep 2004; 4:187–92.
9. Kanpolat Y, Savas A, Ugur HC, Bozkurt M. The trigeminal tract and nucleus procedures in treatment of atypical facial pain. Surg Neurol 2005; (64 Suppl 2):S96–100; discussion S100–1.
10. ICHD. The International Classification of Headache Disorders, 2nd Ed., 1st revision, 2005. Accessed August 2006 at http://www.i-h-s.org/ (under "Guidelines").
11. Schreiber CP, Hutchinson S, Webster CJ, Ames M, Richardson MS, Powers C. Prevalence of migraine in patients with a history of self-reported or physician-diagnosed "sinus" headache. Arch Intern Med 2004; 164(16):1769–72.
12. Tarabichi M. Characteristics of sinus-related pain. Otolaryngol Head Neck Surg 2000; 122:842–7.
13. DelGaudio JM, Wise SK, Wise JC. Association of radiological evidence of frontal sinus disease with the presence of frontal pain. Am J Rhinol 2005; 19:167–73.
14. Benninger MS, Ferguson BJ, Hadley JA, et al. Adult chronic rhinosinusitis: definitions, diagnosis, epidemiology, and pathophysiology. Otolaryngol Head Neck Surg 2003; 129 (3 Suppl.):S1–32.
15. Ozturk O, Oz F, Karakullukcu B, Oghan F, Guclu E, Ada M. Hoarseness and laryngopharyngeal reflux: a cause and effect relationship or coincidence? Eur Arch Otorhinolaryngol 2006 Jul 1; 17 [Epub ahead of print].
16. Lanza DC, Kennedy DW. Adult rhinosinusitis defined. Otolaryngol Head Neck Surg 1997; 117(3 Pt 2):S1–7.
17. Hessler JL, Piccirillo JF, Fang D, et al. Clinical outcomes of chronic rhinosinusitis in response to medical therapy: results of a prospective study. Am J Rhinol. 2007; 21(1):10–18.
18. Meltzer EO, Hamilos DL, Hadley JA, et al. Rhinosinusitis: establishing definitions for clinical research and patient care. Published simultaneously in the J Allergy Clinical Immunol 2004; 114(6 Suppl):155–212 and Otolaryngol Head Neck Surg 2004; 131 (6 Suppl.):S1–62.
19. Banerji A, Piccirillo JF, Thawley SE, et al. Chronic rhinosinusitis patients with polyps or polypoid mucosa have a greater burden of illness. Am J Rhinol 2007 Jan-Feb; 21(1):19–26.
20. Bachert C, Gevaert P, Holtappels G, Cuvelier C, van Cauwenberge P. Nasal polyposis: from cytokines to growth. Am J Rhinol 2000; 14:279–90.
21. Lund VJ, Mackay IS. Staging in rhinosinusitis. Rhinology 31:183–4.
22. Senior BA, Kennedy DW, Tanabodee J, et al. Long-term results of functional endoscopic sinus surgery. Laryngoscope 1998; 108:151–7.
23. Stankiewicz JA. Management of endoscopic sinus surgery failures. Cur Opin Otolaryngol Head Neck Surg 2001; 9:48–52.
24. Deal RT, Kountakis SE. Significance of nasal polyps in chronic rhinosinusitis: Symptoms and surgical outcomes. Laryngoscope 2004; 114:1932–5.
25. Subramanian HN, Schechtman KB, Hamilos DL. A retrospective analysis of treatment outcomes and time to relapse after intensive medical treatment for chronic sinusitis. Am J Rhinol 2002; 16:303–12.
26. Bhattacharyya N. Clinical and symptom criteria for the accurate diagnosis of chronic rhinosinusitis. Laryngoscope 2006; 116(7 Suppl. Part 2):1–22.
27. Giacomini PG, Alessandrini M, DePadova A. Septoturbinal surgery in contact point headache syndrome: long-term results. Cranio 2003; 21:130–5.
28. Pinto A, De Rossi SS, McQuone S, Sollecito TP. Nasal mucosal headache presenting as orofacial pain: a review of the literature and a case report. Oral Surg Oral Med Oral Pathol Oral Radiol Endod 2001; 92:180–3.

2 Impact of Chronic Rhinosinusitis on Quality of Life and Health Care Expenditure

Valerie J. Lund
Professorial Unit, Institute of Laryngology and Otology, University College London, London, U.K.

INCIDENCE

Chronic rhinosinusitis (CRS) is estimated to affect 5–15% of the urban population (1). Its estimated prevalence of 146:1000 of the population exceeds that of any other chronic condition in patients below the age of 45 (2). As one of the more common conditions seen by primary care physicians and specialists alike, it is surprising that even the definition and classification of the condition have remained a source of debate (3). It would appear that one-third to one half of all patients seen by family practitioners suffer from some form of rhinosinusitis, and this figure appears to be rising (3). Relatively little data are available from Europe, though epidemiology initiatives through the European Academy of Allergy and Clinical Immunology hope to address this need in the near future (4). As an indication, a recent Danish study shows nasal polyposis, which is often included in the generic term CRS, has an overall estimated symptomatic incidence of 0.63 patients per 1000 per year (5).

FINANCIAL COSTS
Direct Costs

It is clear from quality of life (QOL) studies that CRS carries a major impact on general well being and thus is associated with major socio-economic costs, again, published data are sparse but Ray et al. (6) estimated the total direct cost of treating sinusitis to be $5.78 billion in the United States, a figure extrapolated from government surveys such as the National Healthcare Survey and Medical Expenditure Data. The cost of physician visits alone, without taking account of investigation or treatment, was an estimated $3.39 billion. Other North American studies from both Canada and United States have underscored the impact of rhinosinusitis on healthcare delivery in general (7,8).

Murphy et al. (9) evaluated the cost of CRS in a single health maintenance organization (HMO) comparing the costs of health care for members with this diagnosis to those without during 1994. In this study, patients with CRS made 43% more outpatient and 25% more urgent care visits than the general population (P = 0.001) and filled 43% more prescriptions. Ultimately, the total cost of treatment was 6% more than that for the average adult in the HMO, or $206 per year, which included the costs of imaging, medication, and hospitalization. Based on the 1994 statistic of just under 21 million individuals seeking care for CRS, this results in a calculated annual direct cost of $4.3 billion. If the figure of those affected is closer to 32 million as indicated by Blackwell and Coles (10) the annual sum would increase to a massive $6.59 billion. It is also worth remembering that rhinosinusitis is often associated with co-morbidities such as asthma, otitis media, and allergic rhinitis. Ray et al. (6) suggested that 10–15% of the cost of these other diseases could be attributable to rhinosinusitis, thus increasing their estimate from $5.78 billion to close to this figure.

Many consensus guidelines have been published outlining the medical management of CRS. These have recommended a wide range of treatments, notably antibiotics and corticosteroids (11,12). An evaluation of CRS treatment in the USA revealed that patients with CRS received an average of 2.7 antibiotic courses, nasal steroids for 18.3 weeks, and prescription antihistamines for 16.3 weeks during a 12-month period despite a considerable paucity of evidence to support their clinical effectiveness. Gliklich and Metson (13) reported an annual expenditure of $1220 per person comprising over-the-counter medications ($198), nasal sprays ($250), and antibiotics ($772). Again, little evidence is available from Europe though a study from Holland looked at the costs of treatment in refractory CRS (14) estimating direct costs to be €1861 per year. This has resulted in an estimate of between 200 and 2000 Euros as an average of the annual direct costs of CRS per patient (4).

Indirect Costs

When the indirect costs of absenteeism and reduced productivity are factored into the equation, the total cost of CRS increases considerably particularly in light of the fact that the majority of patients are of employable age (between 18 and 65 years) (10). As in allergic rhinitis, health economic models may be used to estimate this cost. An alternative is to track insurance claims through employee health insurance looking at time off work and short-term disability claims which give a more accurate indication of the correlation with a particular disease. In a large sample size of 375,000, total healthcare payments were found to be $60.17 per employee per year for both acute and (CRS), just under half of this cost coming from absenteeism and disability (8). As a consequence of this study, rhinosinusitis was named one of the top ten most costly health conditions to US employers (8).

Bhattacharyya (15) calculated the cost of treating CRS per patient at $1539 per year based on patient-completed surveys assessing symptoms, medication use, and days off work attributable to this condition. Of this sum, 40% was attributable to missed work with an average of 4.8 missed work days per year in this cohort of 322 patients. Using this estimate, the annual cost of CRS in the USA could be as great as $47 billion, although this is almost certainly an overestimate as it considers the more severe cases who have required referral to an otolaryngologist.

If the effects of decreased productivity are considered, the 1994 National Health Interview Survey (6) estimated that in addition to 12.5 million work days lost due to rhinosinusitis there were an additional 58.7 million days of restricted activity providing an additional economic loss.

QUALITY OF LIFE
Methods of Assessing Quality of Life

Objective assessment of nose and sinus disease has proved difficult, partly due to a paucity of validated techniques and partly due to the dynamic nature of the area. Even semi-quantitative assessment of symptoms using visual analog scores can only really be applied on an individual basis to demonstrate sequential change (16). However, there is a growing awareness that from a patient's perspective the impact of the disease on daily functioning is of considerable relevance, and during the last decade attention has been paid not only to symptoms but also to patient's

QOL (17). However, it is of interest that the severity of nasal symptoms does not always correlate with QOL scales (18) and correlations between conventional clinical markers of nasal inflammation and a patient's rhinoconjunctivitis-specific QOL are only weak to moderate (19,20).

Quality of life may be measured as the difference, or gap, between expectation and experience (21). Health-related quality of life (HRQL) is the component of overall QOL that is determined primarily by the patient's health and that can be influenced by clinical intervention. Specifically it has been characterized as "the functional effects of an illness and its consequent therapy upon a patient as perceived by the patient" (22). Traditionally, medicine has relied on assessment of change using laboratory or clinical tests, but HRQL is increasingly recognized as an important alternative outcome measure. HRQL measurement has been used in a wide range of medical conditions including rheumatoid arthritis, vascular disease, and respiratory tract diseases such as asthma and cystic fibrosis, but only relatively recently has it been applied to sinonasal disease. QOL questionnaires can provide either general, generic, or disease-specific health assessments.

General Health Status Instruments

Generic measurements enable the comparison of patients suffering from CRS with other patient groups. Of these the Medical Outcomes Study Short Form 36 (SF36) (23) is by far the most widely used and well validated. This instrument has been used both pre- and postoperatively in CRS (24,25). It includes eight domains: physical functioning, role functioning physical, bodily pain, general health, vitality, social functioning, role-functioning emotional, and mental health. Many other generic measurements are also available (26). These include the European Quality of Life Measure (EuroQol 1996), Nottingham Health Profile (27), and the Sickness Impact Profile (28).

The advantage of generic instruments such as the SF-36 is that the impact of illness can be compared between different medical conditions. However, being broad, they lack depth and cannot encompass individual weighting of specific domains that may be of greater importance to the patient. Consequently different results may be obtained after the same intervention in the same patient cohort. Klassen et al. (29) found markedly different results in the same patients undergoing cosmetic rhinoplasty using the SF-36 and EuroQol measures.

This has led to the development of individualized measures of QOL that are receiving increased attention but also have their own intrinsic problems (30). Some, such as the Schedule for the Evaluation of Individualized Quality of Life (31) and the Patient Generated Index (32) are administered by an interviewer and use visual analog scales to assess the five areas which the patient identifies as being the most important to them. However, both the completion and analysis of these assessments can be quite complex, and their applicability in severely ill patients may be limited. There is clearly a need for multilingual and multidimensional QOL assessments which are sensitive to the importance of certain areas on an individual basis.

Disease-Specific Health Status Instruments

Several disease-specific questionnaires for evaluation of QOL in CRS have been published. In these questionnaires, specific symptoms for rhinosinusitis are included. Such areas include headache, facial pain or pressure, nasal discharge or postnasal drip, and nasal congestion.

Rhinosinusitis Outcome Measure (RSOM)
This instrument contains 31 items classified into seven domains and takes approximately 20 minutes to complete (33). A modified instrument referred to as the Sinonasal Outcome Test-20 (SNOT-20) is validated, easy to use and allows patients to identify their most important symptoms (34). This has been used in a number of studies, both medical and surgical (24,35).

The Sinonasal Outcome Test 16 (SNOT-16) is also a rhinosinusitis-specific QOL health-related instrument (36) as is the 11-point Sinonasal Assessment Questionnaire (SNAQ-11) (37).

Chronic Sinusitis Survey (CSS)
This is a six-item duration-based monitor of sinusitis-specific outcomes which has both systemic and medication-based sections (38). In common with other disease-specific questionnaires, it is better at determining the relative impact of CRS compared to other diseases than as a measure of improvement following therapeutic intervention, but can be a useful tool (17,39).

Rhinosinusitis Disability Index
In this 30-item questionnaire the patient is asked to relate nasal and sinus symptoms to specific limitations on daily functioning (40,41). It is similar to the RSOM 31 in the types of questions contained. It can be completed easily and quickly but does not allow the patient to indicate their most important symptoms. It also contains some general questions similar to the SF-36.

The CRS Type Specific Questionnaire
This test contains three forms. Form 1 collects data on nasal and sinus symptoms prior to treatment, form 2 collects data on the clinical classification of sinus disease and form 3 collects data on nasal and sinus symptoms after sinus surgery. Though it is somewhat time consuming to complete, Hoffman et al. used this instrument in combination with an SF-36 to look at CRS patient outcomes after sinus surgery (42).

Rhinoconjunctivitis Quality of Life Questionnaire
This is the best-validated questionnaire for allergic conditions in the upper respiratory tract. However, it specifically focuses on allergy and is therefore of less relevance to CRS and nasal polyposis (20).

Utilities
A further refinement popular with health economists is the measurement of utilities. The utilities represent the value that either patients or society place on various health states. From these, quality-adjusted life years (43) may be derived but there are difficulties in applying these measurements to non-life threatening conditions such as rhinitis or rhinosinusitis.

Rhinitis Symptom Utility Index (RSUI)
An RSUI (44) has been developed in an attempt to measure the value that society places on the condition. It consists of 10 questions on the severity and frequency

of ENT symptoms with an algorithm based on societal responses to various nasal and ocular symptom occasions or events using the Standard Gamble and Rating scale (43). However, this does not take into account the value patients place on rhinitis-induced QOL impairment such as sleep disturbance.

The RSUI consists of 10 questions on the severity and frequency of a stuffy or blocked nose, runny nose, sneezing, itching, watery eyes, and itching nose or throat. The two-week reproducibility of the RSUI was weak, probably reflecting the day-to-day variability of rhinitis (44).

Symptom Scoring

In this self-administered test, patients mark on a 10-cm line (between 0 and 10) where symptom severity falls for five sinonasal symptoms (facial pain or pressure, headache, nasal blockage or congestion, nasal discharge, and olfactory disturbance; 10 indicates the greatest severity) (16). The relative length from the origin of the line is measured and rounded to the nearest integer. Patients are also asked to rank in order of severity their three worst symptoms allowing distinction between symptoms given the same visual analog score.

Most questionnaires concentrate on the duration of the symptoms and not on the severity of the symptoms. A QOL questionnaire developed by Damm et al. includes a severity rating of the symptom scale (45). The domains in the questionnaire are the overall QOL, nasal breathing obstruction, post-nasal drip or discharge, dry mucosa, smell, headache, and asthmatic complaints.

Limitations of QOL Instruments

There are problems regarding the reporting of QOL studies (46,47). These include the use of unfamiliar scales, failure to explain the clinical importance of the instrument, failure to describe a minimal clinically important difference, failure to differentiate between inferences for individuals and for individuals versus groups, documenting the responsiveness to change, identifying the sample size requirements and statistical power and the use of multiple QOL end points. Establishing a "minimal clinically important difference" in terms of a QOL measure helps assure that measured changes have clinical relevance. Anchor-based strategies have been developed for this purpose (47).

When choosing which QOL measure to use, the following criteria should be considered:

1. Demonstrated test/retest reliability
2. Validity (i.e., whether the test measures what it purports to measure)
3. Responsiveness to change
4. Ease of interpretability of the results
5. Degree of respondent burden
6. Intended purpose of the outcome measure

Ultimately, one's choice of a QOL measure for CRS also depends on one's own prejudice and experience. The instruments discussed above are easy to use, and the point is that one should be selected for use rather than not selecting one at all. Utility tests have not caught on yet in surgical research but Visual Analog Scoring is a well-established method of sequential semi-quantitative monitoring of symptom severity and my most frequently used method of patient assessment. It does not, however, consider QOL, per se.

Impact of CRS on Quality of Life

Using a generic SF-36 survey, patients with CRS were compared with a healthy population in Canada and demonstrated to have a statistically significant difference in seven of the eight domains (48). Gliklich and Metson (49) also demonstrated that patients with CRS had significantly worse scores for social functioning, body pain, vitality and general health when compared with the general population, with impairments similar to those experienced by patients with back pain, chronic obstructive pulmonary disease, and angina. Winstead and Barnett (25) found similar results as did Khalid et al. (49) in a long-term QOL study after endoscopic sinus surgery (ESS).

Radenne et al. (18) looked specifically at nasal polyposis with the SF-36 and showed a greater impairment in QOL than with perennial rhinitis. This, in tandem with symptoms, was significantly improved by endoscopic surgery. Similar findings have been reported by Alobid et al. (51) when compared with the normal Spanish population.

Improvement in Quality of Life from Medical and Surgical Treatment

Although CRS has a significant impact on general well-being, its very chronicity may mitigate against demonstration of dramatic improvement with therapeutic intervention when compared with seasonal allergic rhinitis (51). Nonetheless, several surgical studies have been able to show significant change. In the Winstead and Barnett (25) study, a return to normality in all eight domains of the SF-36 was shown at six months post-operatively, and was maintained at 12 months. Similar improvements were shown by Gliklich and Metson (39) with significant improvement to near normative levels in general health status occurring in six of the eight categories. Significant improvements in symptoms and medication requirements were also demonstrated.

In a recent prospective study using the SF-36 in 150 patients with CRS, a significant improvement in all six of the eight domains initially affected was demonstrated at a mean of three years follow-up after functional ESS. QOL scores returned to within the published norms for the general population (50).

Disease-specific questionnaires may be more sensitive as shown in another study by Damm et al. (45). Three-quarters of the patients reported relief of symptoms after ESS. Metson and Gliklich (53) using the CSS demonstrated a significant improvement in symptoms of pain, congestion and mucous drainage as well as use of medications one year after endoscopic frontal sinus surgery. Improvements following surgery were not exclusive to ESS, however; and the CSS was also used to assess patients after osteoplastic frontal sinus obliteration (54) confirming improvement in patient scores, reduction in clinic visits, and medication usage.

The Royal College of Surgeons of England's National Comparative Audit of Surgery for Nasal Polyposis and CRS utilized a slightly modified SNOT-20 (SNOT-22) as the main outcome measure to assess over 3000 patients undergoing surgery. Interestingly in this study females reported higher preoperative SNOT-22 scores than men despite less extensive disease on cross-sectional imaging. This gender difference has been found with other QOL assessment tools such as the SF-36 and may represent a systematic difference in response style rather than a reflection of underlying disease severity (55). There was a small but significant difference between the polyp and non-polyp patients with preoperative symptoms higher in the polyp patients. Older patients (>60 years) had lower preoperative SNOT-22 scores in those patients undergoing polypectomy. However, there was a small increase in preoperative scores in patients with increased stages of polyposis, though, as anticipated, the correlation with the computerized tomography (CT) score was poor. Patients who had suffered their sinonasal symptoms for longer periods and those who had undergone previous surgery reported significantly higher pre-operative scores. The patients who were smokers or asthmatic had higher scores compared to patients without these risk factors. The patients underwent a range of surgical procedures from simple polypectomy to complete endoscopic clearance of the sinuses. Irrespective of the surgical procedure, there was an overall high level of satisfaction with the surgery, and clinically significant improvement in the SNOT-22 scores at 3 and 12 months that was generally maintained up to three years.

Fewer studies have been performed to assess QOL responses to medical treatment in CRS. In a recent prospective study of patients with CRS and/or nasal polyps, patients were randomized to either ESS or three months' treatment with a macrolide antibiotic such as erythromycin (24). The patients were followed up at 6 and 12 months with a variety of parameters including visual analog scores of nasal symptoms, SNOT-20, SF-36, nitric oxide measurements of both the upper and lower respiratory tract expired air, acoustic rhinometry, saccharin clearance, and nasal endoscopy. Ninety patients were randomized with 45 in each arm; at the end of one year 38 were available for analysis in the medical arm and 40 in the surgical arm. The study demonstrated a significant improvement in all subjective and objective parameters but there was no difference between the medical and surgical groups except that total nasal volume as measured by acoustic rhinometry was greater in the surgical group. Uri et al. (56) considered both lower and upper respiratory tract symptoms in patients with massive nasal polyposis and demonstrated both subjective and objective improvement including QOL following sinus surgery.

Improvement in QOL with both medical and surgical treatment was also shown in a cohort of 109 patients with polyps using SF-36 with one year follow-up (51). Although van Agthoven et al. were able to demonstrate improvement in QOL in refractory CRS treated with filgrastim, it was not possible to show improvement in QOL when less severe patients were treated with three months of topical budesonide, despite improvement by objective airway assessment and symptom scores (57). Aside from these studies, there have been few prospective studies assessing the effects of medical treatment on qualify of life in CRS patients (58). In large part, this reflects the lack of studies of medical treatment for this condition.

CONCLUSION

Chronic rhinosinusitis is one of the most common chronic health problems and is associated with a huge socio-economic cost and impact on patient's perception of well-being and functional status. Its impact on QOL has only recently been appreciated and examined in the context of surgical or medical management. Going forward, QOL assessment should be regarded as an invaluable tool for measurement of patients' outcomes that should be incorporated in most, if not all, future clinical studies (4,47).

REFERENCES

1. Mélen I. Chronic sinusitis: clinical and pathological aspects. Arch Otolaryngol 1994; 515(Suppl.):45–48.

2. Williams JW Jr. Sinusitis—beginning a new age of enlightenment? West J Med 1995; 163:80–2.
3. Lund VJ, Gwaltney J, Baquero F, et al. Infectious rhinosinusitis in adults: classification, etiology and management. ENT J Suppl 1997; 76:1–22.
4. Fokkens W, Lund VJ, et al. EPOS: EAACI position paper on rhinosinusitis and nasal polyps. Allergy 2005; 60:583–601.
5. Larsen K, Tos M. The estimated incidence of symptomatic nasal polyps. Acta Otolaryngol 2002; 122:79–182.
6. Ray NF, Baraniuk JN, Thamer M, et al. Healthcare expenditures for sinusitis in 1996: contributions of asthma, rhinitis, and other airway disorders. J Allergy Clin Immunol 1999; 103(3 Pt 1):408–14.
7. Durr DG, Desrosiers MY, Dassa C. Impact of rhinosinusitis in health care delivery: the Quebec experience. J Otolaryngol 2001; 30:93–7.
8. Goetzel RZ, Hawkins K, Ozminkowski RJ, et al. The health and productivity cost burden of the 'top 10' physical and mental health conditions affecting six large U.S. employers in 1999. J Occup Environ Med 2003; 45:5–14.
9. Murphy MP, Fishman P, Short SO, et al. Health care utilization and cost among adults with chronic rhinosinusitis enrolled in a health maintenance organization. Otolaryngol Head Neck Surg 2002; 127:367–76.
10. Blackwell DCJ, Coles R. Summary health statistics for US adults: National Health Interview Survey 1997. National Center for Health Statistics. Vital Health Stat 2002; 10:15.
11. New guidelines for sinusitis target prescribing practices. Dis Manag Advis 2004; 10:27–30.
12. Anon JB, Jacobs MR, Poole MD, et al. Antimicrobial treatment guidelines for acute bacterial rhinosinusitis. Otolaryngol Head Neck Surg 2004; 130(1 Suppl.):1–45.
13. Gliklich RE, Metson R. Economic implications of chronic sinusitis. Otolaryngol Head Neck Surg 1998; 118(3 Pt 1):344–9.
14. van Agthoven M, Uyl-de Groot CA, Fokkens WJ, et al. Cost analysis of regular and filgrastim treatment in patients with refractory chronic rhinosinusitis. Rhinology 2002; 40:69–74.
15. Bhattacharyya NI. The economic burden and symptom manifestations of chronic rhinosinusitis. Am J Rhinol 2003; 17:27–32.
16. Lund VJ, Holmstrom M, Scadding GK. Functional endoscopic sinus surgery in the management of chronic rhinosinusitis: an objective assessment. J Laryngol 1991; 105:832–5.
17. Metson RB, Gliklich RE. Clinical outcomes in patients with chronic sinusitis. Laryngoscope 2000; 110(3 Pt 3):24–8.
18. Radenne F, Lamblin C, Vandezande LM, et al. Quality of life in nasal polyposis. J Allergy Clin Immunol 1999; 104:79–84.
19. de-Graaf in-'t-Veld T, Koenders S, Garrelds IM, et al. The relationships between nasal hyper-reactivity, quality of life, and nasal symptoms in patients with perennial allergic rhinitis. J Allergy Clin Immunol 1996; 98:508–13.
20. Juniper EF, Guyatt GH. Development and testing of a new measure of health status for clinical trials in rhinoconjunctivitis. Clin Exp Allergy 1991; 21:77–83.
21. Calman KC. Quality of life in cancer patients—an hypothesis. J Med Ethics 1984; 10:124–7.
22. Schipper H, Clinch J, Powell V. ??? In: Spilker B, ed. Definitions and Conceptual Issues. Quality of Life Assessment in Clinical Trials. New York: Raven Press Ltd 1990:11–24.
23. Ware JE, Sherbourne CD. The MOS 36 Item Short-Form Health Survey (SF-36). I. Conceptual framework and item selection. Med Care 1992; 30:473–83.
24. Ragab SM, Lund VJ, Scadding G. Evaluation of medical and surgical treatment of chronic rhinosinusitis: a prospective randomised control trial. Laryngoscope 2004; 114:923–30.
25. Winstead W, Barnett SN. Impact of endoscopic sinus surgery on global health perception: an outcomes study. Otolaryngol Head Neck Surg 1998; 119:486–91.
26. Anderson RT, Aaronson NK, Wilkin D. Critical review of the international assessments of health-related quality of life. Qual Life Res 1993; 2:369–95.

27. Hunt SM, McEwan J, McKenna SP. Measuring Health Status. Beckenham: Croom Helm, 1986.
28. Bergner M, Bobbitt RA, Carter WB, Gilson BS. The sickness impact profile: development and final revision of a health status measure. Med Care 1981; 19:787–805.
29. Klassen A, Fitzpatrick R, Jenkinson C, Goodrace T. Contrasting evidence for the effectiveness of cosmetic surgery from two health related quality of life measures. J Epidemiol Community Health 1999; 53:440–1.
30. Carr AJ, Higginson IJ. Are quality of life measures patient centred? BMJ 2001; 322:1357–60.
31. Bernheim JL. How to get serious answers to the serius question: 'How have you been?' Subjective quality of life (QOL) as an individual experimental emergent construct. Bioethics 1999; 13:272–87.
32. Skevington S. Measuring quality of life in Britain. Introducing the WHOQOL-100. J Psychsom Res 1999; 47:449–59.
33. Piccirillo JF, Haiduk A, et al. Psychometric and clinimetric validity of the 3-item rhinosinusitis outcome measure (RSOM-31). Am J Rhinol 1995; 9:297–306.
34. Piccirillo JF, Merritt MG Jr, Richards ML. Psychometric and clinimetric validity of the 20-Item Sino-Nasal Outcome Test (SNOT-20). Otolaryngol Head Neck Surg 2002; 126:41–7.
35. Browne JP, Hopkins C, Slack R, et al. Health-related quality of life after polypectomy with and without additional surgery. Laryngoscope 2006; 116:297–302.
36. Anderson ER, Murphy MP, Weymuller EA Jr. Clinimetric evaluation of the Sinonasal Outcome Test-16. Student Research Award 1998. Otolaryngol Head Neck Surg 1999; 121:702–7.
37. Fahmy FF, McCombe A, McKiernan DC. Sinonasal assessment questionnaire, a patient focused, rhinosinusitis specific outcome measure. Rhinology 2002; 40:195–7.
38. Gliklich RE, Metson R. Techniques for outcomes research in chronic sinusitis. Laryngoscope 1995; 105(4 Pt 1):387–90.
39. Gliklich RE, Metson R. Effect of sinus surgery on quality of life. Otolaryngol Head Neck Surg 1997; 117:12–7.
40. Benninger MS, Senior BA. The development of the Rhinosinusitis Disability Index. Arch Otolaryngol Head Neck Surg 1997; 123:1175.
41. Senior BA, Glaze C, Benninger MS. Use of the Rhinosinusitis Disability Index (RSDI) in rhinologic disease. Am J Rhinol 2001; 15:15–20.
42. Hoffman SR, Mahoney MC, Chmiel JF, Stinziano GD, Hoffman KN. Symptom relief after endoscopic sinus surgery: an outcomes-based study. Ear Nose Throat J 1993; 72:413–4, 419–20.
43. Torrance GW. Measurement of health state utilities for economic appraisal. J Health Econom 1996; 5:1–30.
44. Revicki DA, Leidy NK, Brennan Diemer F, et al. Development and preliminary validation of the multiattribute Rhinitis Symptom Utility Index. Qual Life Res 1998; 7:693–702.
45. Damm M, Quante G, Jungehuelsing M, et al. Impact of functional endoscopic sinus surgery on symptoms and quality of life in chronic rhinosinusitis. Laryngoscope 2002; 112:310–5.
46. Yueh B, Feinstein AR. Abstruse comparisons: the problems of numerical contrasts of two groups. J Clin Epidemiol 1999; 52:13–8.
47. Meltzer EO, Hamilos DL, Hadley JA, et al. Rhinosinusitis: establishing definitions for clinical research and patient care. J Allergy Clin Immunol Suppl 2004; 114:S155–212.
48. Durr DG, Desrosiers MY, Dassa C. Quality of life in patients with rhinosinusitis. J Otolaryngol 1999; 28:108–11.
49. Gliklich RE, Metson R. The health impact of chronic sinusitis in patients seeking otolaryngologic care. Head Neck Surg 1995; 113:104–9.
50. Khalid AN, Quraishi SA, Kennedy DW. Long-term quality of life measures after functional endoscopic sinus surgery. Am J Rhinol 2004; 18:131–6.
51. Alobid I, Benítez P, Bernal-Sprekelsen M, et al. Nasal polyposis and its impact on quality of life: comparison between the effects of medical and surgical treatments. Allergy 2005; 60:452–8.

52. Bousquet J, Lund VJ, Van Cauwenberge P, et al. Implementation of guidelines for seasonal allergic rhinitis. A randomised controlled trial. Allergy 2003; 58:733–41.
53. Metson R, Gliklich RE. Clinical outcome of endoscopic sinus surgery for frontal sinusitis. Arch Otolaryngol Head Neck Surg 1998; 124:1090–6.
54. Alsarraf R, Kriet J, Weymuller EA Jr. Quality of life outcomes after osteoplastic frontal sinus obliteration. Otolaryngol Head Neck Surg 1999; 121:435–40.
55. Ware JE, Kosinski M, Dewey JE. How to Score Version of SF-36 Health Survey. Lincoln, RI: Quality Metric Incorporate, 2000.
56. Uri N, Cohen-Kerem R, Barzilai G, et al. Functional endoscopic sinus surgery in the treatment of massive polyposis in asthmatic patients. J Laryngol Otol 2002; 116:185–9.
57. van Agthoven M, Fokkens WJ, van de Merwe JP, et al. Quality of life of patients with refractory chronic rhinosinusitis: effects of filgrastim treatment. Am J Rhinol 2001; 15:231–7.
58. Lund VJ, Black SA, Laszloz S, et al. Randomised trial of efficacy and tolerability of budesonide aqueous nasal spray in patients with chronic rhinosinusitis. Rhinology 2004; 42:57–62.

3 Environmental and Allergic Factors in Chronic Rhinosinusitis

Jayant M. Pinto and Robert M. Naclerio
Section of Otolaryngology–Head and Neck Surgery, Department of Surgery, University of Chicago, Chicago, Illinois, U.S.A.

INTRODUCTION
Determination of Important Factors

A host of factors influence the development and pathogenesis of chronic rhinosinusitis (CRS) (1,2). Although these factors have been suggested based on clinical observations and, in some circumstances, have been studied experimentally, there is a paucity of knowledge of how or even whether these factors have any bearing on the disease. We can consider existing data by using the framework of Koch's postulates by first examining epidemiologic evidence: what factors are associated with CRS? Second, is there a plausible mechanism to explain the factor's role in either the etiology or the pathophysiology of CRS? And third, does alteration of the proposed factor cause a change in disease expression: what is the response to treatment? These critical questions are difficult to answer in the current state of CRS research, but to achieve progress in this field, we must attack this problem by using this mindset.

In this chapter, we review the effects of environmental factors on CRS including pollution and allergy. We also review existing animal and human models of sinus disease with an aim toward developing systems for testing proposed factors that influence CRS.

ENVIRONMENTAL
Pollution

Perhaps the gases and particulates that pass through the sinonasal tract have the most obvious influence on the development of rhinosinusitis (3). Pollutants can be broadly classified into primary (emitted directly into the atmosphere) and secondary (formed in the air as a result of chemical reactions with other pollutants and gases); they can also be divided based on the location of exposure (indoor or outdoor) or the molecular state (gaseous, particulate, or organic) (4). A variety of pollutants may cause detrimental effects in the nose and sinuses. Although the passage of these pollutants from the nose into the sinuses has not been clearly demonstrated, their effects on the nasal mucosa may affect sinus physiology through sinonasal reflexes, mucociliary clearance, epithelial damage, immune responses, ostial obstruction, and changes in nasal airflow.

Despite the importance of the effects of air pollution on the sinuses, there have been essentially no studies directly addressing this topic. There has been limited work on the possibility of particles entering the sinuses directly from the nose. For example, Adkins et al. showed that inhaled radiolabeled ragweed pollen did not enter the sinus cavities (5). In contrast, fungal spores have been found in sinus biopsy specimens. Whether gases or pollutants of smaller size can enter the sinuses directly has not been assessed. However, analysis of the composition of air within the maxillary sinuses suggests there is limited gaseous exchange between the nose and the sinuses (6). Additionally, Gwaltney et al. demonstrated that blowing of the nose leads to entry of secretions into the sinuses, suggesting that pollutants could gain entry in this fashion (7).

Other data that support air exchange between the nose and sinuses include studies of nitric oxide. Nitric oxide is a gas endogenously produced in the upper airways (8) that plays a role in immunity, host defense, and ciliary motility (9). Lundberg et al. demonstrated that nitric oxide is produced in humans constitutively by sinus epithelial cells in very high concentrations (10). These levels can be assessed in the nose, suggesting the possibility of gaseous exchange between the sinus cavities and the nose and highlighting that other pollutant gases may cross these spaces.

Most of the limited studies in this field have focused on nasal responses, probably because of easier access to the nose and more facile epidemiologic and clinical assessment. We will briefly review these nasal studies.

Pathophysiologic Effects of Pollutants

Pollutants may promote airway disease through a number of mechanisms, including induction or modulation of inflammatory responses, stimulation of nervous system reactivity or direct toxic effects (4). The nature of air pollution, its effects on airway inflammation and allergy, and genetic susceptibility to these effects are the subjects of intense research interest (11). In the nose, these mechanisms might potentially lead to the development of (CRS). First, responses likely to be mediated by the trigeminal nerve exist for many substances that have been found to cause nasal irritation. These include paper, coffee, borax, and fiberglass dust (12). Such responses could trigger reflex neurogenic inflammation which sets the stage for a chronic mucosal disease state. Second, air flow effects can alter sinonasal physiology; for example, resistance to nasal airflow is increased with exposure to sulfur dioxide (SO_2) and also to tobacco smoke in sensitive patients (13). It is not clear whether this is due to reflex or vascular mechanisms, toxic effects or inflammatory effects. Cigarette smoke, nicotine, capsaicin, ether, and formaldehyde can cause the release of neuropeptides, such as substance P from the nasal mucosa, with resultant inflammation (3). Cigarette smoke has also been shown to inhibit neutral endopeptidase, an enzyme involved in the degradation of neuropeptides in lung tissue, possibly leading to increased or chronic inflammation (14). Third, many substances [cigarette smoke, grain dust, ozone (O_3), cadmium, SO_2, hair spray, and wood dust] impair mucociliary clearance, another factor predisposing to stasis of secretions (12). Fourth, direct toxic effects on the sinonasal epithelium represent another mechanism leading to the development of disease in the sinonasal tract. Immunotoxic effects of pollutants include compromised phagocytic and killing ability possibly leading to chronic infection or inflammation (15,16). Fifth, certain pollutants, such as diesel exhaust particles (DEP) have been shown to augment allergen-induced inflammation, and this may indirectly potentiate the development of rhinosinusitis (see "Allergy and CRS").

Indoor Pollutants

In the developed world, because people spend the majority of their time indoors, exposure to indoor pollutants remains an important concern. The most common indoor pollutants include nitrogen dioxide (NO_2), formaldehyde, SO_2, aromatic hydrocarbons, and tobacco smoke (considered separately because of its importance). Organic substances such as molds and bacterial endotoxins in ventilation systems also influence the development of rhinosinusitis. A statistically significant inhibition of ciliary beat frequency caused by *Aspergillus fumigatus* and *Alternaria alternata* was demonstrated in vitro, suggesting a link between mold exposure and chronic sinusitis (17).

NO_2

Nitrogen dioxide, produced by the combustion of household cooking gas, is an indoor pollutant that has been found to be associated with respiratory illness in epidemiologic studies (18–21). High NO_2 exposure can cause lung injury and a decrease in defense mechanisms of the lungs (22). Although the threshold of such effects is unknown, subtle effects in susceptible subjects are possible. Interestingly, it has been demonstrated that exposure to NO_2 can potentiate the effect of exposure to allergens (23) and recent experimental studies suggest an interaction between NO_2 exposure and indoor allergens (23,24), emphasizing a possible relationship between the two etiologic factors involved in CRS.

Formaldehyde

Formaldehyde is commonly used in construction materials such as insulation, carpet adhesive, and plywood. It has been implicated in carcinogenesis as well as the sick building syndrome; it is also known to irritate mucous membranes (3). There are a number of potential mechanisms by which formaldehyde could be involved in the pathogenesis of CRS. Chronic exposure has been shown to be associated with immune system activation, potentially leading to a chronic inflammatory state (25). Indeed, individuals exposed even to low concentrations of formaldehyde present nasal hyperreactivity and edema (26). Alternatively, formaldehyde exposure could have other immunomodulatory effects such as immunosuppression that could lead to chronic infection (27). Formaldehyde also has direct toxic effects on the nasal epithelium and reduces mucociliary clearance (28). Finally, formaldehyde significantly reduces the ciliary beat frequency in isolated respiratory epithelial cells (29).

Outdoor Pollutants

Pollutants in the ambient outdoor air also have a potentially important role in CRS. The association of respiratory illnesses with air pollution, such as asthma and bronchitis, has been well documented and will not be reviewed here. However, there is intense interest in determining how pollutants interact with the airways to modulate immune responses and cause disease (11). Chemical reactions in the atmosphere involving sunlight and byproducts from petroleum combustion result in production of ozone and NO_2. Additionally, SO_2 emissions, primarily from power plants, and also from indoor kerosene heaters, are another important pollutant. A large-scale questionnaires study in Brazil comparing children from polluted and non-polluted areas demonstrated an increased incidence of rhinosinusitis (12% vs. 8%) and rhinitis (7% vs. 4%) in those exposed to pollutants (30). Indeed, compared to control groups, according to questionnaires mail carriers who work in an outdoor environment have been shown to have an increased prevalence of CRS, with smoking being an additional negative factor (31). Studies of sanitation workers exposed to pollutants demonstrated significant sinonasal symptoms as well as increases in nasal inflammation (32,33). Airway inflammation correlating with endotoxin and B1-3-glucan exposure has also been demonstrated in sanitation workers exposed to organic waste (34).

Ozone

Ozone is a naturally occurring, highly reactive, irritating gas that is recognized by the Environmental Protection Agency as an important public health hazard. O_3 has been shown to cause respiratory symptoms, alterations in pulmonary function, and lower-airway inflammation (35–40). Inflammatory effects include an influx of neutrophils, epithelial damage, upregulated adhesion molecules (39–44), increased number of mast cells (45), and cytokine alterations (39,40,46,47). Other effects include reduced mucociliary clearance (48). These pathologic effects have been bolstered by epidemiologic data linking increases in O_3 concentration to impaired lung function and bronchial hyperreactivity (49–51). Analogous pathologic effects on the nose and sinuses have not been well studied.

Although nasal studies are limited, O_3 elicits similar effects in the upper airways. Graham found increased numbers of neutrophils after exposure to O_3 (52). Other inflammatory markers have been found to be elevated in nasal lavage when ambient O_3 levels were elevated (53). Population studies have also demonstrated structural changes in the nasal epithelium in subjects exposed to high or prolonged O_3 levels (54,55). The deleterious effects of O_3 on the nose include epithelial disruption and increased permeability, inflammatory cell influx, and proliferative and secretory responses, release of cytokines, cyclooxygenase, and lipoxygenase products, decreased mucociliary clearance, as well as a priming effect on the late-phase response to allergen challenge (56). Interestingly, allergic asthmatic patients challenged intranasally with dust mite allergen and exposed to O_3 showed increased eosinophils and inflammatory cytokines after four hours (57). Given the wide range of physiologic processes impaired by O_3 in the nose as well the as extensive data on the lung, it is certainly plausible that O_3 plays a role in CRS.

NO_2

Besides cooking on gas stoves, NO_2 is let out into the atmosphere by the combustion of fossil fuels, with peak concentrations in cities during the commuting hours (58). At certain doses, NO_2-induced airway inflammation elicits an increase in the number of mast cells and lymphocytes in the lower airways (59,60), as well as increases in interleukin-8 levels (61). Challenge studies also showed that exposure to NO_2 induces airway inflammation, including neutrophil influx and a reduction in lymphocyte subpopulations (59,62). Studies of the lung have revealed neutrophilic inflammation with an increase in myeloperoxidase, suggesting both migration and activation of neutrophils in the lower airways (63). NO_2 might act as a sensitizing agent to inhaled allergens, because exposure to NO_2 enhanced both immediate- and late-phase allergenic responses (64,65). There are limited data on the role of NO_2 in outdoor settings in CRS. Interestingly, a recent longitudinal study in reunified Germany suggested that improvement in air quality might account for a decrease in respiratory diseases including rhinosinusitis (66,67).

SO_2

Sulfur dioxide has long been known to induce bronchoconstriction, and short-term exposures lead to increased nasal airway resistance (68). Epidemiologic studies have found on association between the concentration of SO_2 and respiratory symptoms and functions in urban areas (69,70). SO_2 and related compounds comprise a complex group of air pollutants that are associated with a number of health-related problems (71). SO_2 also contributes to the production of sulfuric acid, another airborne pollutant that has respiratory effects (72,73). The problem of SO_2 pollution is significant in developing countries where coal with high sulfur content is used for power generation.

Environmental chamber studies have shown increased alveolar macrophage activity as well as a delayed increase in the number of macrophages and lymphocytes upon exposure to SO_2 (74). Inhalation of SO_2 produced a significant decrease in nasal as well as lower airway effects, suggesting effects on nasal congestion (75).

As influx of inflammation cells influx has been observed in the lower airways after exposure to SO_2 (76) which may be related to increased susceptibility to cellular injury by pollutants and/or epithelial cell release of inflammatory mediators after exposure (77). However, in a study of eight subjects, brief exposure to SO_2 did not cause significant nasal dysfunction, suggesting that the responsiveness may be different in the upper airways (78). In vitro studies of cultured cells derived from human nasal turbinate tissue show that, compared to normal air exposure to SO_2 significantly inhibits ^{3}H-leucine incorporation in a dose-dependent fashion (79). Some researchers have suggested that SO_2 activates mast cells in the airways, causing release of mediators that induce both direct and parasympathetically mediated reflex bronchoconstriction (80,81). The release of these mediators may cause eosinophil chemoattraction, activation, and recruitment into the airways (77,82,83). Kienast et al. demonstrated a strong correlation between SO_2-modified pH values and ciliary beat frequency (CBF) (84). Indeed, inhaled sulfuric acid compounds have been shown to decrease mucociliary clearance (85,86). These events have parallels to the pathophysiology of CRS. The fact that metabolites in nasal lavage can be used as a biomarker for exposure suggests a promising avenue for further sinonasal studies (87).

Tobacco Smoke

Alhough 4000 chemicals have been identified in tobacco smoke, the actual number may be greater than 100,000 (88). At least 60 are carcinogens, including formaldehyde. Others, such as nicotine and carbon monoxide, interfere with normal cell development (89,90). In microgram quantities, irritants such as acrolein, formaldehyde, ammonia, nitrogen oxides, toluene, phenol, and pyridine are also present in every cigarette (91). The amount of smoke inhaled into the nasal cavity will be a proportion of the side-stream smoke (inhaled from smoke emanating from the burning tip into the atmosphere instead of through the cigarette into the mouth); the amount may vary because some subjects exhale smoke through the nostrils.

Cigarette smoke is associated with a statistically significant increase in nasal airway resistance in subjects reporting sensitivity to the smoke (13). As early as 1964, studies indicated that cigarette smoke may affect mucociliary clearance (92). Carson et al. suggested that cigarette smoke disrupts ciliary activity by both alterations in mucus and direct effects on cilia (93). Interestingly, there were no significant differences in mean CBF or mean nasal mucociliary clearance time after 10 healthy non-smoking volunteers had smoked two cigarettes each, exhaling the smoke through their nostrils. It is possible that the defective clearance seen in chronic smokers may be due to mucosal changes rather than a slowed CBF barring a prompt reversal of any ciliotoxic effect missed when cilia are examined in vitro (94). The effects of smoking on the airway mucosa of the lungs have been better studied than those on the nasal epithelium; a detailed review of these studies is beyond the scope of this chapter. Smoke inhalation results in increased goblet cell and submucosal gland hyperplasia in the lungs, leading to excessive mucus production (95). Inouye et al. found histologic features similar to those found in perennial allergic rhinitis (96).

Despite the minimal data regarding the effects of tobacco smoke on CRS, there is a long-established association of smoke exposure with nasal symptoms. Surveys of airline crew and passengers, performed when smoking was allowed, cite significant complaints related to the nose, sinuses, and throat that are common among participants (97,98). Mattson et al. studied symptoms and nicotine exposures and found that ocular and nasal symptoms were related to nicotine exposure and reflected in urinary cotinine measurements (99). In one epidemiologic study, Lieu et al. used the Third National Health and Nutrition Examination Survey to assess active and passive smoking and self-reported rhinosinusitis or sinus problems. Active smoking was associated with a slightly increased risk of sinus disease (relative risk 1.22, 95% confidence interval 1.05–1.39), with some evidence of a dose response, while passive smoking was not (100). These effects may be analogous to effects in the ear as seen in extensive studies linking smoking to chronic otitis media in children, given that both are mucosal inflammatory diseases (101). Exposure studies of police from Hong Kong indicate that environmental tobacco smoke is associated with respiratory symptoms, including a blocked or runny nose, and physician consultation (102). A dose-dependent effect was suggested. Thus, a limited data set suggests that smoking may influence CRS.

Bascom et al. showed that subjects sensitive to smoke reported increased rhinorrhea and other nasal symptoms after exposure to smoke as compared to non-sensitive subjects. Nasal resistance was also noted to increase more in the sensitive subjects, but mediators of inflammation in the nasal lavage were unchanged by smoke exposure (13). In a similar inhalation challenge experiment, Wilkes et al. showed that after exposure to smoke, irritation and rhinitis symptoms increased, nasal resistance rose, and specific airway conductance decreased; total cell counts, neutrophils, and albumin values were unchanged. They concluded that healthy normal subjects demonstrate nasal congestion with exposure to moderate levels of smoke without evidence of increased nasal vascular permeability (103). Other studies by this group have attempted to determine the biologic variables that mediate these effects (104–106).

Smoke may have direct effects on the sinonasal epithelium. Nicotine has been shown to affect ion transport in cultured nasal epithelial cells (107). This effect could influence mucus viscosity, air conditioning, or the epithelial cell barrier function, with resultant pathologic effects. A small-scale study failed to show increased nasal epithelial permeability in smokers in vivo (108). However, other studies suggest effects on the transmembrane potential difference of the nasal mucosa in moderate- to heavy–smokers (109). Effects on capillary and membrane permeability remain uncertain. Some studies have failed to replicate these findings, though a lack of quantification of smoke inhaled may explain the wide differences in data.

Cigarette smoke is known to have immunomodulatory effects on the lower airways (110). Indeed, a number of studies have demonstrated effects on the innate immune system, adaptive immunity, and neuroimmunology (111). These effects have important and direct parallels to rhinosinusitis, however no definitive studies have been performed in this area. Interestingly, exposure to smoke has also been noted to be a negative factor in mucosal recovery after endoscopic sinus surgery in both adults and children (112–115). Measured by use of validated outcome tools, active but not passive smokers also have elevated symptoms after sinus surgery, even accounting for confounding factors (114). The mechanism behind these effects has not yet been identified.

ALLERGY AND CRS
Epidemiology
In population-based studies, allergic inflammation has been identified consistently as one factor contributing to both acute and CRS (116–122). Although no adequately controlled studies of the incidence of CRS in patients with allergic rhinitis have been conducted, data from a number of clinical studies support this association. In an otolaryngology clinic setting, 54% of patients with CRS also had allergic rhinitis (123). In various studies, patients undergoing sinus surgery were found to have between 50% and 94% incidence of atopy. The results were similar in pediatric studies (124–130) Recently, a large Canadian population-based study using survey data demonstrated a higher incidence of rhinosinusitis in persons having a history of allergies (131). However, these data are confounded by referral pattern bias and no rigorous controlled studies have been performed. Nevertheless, data suggest a significant clinical overlap of allergic rhinitis and CRS.

Complementing these findings are studies showing a high prevalence of sinus disease in patients with allergic rhinitis. A number of radiologic studies which document inflammatory changes in the sinus epithelium corroborate this association. Sixty percent of subjects with rhinitis due to ragweed pollen during the pollen season have sinus mucosal abnormalities as evidenced by computed tomography (CT) scan (132). Analysis by other methods, such as magnetic resonance imaging (MRI), has also demonstrated increased evidence of sinus mucosal abnormalities during major pollen seasons (133).

Savolainen found the incidence of allergy to be 25% in a group of 224 patients with acute maxillary rhinosinusitis, which was significantly greater than a 16% incidence in a control group (117). Holzmann et al. reported an increased prevalence of allergic rhinitis in children who had orbital complications of acute rhinosinusitis, and these complications occurred especially during the pollen seasons (134). In a study involving 8723 children, Chen and colleagues found the prevalence of rhinosinusitis to be significantly higher in children with allergic rhinitis than in those without allergy (135).

Another example of a link between allergy and CRS is the correlation between data and disease severity, as documented by imaging with markers of allergy including eosinophilia and specific IgE to inhalant allergens (136). A follow-up study showed a highly significant correlation between peripheral eosinophil counts and extent of disease (137). These data suggest that the sinus inflammation documented by imaging was correlated with known mediators of allergic inflammation.

Common Pathophysiologic Mechanisms
Despite the high co-prevalence of allergic rhinitis and rhinosinusitis and the enormous public health impact of these diseases, there are very few data on the mechanisms by which allergic rhinitis leads to CRS. We will briefly review some possible mechanisms and the data that support these mechanisms.

Ostial Obstruction
Perhaps the classic explanation of how allergic rhinitis causes alterations in sinus physiology leading to disease is ostial obstruction. Under this explanation,

mucosal edema caused by allergic responses leads to ostial obstruction. This blockage prevents normal drainage and ventilation from the sinuses, leading to accumulation of mucus, serum transudation, and decreased oxygenation within the sinuses, with resultant impairment of mucociliary transport, stasis of secretions, and growth of bacteria. A cycle of such effects may lead to a chronic inflammatory state.

Evidence to support this theory in humans is limited. Sinus mucosal thickening in allergic patients has been documented: a number of imaging studies, including our own, have demonstrated mucosal thickening in the sinuses of allergic patients both in challenge and seasonal models (138–140) Additionally, in some cases, epithelial thickening could be demonstrated in the absence of ostial obstruction. These changes did not resolve even after treatment. Impaired mucociliary movement could reduce the clearance of bacteria, leading to detrimental effects (141) However, the effects of allergic rhinitis on mucociliary transport have been studied with no consensus on these effects (142). Despite proposals that negative pressure created by ostial obstruction could cause pathogenic flora to move from the nose into the sinuses (141,143), there is no experimental evidence to support this mechanism in human subjects. Studies of ostial obstruction in animal models have primarily focused on acute rhinosinusitis, with no clear results (see "Experimental Models of Rhinosinusitis" below).

Direct Effects of Pollen

Studies of the effects of pollen on the sinuses are limited because of problems of access. However, fungal elements including spores and hyphae have been documented in the sinuses, suggesting that mucosal inflammation in the sinuses could be a direct response to allergens. In support of this theory, contrast material instilled into the nasopharynx can be blown into the sinuses, suggesting that polyps can be blown into the sinus (7). A major problem with this hypothesis is that the openings of the sinuses are connected to the nose by narrow passages. For example, Adkins et al. showed that inhaled radiolabeled ragweed pollen did not directly enter thesinus cavities (5). Furthermore, histologic studies found dust mite-specific IgE antibodies in the nasal mucosa of dust-sensitive patients, but levels in the sinus mucosa were similar to those in non-allergic patients with rhinitis (144). The lack of specific IgE against an inhalant allergen in the sinus mucosa does not support a simultaneous allergic process occurring in the sinuses. Finally, mucociliary transport carries mucus out of the sinuses; thus, allergens deposited near the sinus ostia would be cleared away from the sinuses (145). These effects should be reviewed in the context of data suggesting that immune responses to fungi may explain CRS (see Chapter 11).

Viral Infection

Studies linking viral infection to airway disease support the theory that viral infections can predispose to chronic mucosal inflammation (146–148). For example, in the lung, epidemiologic studies have suggested a strong link between severe respiratory syncytial virus-induced bronchiolitis in infancy and asthma later in life (149). Sotir et al. reported that allergy was associated with upper respiratory infection and caused wheezing (150). Whether disease relationships that are analogous to these observations exist in the sinuses is unknown and is a promising area of future study.

Chronic Inflammatory Effects

Inflammatory cells and their mediators are important for orchestrating the inflammatory and immunologic response in both CRS and allergic rhinitis. Similar perturbations of the immune system could explain the association between the diseases. Allergic rhinitis and CRS share similar inflammatory cell infiltrates, especially eosinophils, mast cells, and T lymphocytes, the major effector cells in these diseases. Eosinophils, long known to be involved in allergic inflammation, have been found to be the predominant inflammatory cell type in studies of sinus tissue from patients with CRS (151–156). Inflammatory mediators, such as major basic proteins and eosinophil cationic proteins released by eosinophils, have toxic effects on epithelial cells and ciliary structure. Damage to the sinus epithelium caused by these mediators could lead to CRS. In contrast, however, our group did not find a significant difference in the number of eosinophils in the sinus mucosa between children with allergic and non-allergic rhinitis with CRS (157).

Lymphocytes are thought to be important components of the inflammatory response in CRS. Driscoll et al. found significantly more CD4+, but not CD8+, cells in the sinus mucosa of children with CRS than in control patients (157). T-helper (Th)-cell subsets have been identified as important contributors to sinus pathophysiology, and allergic rhinitis and CRS share some of these mechanisms. These cells are characterized by distinct cytokine patterns: Th1 responses induce a cell-mediated immune response by producing interferon (IFN)-γ and interleukin (IL)-2, whereas Th2 responses induce eosinophil-mediated inflammatory responses such as IL-4, IL-5, and IL-13 and counter-regulatory cytokines such as IL-10 (158). The immunopathologic response of CRS has been related to the effects of Th2 cytokines in allergic patients (159). For example, higher levels of IL-5 are present in the sinus effusion of patients with allergic rhinitis and CRS than in those with non-allergic CRS (153). Hamilos et al. demonstrated that allergic patients had significantly higher IL-4 and IL-5, but lower IFN-γ levels compared to non-allergic patients (155,156). In contrast, high IL-13 expression was found in the tissues of both allergic and non-allergic CRS patients (159). IL-4 expression was significantly higher in allergic patients with CRS than in non-allergic patients or normal controls. A number of other studies suggest that alterations in the balance of Th1 and Th2 responses in the sinuses may affect disease expression; this idea of CRS as a Th2 disease marks a commonality with allergic rhinitis (158–160). Data from studies of children with refractory CRS showed significantly more CD4+ cells in the sinus mucosa of patients compared with control tissue. The involvement of T lymphocytes in sinus inflammation suggests that polarization of these cells into Th1 and Th2 effectors may influence progress of the disease. The similar repertoire of immune responses implicated in allergic disease and CRS suggests that similar mechanisms may be involved in the pathology. Current data support the concept that rhinosinusitis is a type of Th2-mediated disease process.

EXPERIMENTAL MODELS OF RHINOSINUSITIS

Significant progress in unraveling the pathophysiology of CRS in human subjects has been hampered by the difficulties of performing studies in human subjects particularly given the difficulty in accessing the sinuses. This physical limitation has resulted in investigations being restricted to puncture studies of the maxillary sinus during episodes of acute rhinosinusitis and biopsy studies of patients undergoing sinus surgery. These are limited both by single time-point analysis as well as examination of the end-stage of the disease in patients undergoing surgery. Hence, there is a great need for other avenues of generating data on the etiology of this disease. For example, recent studies of the effects of fungi, local IgE production, and peripheral blood cells on the pathophysiology of CRS are new approaches to solving this problem (see other chapters in this text) (161–164).

In addition to the challenges posed by human studies, one major obstacle to definitive studies of the pathophysiology of CRS is the lack of adequate animal models. Development of an animal model would make it possible to test a variety of etiologic factors, including environmental and genetic influences on the development and expression of the disease. To date, there are few reported animal models of CRS although a number of models exist for acute rhinosinusitis. We will review the various animal models of rhinosinusitis focusing on those for which a significant body of literature exists. Sporadic reports exist on studies of other animals (165,166).

Sheep

A sheep cadaver head model was developed to allow trainees in nasal and sinus endoscopy to develop their skills without risk to patients (167). More recently, this experimental model has been employed for the study of aspects of postoperative healing after endoscopic sinus surgery. The benefits of the sheep model include a useful representation of sinus anatomy and large passages permitting a range of surgical manipulation. Sheep develop sinonasal diseases similar to those in humans, including allergic rhinitis, nasal polyposis, and CRS (168).

Studies using this model have been confined to packing materials, anatomic abnormalities, and surgical techniques, with limited relevance to the pathobiology of CRS. In a comparison of nasal packing materials, Shaw et al. demonstrated significant mucosal injury with loss of cilia when they used both gauze and neuropatties, potentially influencing mucociliary clearance (169). Similar studies with microscopic assessment suggested that hyaluronic acid-based packing had positive effects on re-epithelialization of the nasal mucosa; however, ciliary function remained impaired (170). The addition of prednisolone to this regimen did not improve mucosal healing in a model of infection (171). A similar study with insulin-like growth factor-1-impregnated hyaluronic packs showed improvement in mucosal healing in healthy sheep after 4 weeks, but not in those with rhinosinusitis. Ciliary function was impaired in the rhinosinusitis group as compared to that in healthy sheep (172). Interestingly, this group utilized *Oestrus ovis*, a botfly parasite which produces an eosinophilic chronic inflammatory response to model CRS, similar to the use of schistosoma eggs in animal models for asthma generating Th2 responses (173,174). Details of the model were not clearly provided, including the time course of infection and the histology of the response. Nevertheless, this approach appears promising.

The same group also employed a sheep model to study surgical technique. Animals underwent modified endoscopic lothrop (MEL) procedures on the frontal sinuses, with some animals randomized to undergo frontal sinus trephination and irrigation. Frontal sinus irrigation in the immediate postoperative period showed a trend toward improved postoperative mucociliary function, with no adverse effects seen from the MEL on mucociliary clearance, as assessed by nuclear medicine gamma-scintigraphy of the frontal sinus three months postoperatively (175). A similar study examined osteoneogenesis and restenosis of the frontal duct (175).

The sheep model has also been employed in a study of sinus ventilation in which xenon gas and CT scanning were used (176). Comparing large and small antrostomies, Brummund et al. found no additional benefit in gas exchange to enlargement of the antrostomy beyond the smallest opening (176).

Rabbit

Rabbit sinus anatomy shows similarities to human anatomy both macroscopically and microscopically (177–179). There is significant experience using the rabbit model to study acute rhinosinusitis. The large size of the rabbit sinuses allows easy surgical manipulation (180) and disease assessment by CT scan or MRI (181,182). Additionally, related diseases such as pneumonia (181), otitis media (183), asthma (184,185) and dacrocystitis (181) can be studied in these animals.

Early studies focused on closure or obstruction of the natural ostia with subsequent administration of bacteria into the sinus (186–192). Other protocols focused on the delivery of a bacterial load to the sinuses by using absorbable materials intranasally (178–181,193). A host of other aspects of acute rhinosinusitis have been examined including the response to steroids and antibiotics (194), sinus leukotriene levels (195), therapeutic response to anti-inflammatory agents (196,197), the sugar xylitol (198), decongestants (199,200), and antibiotics (201). As with the sheep, surgical techniques have been evaluated including the effects of surgery on facial bone growth (202), antrostomy technique (203,204), and length of obstruction of the maxillary ostia (205,206). Physiologic measures have been assessed, including pressure measurement in the sinus (207), epithelial turnover (208), neuropeptide release (209), as well as mucosal changes and ciliary function (210). Besides the study of bacteria, fungal disease has also recently been studied (211). To mimic the clinical problem of foreign bodies causing rhinosinusitis in patients, the effects of nasotracheal and nasogastric tubes have also been studied (212,213).

Most studies of the rabbit model have relied on mechanical obstruction of sinus ostia and focused on acute rhinosinusitis (214). Some authors attempted to simulate CRS in humans (215,216), especially after lengthy ostial obstruction (217), but these models do not give an accurate picture. Additionally, these models also suffer from a lack of immunologic reagents and genetically modified animals.

Mouse

A murine model of rhinosinusitis offers a number of advantages over models using larger animals. Though surgical manipulation is limited due to size, understanding of the mouse immune system is advanced, allowing for a wide range of immunologic manipulation, including use of monoclonal antibodies, cytokines, and biologic agents. Genetic manipulation is also easy, enabling the study of knockouts, transgenics, and strain-specific responses. Moreover, the mouse model affords the opportunity to study related diseases, such as atopy and asthma in conjunction with rhinosinusitis.

Our group developed a mouse model of acute bacterial rhinosinusitis (218). Mice were inoculated intranasally with *Streptococcus pneumoniae*, the most commonly cultured organism from clinical puncture studies in humans. A known time course of infection was shown, with the inflammatory infiltrate peaking on day 5 and resolving by day 14. This culture data paralleled the infiltrate data. Hence, this model mimics the clinical course of acute bacterial rhinosinusitis in humans. This model was used for the study of a number of parameters affecting the pathophysiology of rhinosinusitis. In one study, C57BL/6 mice were inoculated intranasally with a susceptible strain of *S. pneumoniae,* and the effect of trimethoprim-sulfamethoxazole on acute rhinosinusitis was examined (219). The mice were sacrificed on day 5 and examined histologically. Trimethoprim-sulfamethoxazole decreased the number of neutrophil clusters in the sinus cavities, the number of neutrophils infiltrating the sinus mucosa, and bacterial growth. This study demonstrated the utility of this model for the study of the pharmacologic treatment of acute rhinosinusitis.

This model was also used to examine the relationship between allergy and rhinosinusitis (220). Mice were sensitized to ovalbumin (OVA) via intraperitoneal injection and then inoculated with *S. pneumoniae*, either with or without concomitant intranasal administration of OVA. A control group was infected without prior sensitization. Animals were sacrificed at various time points and evaluated histologically for inflammation and bacterial growth in culture. Sensitized mice exposed to intranasal OVA had significantly more inflammatory cells (neutrophils, monocytes, and eosinophils) in the sinus mucosa than did controls. Cultures demonstrated increased bacterial counts at sacrifice in sensitized/allergen-exposed animals compared to non-sensitized, infected mice. Compared to controls, the percentage of the sinus occupied by neutrophil clusters and the number of neutrophils per square millimeter of sinus mucosa were significantly higher in the sensitized/allergen-exposed mice. A comparison group of mice sensitized, but challenged with aerosolized allergen to target the lower, rather than the upper, airways, did not show augmented inflammation or infection in the sinuses. This study suggested that local allergic inflammation plays an important role in the expression of rhinosinusitis, with allergic responses causing more severe disease. This parallels the anecdotal clinical data suggesting that the expression of acute and CRS is worse in allergic individuals. The mechanism of these effects is not clear, but could be related to altered cellular infiltrates, inflammatory mediators, ciliary dysfunction, or lymphocyte ratios.

In a follow-up study, we focused on the importance of Th2 cells given the hypothesis that CRS is a Th2-mediated disease. BALB/c mice were sensitized to OVA by adoptive transfer of OVA-specific Th2- or Th1-skewed cells (221). Passive sensitization with Th2 cells followed by intranasal OVA challenge showed a five-fold increase in local eosinophilic response compared with that seen in mice that only received Th2 passive sensitization ($P < 0.001$). Mice with Th2 passive sensitization and intranasal OVA exposure followed by infection with *S. pneumoniae* showed an increase in the number of recovered bacteria ($P < 0.05$) and an increase in sinus inflammation compared with mice subjected to infection alone ($P < 0.01$). This represents an excellent model of the clinical picture in humans in which allergic individuals are exposed intranasally to allergens. This is the first set of data supporting the widely held clinical observation that allergy worsens acute rhinosinusitis.

The alternative arm of this experiment also provided some insight into the immunopathology of rhinosinusitis. Mice passively sensitized with OVA-specific Th1 cells followed by intranasal OVA exposure and infection showed no significant increase in the recovery of *S. pneumoniae* or sinus inflammation compared with those that had infection alone. This suggested that the prolongation of infection and the increased inflammation seen in sinus disease may be related to Th2 cell function, rather than the bacterial clearance function of Th1 cells.

Overall, these data support the importance of antigen-stimulated Th2 cells in the augmented response to infection in allergic mice. The mechanism underlying these differences remains to be explored and may relate to the direct effects of Th2 cells, released cytokines, and/or subsequent recruitment of other cells such as eosinophils. Perhaps the local mucosal response to infection involving Th1 cells is hindered by an ongoing local mucosal response to allergens involving Th2 cells. In other disease states, polarization of T lymphocytes into Th1 or Th2 cells has been shown to influence the course of the disease. This animal model of acute rhinosinusitis simulates the clinical situation of an allergic individual who develops an infection and supports the epidemiologic data presented earlier.

In another experiment designed to mimic the clinical setting in humans, we performed a treatment trial to test whether an H1 receptor antagonist, desloratadine, could reduce the augmenting effect of an ongoing allergic reaction on acute bacterial rhinosinusitis (222). We compared the responses of four groups of mice: (i) infected and allergic mice treated with desloratadine, (ii) infected and allergic mice treated with placebo, (iii) infected mice, and (iv) uninfected, non-sensitized mice as a control. Nasal allergic symptoms were observed by counting nasal rubbing and sneezing for 10 minutes after OVA or control nasal challenge. On day 5 after infection, bacterial cultures were obtained by nasal lavage, and inflammatory cells in the sinuses were evaluated by flow cytometry. More *S. pneumoniae* and phagocytes were recovered from mice that were made allergic, infected, and treated with placebo than from mice that were only infected. The former mice also manifested allergic symptoms and eosinophil influx into the sinuses. Desloratadine treatment during allergen exposure or challenge reduced allergic symptoms and sinonasal infection ($P < 0.05$). This study suggested that histamine contributes to the augmentation of infection in mice that have an ongoing allergic reaction. Follow-up studies in humans may confirm this effect.

Furthermore, to examine the role of T lymphocytes in the resolution of acute rhinosinusitis, we examined the importance of the adaptive and innate immune responses in the resolution of acute infection (223). Recombinase-activating gene knockout [RAG-1(−/−) or KO] (which have no lymphocytes) and C57BL/6 (wild-type) mice were infected with *S. pneumoniae*. For isolation of the key cells involved in the eradication of infection, lymphocytes were adoptively transferred into RAG-1(−/−) from C57BL/6 (wild-type) mice. The degrees of infection and inflammation were determined by the quantitative culture of *S. pneumoniae* from nasal lavage and analysis of sinus tissue, respectively. In C57BL/6 mice (wild-type), both the infection and inflammation resolved in 21 days, whereas neither resolved in RAG-1(−/−) mice. When C57BL/6 lymphocytes were adoptively transferred into RAG-1(−/−) mice, resolution of the infection and inflammation occurred. Mice without B cells were able to clear the infection, whereas mice without T cells could not clear it.

These studies demonstrated that T cells are essential in clearing acute *S. pneumoniae* bacterial sinus infection (223), RAG-1(−/−) mice with innate immunity (but no lymphocytes) contain but cannot clear a bacterial sinus infection. The RAG-1 KO mice had the same initial response to infection as did their wild-type counterparts, suggesting that the innate immune system is the key element in limiting the *S. pneumoniae* infection to the sinus cavity. However, the wild-type mice went on to resolve the infection, whereas the RAG-1 KO mice did not eliminate the infection and continued to have measurable infection and inflammation after 21 days. We then adoptively transferred lymphocytes from wild-type mice into RAG-1 KO mice and restored their ability to eliminate the infection and related inflammation. Similar results have been obtained by another group (224).

These data suggested that alterations in T-lymphocyte function, (in the extreme case, absence) could lead to persistent sinus inflammation.

We propose that these T-cell-deficient mice which have persistent inflammation represent one model of CRS. The tissue environment, signals, cytokines, and structural changes needed for developing and maintaining such inflammation are not yet clear, but this model represents a novel way of approaching the study of CRS. Determining how an immune-competent host resolves an acute sinus infection may provide new strategies for shortening the duration of an acute infection and preventing the development of CRS. Whereas the inflammatory response to *S. pneumoniae* infection is necessary for clearing it, it may also cause collateral damage to the host (e.g., as occurs in the hearing loss that follows *S. pneumoniae*-induced meningitis) or dysregulation of normal immune-system processes.

Another area where this mouse model might prove a useful tool is in the study of viruses. Viral infection is a major factor influencing acute and CRS. Viruses probably affect rhinosinusitis in three ways: (i) they may initiate CRS; (ii) repeated exposure in childhood may prevent or reverse a Th2 response to allergen; or (iii) they may exacerbate chronic airway disease in adults (225). Each of these possibilities represents an important area for future work.

Other groups have reported the successful use of the mouse model to study CRS. Using similar techniques as in the rabbit model (ostial obstruction), Jacob was able to induce persistent sinus inflammation at four weeks in C57BL/6 mice infected with *Bacteroidies fragilis* (employed because anaerobes are frequently cultured from humans with CRS) (226). This inflammation consisted of epithelial thickening, goblet cell hyperplasia, and fibrosis in addition to cellular infiltrates. McCool and Weiser's study of pneumococcal nasal carriage supports our results that B cells and adaptive immunity are not required for containment of infection (227). Lipsitch et al. also studied competition among serotypes of *S. pneumoniae* as regards nasal carriage (228). These studies may also have implications for the study of CRS.

Human Studies

Experimental studies of rhinovirus infection are well established and provide a model for the study of CRS (229,230). Although these studies are complex and require a number of important controls, they have recently been successfully employed in therapeutic trials of *Echinacea* (231). Buchman et al. studied nasal inoculation of healthy, susceptible adult volunteers with respiratory syncytial virus to examine the relationship between viral upper respiratory tract infections and otitis media (232). Similar studies can be envisioned for examining viral effects on acute and CRS. A well-characterized, reproducible human model of viral rhinosinusitis would be a valuable tool.

Another approach to dissecting the disease is to utilize human tissue. Using an explant nasal biopsy model, Fakhri and colleagues studied the interaction of allergen and staphylococcal superantigen on the expression of glucocorticoid receptor expression (233,234). The same group utilized sinus biopsy samples from patients with chronic sinusitis undergoing sinus surgery to monitor gene expression, and they used laser capture microdissection to quantify such effects (235). Similar tissue culture and explant studies might allow for investigation of the effect of topical agents and other molecules on the disease process at the organ or cellular level. Further studies are necessary to advance this field.

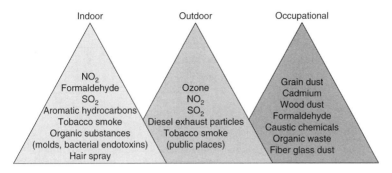

FIGURE 1   Environmental pollutants of potential relevance to rhinosinusitis.

CONCLUSION

A number of environmental effects may be involved in the development and pathophysiology of CRS (Fig. 1). Though only limited studies have been performed on the effects of pollution on sinus physiology, inferences can be made from studies of the nose and lungs that suggest mechanisms that may cause sinus dysfunction. Of particular interest are components of pollution, such as diesel exhaust particles, that augment allergic responses or others, including O_3, SO_2, formaldehyde and cigarette smoke that impair mucociliary clearance or induce mucosal inflammation. Further study is needed on the effects of tobacco smoke, given the widespread exposure of the population both directly and indirectly to this agent. A number of animal models of sinus disease exist (Table 1). Whereas,

TABLE 1   Animal Models of Sinonasal Disease

Animal	Experimental procedures	Sinonasal disease model	Advantages
Sheep	Surgical techniques Postoperative healing Sinus ventilation	Allergic rhinitis Nasal polyposis Chronic rhino- sinusitis	Similarities to human anatomy Amenable to surgical manipulation

Rabbit	Sinus ostial function
	Experimental sinus
	   ostial closure
	Surgical techniques
	Bacterial infection
	Measurement of:
	   – Inflammatory
	      mediators
	   – Response to
	      medications
	   – Mucosal changes
	   – Ciliary function
		Allergic rhinitis
		Acute bacterial
		   rhinosinusitis
		Fungal rhino-
		   sinusitis
			Similarities to human anatomy
			Amenable to surgical manipulation
			Disease assessment by CT or MRI
			Assessment of disease
			   relationships (e.g. relationship
			   between rhinosinusitis
			   and asthma)

Mouse	Bacterial infection
	Allergen sensitization
		Allergic rhinitis
		Acute bacterial
		   rhinosinusitis
			Multiple genetically-defined strains
			Wide range of immunologic
			   manipulation, including
			   studies of transgenic strains
			   and knockout mice

these have focused primarily on acute rhinosinusitis, progress is being made toward developing models of CRS, especially using the mouse model which allows for manipulation of environmental, immunologic, and genetic parameters that may impact on the pathophysiology of this disease.

REFERENCES

1. Kennedy DW. Pathogenesis of chronic rhinosinusitis. Ann Otol Rhinol Laryngol 2004; 193:6–9.
2. Meltzer EO, Hamilos DL, Hadley JA, et al. Rhinosinusitis: establishing definitions for clinical research and patient care. Otolaryngol Head Neck Surg 2004; 131:S1–62.
3. Clerico DM. Environmental influences on sinus disease. In: Kennedy DW, Bolger WE, Zinreich SJ, eds. Diseases of the Sinuses. Hamilton, Ont: BC Decker, 2001:107–18.
4. Bernstein JA, Alexis N, Barnes C, et al. Health effects of air pollution. J Allergy Clin Immunol 2004; 114:1116–23.
5. Adkins TN, Goodgold HM, Hendershott L, et al. Does inhaled pollen enter the sinus cavities? Ann Allergy Asthma Immunol 1998; 81:181–4.
6. Drettner B, Ebbesen A, Nilsson M. Prophylactive treatment with flunisolide after-polypectomy. Rhinology 1982; 20:149–58.
7. Gwaltney JM, Hendley JO, Phillips CD, et al. Nose blowing propels nasal fluid into the paranasal sinuses. Clin Infect Dis 2000; 30:387–91.
8. Djupesland PG, Chatkin JM, Qian W, et al. Nitric oxide in the nasal airway: a new dimension in otorhinolaryngology. Am J Otolaryngol 2001; 22:19–32.
9. Arnal JF, Flores P, Rami J, et al. Nasal nitric oxide concentration in paranasal sinus inflammatory diseases. Eur Respir J 1999; 13:307–12.
10. Lundberg JO, Farkas-Szallasi T, Weitzberg E, et al. High nitric oxide production in human paranasal sinuses. Nature Med 1995; 1:370–3.
11. Saxon A, Diaz-Sanchez D. Air pollution and allergy: you are what you breathe. Nat Immunol 2005; 6:223–6.
12. Leopold DA. Pollution: the nose and sinuses. Otolaryngol Head Neck Surg 1992; 106:713–9.
13. Bascom R, Kulle T, Kagey-Sobotka A, et al. Upper respiratory tract environmental tobacco smoke sensitivity. Am Rev Respir Dis 1991; 143:1304–11.
14. Nadel JA. Neutral endopeptidase modulates neurogenic inflammation. Eur Respir J 1991; 4:745–54.
15. Acton JD, Myrvik QN. Nirogen dioxide effects on alveolar macrophages. Arch Environ Health 1972; 24:48–52.
16. Vojdani A, Ghoneum M, Brautbar N. Immune alteration associated with exposure to toxic chemicals. Toxicol Ind Health 1992; 8:239–54.
17. Cody DT II, McCaffrey TV, Roberts G, et al. Effects of *Aspergillus fumigatus* and *Alternaria alternata* on human ciliated epithelium in vitro. Laryngoscope 1997; 107:1511–4.
18. Garrett MH, Hooper MA, Hooper BM. Respiratory symptoms in children and indoor exposure to nitrogen dioxide and gas stoves. Am J Respir Crit Care Med 1998; 158:891–5.
19. Jarvis D, Chinn S, Luczynska C. The association of respiratory symptoms and lung function with the use of gas for cooking. European Community Respiratory Health Survey. Eur Respir J 1998; 11:651–8.
20. Goren AI, Hellmann S. Respiratory conditions among schoolchildren and their relationship to environmental tobacco smoke and other combustion products. Arch Environ Health 1995; 50:112–8.
21. Wong TW, Tam WS, Yu TS. Associations between daily mortalities from respiratory and cardiovascular diseases and air pollution in Hong Kong, China. Occup Environ Med 2002; 59:30–5.
22. Samet JM, Utell MJ. The risk of nitrogen dioxide: what have we learned from epidemiological and clinical studies? Toxicol Ind Health 1990; 6:247–62.

23. Devalia JL, Rusznak C, Herdman MJ, et al. Effect of nitrogen dioxide and sulphur dioxide on airway response of mild asthmatic patients to allergen inhalation. Lancet 1994; 344:668–71.
24. Tunnicliffe WS, Burge PS, Ayres JG. Effect of domestic concentrations of nitrogen dioxide on airway responses to inhaled allergen in asthmatic patients. Lancet 1994; 344:1733–6.
25. Thrasher JD, Broughton A, Madison R. Immune activation and autoantibodies in humans with long-term inhalation exposure to formaldehyde. Arch Environ Health 1990; 45:217–23.
26. Giordano C, Siccardi E, Fedrighini B, et al. Nasal hyperreactivity and work environment. Acta Otorhinolaryngol Ital 1994; 14:S41–7.
27. Vojani A, Ghoneum M, Brautbar N. Immune alteration associated with exposure to toxic chemicals. Toxicol Ind Health 1992; 8:239–54.
28. Andersen I, Molhave L. Controlled human studies with formaldehyde. In: Gibson JE, ed. Formaldehyde Toxicity. Washington, D.C.: Hemipshere, 1983: p 154–165
29. Schafer D, Brommer C, Riechelmann H, et al. In vivo and in vitro effect of ozone and formaldehyde on human nasal mucociliary transport system. Rhinology 1999; 37:56–60.
30. Sih T. Correlation between respiratory alterations and respiratory diseases due to urban pollution. Int J Pediatr Otorhinolaryngol 1999; 49:S261–7.
31. Zuskin E, Mustajbegovic J, Schachter EN, et al. Respiratory findings in mail carriers. Int Arch Occup Environ Health 2000; 73:136–43.
32. Wouters IM, Hilhorst SK, Kleppe P, et al. Upper airway inflammation and respiratory symptoms in domestic waste collectors. Occup Environ Med 2002; 59:106–12. Erratum in: Occup Environ Med 2002; 59:497.
33. Sigsgaard T, Malmros P, Nersting L, et al. Respiratory disorders and atopy in Danish refuse workers. Am J Respir Crit Care Med 1994; 149:1407–12.
34. Heldal KK, Halstensen AS, Thorn J, et al. Airway inflammation in waste handlers exposed to bioaerosols assessed by induced sputum. Eur Respir J 2003; 21:641–5.
35. Seltzer J, Bigby BG, Stulbarg M, et al. O_3-induced change in bronchial reactivity to methacholine and airway inflammation in humans. J Appl Physiol 1986; 60:1321–6.
36. Kulle TJ, Sauder LR, Hebel JR, et al. Ozone response relationships in healthy non-smokers. Am Rev Respir Dis 1985; 132:36–41.
37. McDonnell WF, Horstman DH, Hazucha MJ, et al. Pulmonary effects of ozone exposure during exercise: dose-response characteristics. J Appl Physiol 1983; 54:1345–52.
38. Jacob A, Faddis BT, Chole RA. Chronic bacterial rhinosinusitis: description of a mouse model. Arch Otolaryngol Head Neck Surg. 2001 June; 127(6): 657–664
39. Devlin RB, McDonnell WF, Mann R, et al. Exposure of humans to ambient levels of ozone for 6.6 hours causes cellular and biochemical changes in the lung. Am J Respir Cell Mol Biol 1991; 4:72–81.
40. Aris RM, Christian D, Hearne PQ, et al. Ozone induced airway inflammation in human subjects as determined by airway lavage and biopsy. Am Rev Respir Dis 1993; 148:1363–72.
41. Balmes JR, Chen LL, Scannell C, et al. Ozone induced decrements in FEV1 and FVC do not correlate with measures of inflammation. Am J Respir Crit Care Med 1996; 153:904–9.
42. Koren HS, Devlin RB, Graham DE, et al. Ozone-induced inflammation in the lower airways of human subjects. Am Rev Respir Dis 1989; 139:407–15.
43. Balmes JR, Aris RM, Chen LL, et al. Effects of ozone on normal and potentially Sensitive human subjects. Part I. Airway inflammation and responsiveness to ozone in normal and asthmatic subjects. Res Rep Health Eff Inst 1997; 78:1–37.
44. Krishna MT, Blomberg A, Biscione GL, et al. Short-term ozone exposure upregulates P-selection in normal human airways. Am J Respir Crit Care Med 1997; 155:1798–803.
45. Hamacher J, Schaberg T. Adhesion molecules in lung diseases. Lung 1994; 172:189–213.

46. Blomberg A, Mudway IS, Nordenhäll C, et al. Ozone-induced lung function decrements do not correlate with early airway inflammatory or antioxidant responses. Eur Respir J 1999; 13:1418–28.
47. Frampton MW, Morrow PE, Torres A, et al. Ozone responsiveness in smokers and nonsmokers. Am J Respir Crit Care Med 1997; 155:116–21.
48. Krishna MT, Madden J, Teran LM, et al. Effects of 0.2 ppm ozone on biomarkers of inflammation in bronchoalveolar lavage fluid and bronchial mucosa of healthy subjects. Eur Respir J 1998; 11:1294–300.
49. Frager NB, Phalen RF, Kenoyer JL. Adaptations to ozone in reference to mucociliary clearance. Arch Environ Health 1979; 34:51–7.
50. Higgins IT, D'Arcy JB, Gibbons DI, et al. Effect of exposures to ambient ozone on ventilatory lung function in children. Am Rev Respir Dis 1990; 141:1136–46.
51. Castillejos M, Gold DR, Damokosh AI, et al. Acute effects of ozone on the Pulmonary function of exercising schoolchildren from Mexico City. Am J Respir Crit Care Med 1995; 152:1501–7.
52. Zwick H, Popp W, Wagner C, et al. Effects of ozone on the respiratory health, allergic sensitization, and cellular immune system in children. Am Rev Respir Dis 1992; 144:1075–79.
53. Graham DE, Koren HS. Biomarkers of inflammation in ozone-exposed humans: Comparison of the nasal and bronchoalveolar lavage. Am Rev Respir Dis 1990; 142:152–6.
54. Frischer TM, Kuehr J, Pullwitt A, et al. Ambient ozone causes upper airway inflammation in children. Am Rev Respir Dis 1993; 148:961–4.
55. Calderon-Garciduenas L, Osorno-Velazquez A, Bravo-Alvarez H, et al. Histopathologic changes of the nasal mucosa in southwest Metropolitan Mexico City inhabitants. Am J Pathol 1992; 140:225–32.
56. Christian DL, Chen LL, Scannell CH, et al. Ozone induced inflammation is attenuated with multiday exposure. Am J Respir Crit Care Med 1998; 158:532–7.
57. Nikasinovic L, Momas I, Seta N. Nasal epithelial and inflammatory response to ozone exposure: a review of laboratory-based studies published since 1985. J Toxicol Environ Health B Crit Rev 2003; 6:521–68.
58. Peden DB, Setzer RW Jr., Devlin RB. Ozone exposure has both a priming effect on allergen-induced responses and an intrinsic inflammatory action in the nasal airways of perennially allergic asthmatics, Am J Respir Crit Care Med 1995; 151:1336–45.
59. Mohsenin V. Human exposure to oxides of nitrogen at ambient and supra-ambient concentrations. Toxicology 1994; 89:301–12.
60. Sandström T, Andersson MC, Kolmodin-Hedman B, et al. Bronchoalveolar mastocytosis and lymphocytosis after nitrogen dioxide exposure in man: a time-kinetic study. Eur Respir J 1990; 3:138–43.
61. Sandström T, Stjernberg N, Eklund A, et al. Inflammatory cell response in bronchoalveolar lavage fluid after nitrogen dioxide exposure of healthy subjects: a dose 60 response study. Eur Respir J 1991; 4:332–9.
62. Blomberg A, Krishna MT, Bocchino V, et al. The inflammatory effects of 2 ppm NO_2 on the airways of healthy subjects. Am J Respir Crit Care Med 1997; 156:2028.
63. Sandstrom T, Ledin MC, Thomasson L, et al. Reductions in lymphocyte subpopulations after repeated exposure to 1.5 ppm nitrogen dioxide. Br J Ind Med 1992; 49:850–4.
64. Blomberg A. Airway inflammatory and antioxidant responses to oxidative and particulate air pollutants—experimental exposure studies in humans. Clin Exp Allergy 2000; 30:310–7.
65. Tunnicliffe WS, Burge PS, Ayres JG. Effect of domestic concentrations of nitrogen dioxide on airway responses to inhaled allergen in asthmatic patients. Lancet 1994; 344:1733–1736.
66. Strand V, Rak S, Svartengren M, et al. Nitrogen dioxide exposure enhances asthmatic reaction to inhaled allergen in subjects with asthma. Am J Respir Crit Care Med 1997; 155:881–887.

67. Heinrich J, Hoelscher B, Frye C, et al. Improved air quality in reunified Germany and decreases in respiratory symptoms. Epidemiology 2002; 13:394–401.
68. Heinrich J, Hoelscher B, Wichmann HE. Decline of ambient air pollution and respiratory symptoms in children. Am J Resp Crit Care Med 2000; 161:1930–6.
69. Sheppard D, Wong WS, Uehara CF. Lower threshold and greater bronchomotor responsiveness of asthmatic subjects to sulfur dioxide. Am Rev Respir Dis 1980; 122:873–8.
70. Shy CM, Goldsmith J R, Hackney JD, et al. Health hazard of sulfur oxide; a serious threat in our growing need for electric power. Am Lung Assoc Bull 1977; 63:2–7.
71. Sunyer J, Spix C, Quenel P, et al. Urban air pollution and emergency admissions for asthma in four European cities: the APHEA Project. Thorax 1997; 52:760–5.
72. Katsouyanni K, Touloumi G, Spix C, et al. Short term effects of ambient sulphur dioxide and particulate matter on mortality in 12 European cities: results from time series data from the APHEA project. BMJ 1997; 314:1658–63.
73. Spektor DM, Leikauf GD, Albert RE, et al. Effects of submicrometer sulphuric acid aerosols on mucociliary transport and respiratory mechanics in asymptomatic asthmatics. Environ Res 1985; 37:174–91.
74. Aris RM, Christian D, Sheppard D, et al. Lack of bronchoconstrictor response to sulphuric acid aerosols and fogs. Am Rev Respir Dis 1991; 143:744–50.
75. Sandström T, Stjernberg N, Anderson MC, et al. Is the short-term limit for sulfur dioxide safe? Effects of controlled chamber exposure investigated with bronchoalveolar lavage. Br J Ind Med 1989; 46:200–3.
76. Koenig JQ, Morgan MS, Horike M, et al. The effects of sulfur oxides on nasal and lung function in adolescents with extrinsic asthma. J Allergy Clin Immunol 1985; 76:813–8.
77. Sanstrom T, Stiernberg N, Andersson MC, et al. Cell response in bronchoalveolar lavage fluid after sulfur dioxide exposure. Scand J Work Environ Health 1989; 15:142–6.
78. Mills PR, Davies RJ, Devalia JL. Airway epithelial cells, cytokines, and pollutants. Am J Respir Crit Care Med 1999; 160:S38-S43.
79. Tam EK, Liu J, Bigby BG, et al. Sulfur dioxide does not acutely increase nasal symptoms or nasal resistance in subjects with rhinitis or in subjects with bronchial responsiveness to sulfur dioxide. Am Rev Respir Dis 1988; 138:1559–64.
80. McManus MS, Altman LC, Koenig JQ, et al. Human nasal epithelium: characterization and effects of in vitro exposure to sulfur dioxide. Exp Lung Res 1989; 15:849–65.
81. American Thoracic Society. Health Effects of Air Pollution. New York: American Thoracic Society, 1978:31.
82. Charles JM, Menzel DB. Ammonium and sulfate ion release histamine from lung fragments. Arch Environ Health 1975; 30:314–6.
83. Henderson WR, Lewis DB, Albert RK, et al. The importance of leukotrienes in airway inflammation in a mouse model of asthma. J Exp Med 1996; 184:1483–94.
84. Jatakanon A, Uasuf C, Maziak W, et al. Neutrophilic inflammation in severe persistent asthma. Am J Respir Crit Care Med 1999; 160:1532–9.
85. Kienast K, Riechelmann H, Knorst M, et al. Combined exposures of human ciliated cells to different concentrations of sulfur dioxide and nitrogen dioxide. Eur J Med Res 1996; 1; 533–6.
86. Spektor DM, Yen BM, Lippma M. Effect of concentration and cumulative exposure of inhaled sulfuric acid on tracheobronchial particle clearance in healthy humans. Environ Health Perspect 1989; 79:167–72.
87. Utell MJ, Morrow PE, Hyde RW, et al. Airway reactivity to sulfate and sulfuric acid aerosols in normal and asthmatic subjects. J Air Poll Control Assoc 1984; 34:931–5.
88. Bechtold WE, Waide JJ, Sandstrom T, et al. Biological markers of exposure to SO_2: S-sulfonates in nasal lavage. J Expo Anal Environ Epidemiol 1993; 3:371–82.
89. U.S. Department of Health and Human Services. Report on Carcinogens. 11th Edition. Research Triangle Park, NC: U.S. Department of Health and Human Services, Public Health Service, National Toxicology Program, 2005. (Accessed 2/14/07, at http://ntp.niehs.nih.gov/ntp/roc/toc11.html.)
90. National Cancer Institute. Cancer Progress Report 2003. Public Health Service, National Institutes of Health, U.S. Department of Health and Human Services,

Bethesda, Marylang, 2004. (Accessed xx xxx xxxx, at http://progressreport.cancer.gov/.)

91. National Cancer Institute. Smoking and Tobacco Control Monograph 10: Health Effects of Exposure to Environmental Tobacco Smoke. Bethesda, MD: NCI, 1999. (Accessed August 30, 2004, at http://cancercontrol.cancer.gov/tcrb/monographs/10/index.html.)

92. US Surgeon-General. The Health Consequences of Smoking: Chronic Obstructive Lung Disease. Washington, D.C.: US Department of Health and Human Services, 1984.

93. US Department of Health, Education, and Welfare, US Public Health Service. Smoking and Health: Report of the Advisory Committee to the Surgeon General of the Public Health Service. Washington, D.C.: US Department of Health, Education, and Welfare, 1964.

94. Carson S, Goldhamer R, Carpenter R. Responses of ciliated epithelium to irritants. Mucus transport in the respiratory tract. Am Rev Respir Dis 1966; 93:S86–92.

95. Stanley PJ, Wilson R, Greenstone MA, et al. Effect of cigarette smoking on nasal mucociliary clearance and ciliary beat frequency. Thorax 1986; 41:519–23.

96. Auerbach O, Stout AP, Hammond EC, et al. Changes in bronchial epithelium in relation to cigarette smoking and in relation to lung cancer. N Engl J. Med 1961; 265:253–67.

97. Inouye T, Nakanoboh M, Tanabe T, et al. Laser surgery for allergic and hypertrophic rhinitis. Ann Otol Rhinol Laryngol 1999; 108:3–19.

98. National Research Council. Committee on Airliner Cabin Environment Safety Committee. The Airliner Cabin Environment: Air Quality and Safety. Washington, D.C.: National Academy Press, 1986: p. 259–269.

99. National Research Council (NRC). Committee on Air Quality in Passenger Cabins of Commercial Aircraft, Board on Environmental Studies and Toxicology. The Airliner Cabin Environment and the Health of Passengers and Crew. Washington, D.C.: National Academy Press, 2002: p. 208–222.

100. Mattson ME, Boyd G, Byar D, et al. Passive smoking on commercial airline flights. JAMA 1989; 261:867–72.

101. Lieu JE, Feinstein AR. Confirmations and surprises in the association of tobacco use with sinusitis. Arch Otolaryngol Head Neck Surg 2000; 126:940–6.

102. Lieu JE, Feinstein AR. Effect of gestational and passive smoke exposure on ear infections in children. Arch Pediatr Adolesc Med 2002; 156:147–54.

103. Lam TH, Ho LM, Hedley AJ, et al. Environmental tobacco smoke exposure among police officers in Hong Kong. JAMA 2000; 284:756–63.

104. Willes SR, Fitzgerald TK, Bascom R. Nasal inhalation challenge studies with side-stream tobacco smoke. Arch Environ Health 1992; 47:223–30.

105. Bascom R, Kesavanathan J, Permutt T, et al. Tobacco smoke upper respiratory response relationships in healthy nonsmokers. Fundam Appl Toxicol 1996; 29:86–93.

106. Bascom R, Kesavanathan J, Fitzgerald TK, et al. Sidestream tobacco smoke exposure acutely alters human nasal mucociliary clearance. Environ Health Perspect. 1995; 103:1026–30.

107. Willes SR, Fitzgerald TK, Permutt T, et al. Acute respiratory response to prolonged, moderate levels of sidestream tobacco smoke. J Toxicol Environ Health A 1998; 53:193–209.

108. Klimek T, Glanz H, Ruckes-Nilges C. Nicotine induced endocytosis of amiloride-sensitive sodium channels in human nasal epithelium. Acta Otolaryngol 2000; 120:286–90.

109. Grieff L, Wollmer P, Andersson MC, et al. Human nasal absorption of 51 Cr- EDTA in smokers and control subjects. Clin Exp Allergy 1994; 24:1036–40.

110. Fischer J, Dahmen K, Jackowski M. Effect of chronic inhaled pollutants (cigarette smoke) on transepithelial measured potential difference of nasal mucosa in the human. Pneumologie 1990; 44:343–4.

111. Sopori ML, Kozak W. Immunomodulatory effects of cigarette smoke. J Neuroimmunol 1998; 83:148–52.

112.
Sopori M. Effects of cigarette smoke on the immune system. Nat Rev Immunol. 2002; 2:372–7.
113. Ramadan HH, Hinerman RA. Smoke exposure and outcome of endoscopic sinus surgery in children. Otolaryngol Head Neck Surg 2002; 127:546–8.
114. Sobol SE, Wright ED, Frenkiel S. One-year outcome analysis of functional endoscopic sinus surgery for chronic sinusitis. J Otolaryngol 1998; 27:252–7.
115. Briggs RD, Wright ST, Cordes S, et al. Smoking in chronic rhinosinusitis: a predictor of poor long-term outcome after endoscopic sinus surgery. Laryngoscope 2004; 114:126–8.
116. Senior BA, Kennedy DW, Tanabodee J, et al. Long-term results of functional endoscopic sinus surgery. Laryngoscope 1998; 108:151–7.
117. Spector SL. The role of allergy in sinusitis in adults. J Allergy Clin Immunol 1992; 90:518–20.
118. Savolainen S. Allergy in patients with acute maxillary sinusitis. Allergy 1989; 44:116–22.
119. Shapiro GG, Virant FS, Furukawa CT, et al. Immunologic defects in patients with refractory sinusitis. Pediatrics 1991; 87:311–6.
120. Rachelefsky G, Goldberg M, Kutz R, et al. Sinus disease in children with respiratory allergy. J Allergy Clin Immunol 1978; 61:310–4.
121. Shapiro GG. Role of allergy in sinusitis. Pediatr Infect Dis 1985; 4:S55-S59.
122. Iwens P, Clement PA. Sinusitis in allergic patients. Rhinology. 1994; 32:65–7.
123. Binder E, Holopainen E, Malmberg H, et al. Clinical findings in patients with allergic rhinitis. Rhinology 1984; 22:255–60.
124. Benninger M. Rhinitis, sinusitis and their relationships to allergies. Am J Rhinol 1992; 6:37–43.
125. Gutman M, Torees A., Keen KJ, et al. Prevalence of allergy in patients with chronic rhinosinusitis. Otolaryngol Head and Neck Surg 2002; 130:545–52.
126. Kirtsreesakul V, Naclerio RM. Role of allergy in rhinosinusitis. Curr Opin Allergy Clin Immunol 2004; 4:17–23.
127. Grove R, Farrior J. Chronic hyperplastic sinusitis in allergic patients. A bacteriologic study of two hundred operative cases. J Allergy 1990; 11:271–6.
128. Friedman WH. Surgery for chronic hyperplastic rhinosinusitis. Laryngoscope 1975; 85, 199–2011.
129. Van Dishoeck H, Franssen M. The incidence and correlation of allergy and chronic maxillary sinusitis. Pract Otolaryngol 1957; 19:502–6.
130. Rachelefsky GS. Chronic sinusitis. The disease of all ages. Am J Dis Child 1989; 143:886–8.
131. Furukawa CT. The role of allergy in sinusitis in children. J Allergy Clin Immunol 1992; 90, 515–7.
132. Chen Y, Dales R, Lin M. The epidemiology of chronic rhinosinusitis in Canadians. Laryngoscope 2003; 113:1199–205.
133. Naclerio RM, deTineo ML, Baroody FM. Ragweed allergic rhinitis and the paranasal sinuses: a computed tomographic study. Arch Otolaryngol Head Neck Surg 1997; 123:193–6.
134. Conner BL, Roach ES, Laster WS, et al. Magnetic resonance imaging of the paranasal sinuses: frequency and type of abnormalities. Ann Allergy 1989; 62:457–60.
135. Holzmann D, Willi U, Nadal D. Allergic rhinitis as a risk factor for orbital complication of acute rhinosinusitis in children. Am J Rhinol 2001; 15:387–90.
136. Chen CF, Wu KG, Hsu MC, et al. Prevalence and relationship between allergic diseases and infectious diseases. J Microbiol Immunol Infect 2001; 34:57–62.
137. Newman LJ, Platts-Mills TA, Phillips C, et al. Chronic sinusitis: relationship of computed tomography findings to allergy, asthma, and eosinophilia. JAMA 1994; 271:363–7.
138. Hoover GE, Newman LJ, Platts-Mills TA, et al. Chronic sinusitis: risk factors for extensive disease. J Allergy Clin Immunol 1997; 100:185–91.

139. Pelikan Z, Pelikan-Filipek M. Role of nasal allergy in chronic maxillary sinusitis-diagnostic value of nasal challenge with allergen. J Allergy Clin Immunol 1990; 86, 484–91.
140. Naclerio RM, deTineo ML, Baroody FM. Ragweed allergic rhinitis and the paranasal sinuses: a computed tomographic study. Arch Otolaryngol Head Neck Surg 1997; 123:193–06.
141. Berrettini S, Carabelli A, Sellari-Franceschini S, et al. Perennial allergic rhinitis and chronic sinusitis: correlation with rhinologic risk factors. Allergy 1999; 54:242–248.
142. Krause HF. Allergy and chronic rhinosinusitis. Otolaryngol Head Neck Surg 2003; 128:14–6.
143. Naclerio RM, Baroody FM, Nalini B, et al. A comparison of nasal clearance after treatment of perennial allergic rhinitis with budesonide and mometasone. Otolaryngol Head Neck Surg 2003; 128:220–7.
144. Parson DS. Chronic sinusitis: a medical or surgical disease? Otolaryngol Clin North Am 1996; 29:1–9.
145. Liu CM, Shun CT, Song HC, et al. Investigation into allergic response in patients with chronic sinusitis. J Formos Med Assoc 1992; 91:252–7.
146. Stammberger H. Endoscopic endonasal surgery—concepts in treatment of recovering rhinosinusitis. Part 1: Anatomic and pathophysiological considerations. Otolaryngol Head Neck Surg. 1986; 94:143–7.
147. Gern JE, Rosenthal LA, Sorkness RL, et al. Effects of viral respiratory infections on lung development and childhood asthma. J Allergy Clin Immunol. 2005; 15:668–74.
148. Arruda LK, Sole D, Baena-Cagnani CE, et al. Risk factors for asthma and atopy. Curr Opin Allergy Clin Immunol 2005; 5:153–9.
149. Ramsey CD, Celedon JC. The hygiene hypothesis and asthma. Curr Opin Pulm Med 2005; 11:14–20.
150. Peebles RS, Hashimoto K, Graham BS. The complex relationship between respiratory syntytial virus and allergy in lung disease. Viral Immunol 2003; 16:25–34.
151. Sotir M, Yeatts K, Shy C. Presence of asthma risk factors and environmental exposures related to upper respiratory infection-triggered wheezing in middle school-age children. Environ Health Perspect 2003; 111:657–62.
152. Harlin SL, Ansel DG, Lane SR, et al. A clinical and pathologic study of chronic sinusitis: the role of the eosinophil. J Allergy Clin Immunol 1988; 81:867–75.
153. Elwany S, Bassyouni M, Morad F. Some risk factors for refractory chronic sinusitis: an immunohistochemical and electron microscopic study. J Laryngol Otol 2002; 116:112–5.
154. Suzuki M, Watanabe T, Suko T, et al. Comparison of sinusitis with and without allergic rhinitis: characteristics of paranasal sinus effusion and mucosa. Am J Otolaryngol 1999; 20:143–50.
155. Hamilos DL, Leung DYM, Wood R, et al. Evidence for distinct cytokine expression in allergic versus non-allergic chronic sinusitis. J Allergy Clin Immunol 1995; 96: 537–44.
156. Hamilos DL, Leung DYM, Wood R, et al. Chronic hyperplastic sinusitis: association of tissue eosinophilia with mRNA expression of granulocyte-macrophage colony-stimulating factor and interleukin-3. J Allergy Clin Immunol 1993; 92:39–48.
157. Hamilos DL, Leung DYM, Wood R, et al. Eosinophil infiltration in non-allergic chronic hyperplastic sinusitis with nasal polyposis (CHS/NP) is associated with endothelial VCAM-1 upregulation and expression of TNF-α. Am J Respir Cell Mol Biol 1996; 15:443–50.
158. Driscoll PV, Naclerio RM, Baroody FM. CD4+ lymphocytes are increased in the sinus mucosa of children with chronic sinusitis. Arch Otolaryngol Head Neck Surg 1996; 122:1071–76.
159. Jyonouchi H, Sun S, Rimell F. Cytokine production by sinus lavage, bronchial lavage, and blood mononuclears in chronic rhinosinusitis with or without atopy. Arch Otolaryngol Head Neck Surg 2000; 126:522–8.
160. Riccio AM, Tosca MA, Cosentino C, et al. Cytokine pattern in allergic and non-allergic chronic rhinosinusitis in asthmatic children. Clin Exp Allergy 2002; 32:422–6.

161. Wright ED, Frenkiel S, Al-Ghamdi K. Interleukin-4: interleukin-5: and granulocyte-colony-stimulating factor receptor expression in chronic sinusitis and response to topical steroids. Otolaryngol Head Neck Surg 1998; 118:490–95.
162. Bachert C, Gevaert P, Holtappels G, et al. Total and specific IgE in nasal polyps is related to local eosinophilic inflammation. J Allergy Clin Immunol 2001; 107:607–14.
163. Bachert C, van Zele T, Gevaert P, et al. Superantigens and nasal polyps. Curr Allergy Asthma Rep 2003; 3:523–31.
164. Jyonouchi H, Sun S, Le H, et al. Evidence of dysregulated cytokine production by sinus lavage and peripheral blood mononuclear cells in patients with treatment-resistant chronic rhinosinusitis. Arch Otolaryngol Head Neck Surg 2001; 127:1488–94.
165. Sasama J, Sherris DA, Shin SH, et al. New paradigm for the roles of fungi and eosino-phils in chronic rhinosinusitis. Curr Opin Otolaryngol Head Neck Surg. 2005; 13:2–8.
166. Neel HB, Whicker JH, Lake CF. Thin rubber sheeting in frontal sinus surgery: animal and clinical studies. Laryngoscope 1976; 86:524–36.
167. McNeil RA. An obliteration operation for chronic maxillary sinusitis. A preliminary report. J Laryngol Otol 1966; 80:953–6.
168. Gardiner Q, Oluwole M, Tan L, et al. An animal model for training in endoscopic nasal and sinus surgery. J Laryngol Otol 1996; 110:425–8.
169. McIntosh D, Cowin A, Adams D, et al. The effect of a dissolvable hyaluronic acid-based pack on the healing of the nasal mucosa of sheep. Am J Rhinol 2002; 16:85–90.
170. Shaw CL, Dymock RB, Cowin A. Effect of packing on nasal mucosa of sheep. J Laryngol Otol 2000; 114:506–9.
171. McIntosh D, Cowin A, Adams D. The effect of a dissolvable hyaluronic acid-based pack on the healing of the nasal mucosa of sheep. Am J Rhinol 2002; 16:85–90.
172. Robinson S, Adams D, Wormald PJ. The effect of nasal packing and prednisolone on mucosal healing and reciliation in a sheep model. Rhinology 2004; 42:68–72.
173. Rajapaksa S, McIntosh D, Cowin A, et al. The effect of insulin like growth factor 1 incorporated into a hyaluronic acid-based nasal pack on nasal mucosal healing in a healthy sheep model and a sheep model of chronic sinusitis. Am J Rhinol 2005; 19:251–6.
174. Padrid PA, Mathur M, Li X, et al. CTLA4Ig inhibits airway eosinophilia and hyperresponsiveness by regulating the development of Th1/Th2 subsets in a murine model of asthma. Am J Respir Cell Mol Biol 1998; 18:453–62.
175. Ramalingam TR, Reiman RM, Wynn TA. Exploiting worm and allergy models to understand Th2 cytokine biology. Curr Opin Allergy Clin Immunol 2005; 5:392–8.
176. Brumund KT, Graham SM, Beck KC. The effect of maxillary sinus antrostomy size on xenon ventilation in the sheep model. Otolaryngol Head Neck Surg 2004; 131:528–33.
177. Kelemen G. The nasal and paranasal cavities of the rabbit in experimental work. Arch Otolaryngol 1955; 61:497–512.
178. Marks SC. Acute sinusitis in the rabbit: a new rhinogenic model. Laryngoscope. 1997; 107, 1579–85.
179. Marks SC. Acute sinusitis in the rabbit model: histologic analysis. Laryngoscope. 1998; 108:320–5.
180. Kara CO, Cetin CB, Demirkan N, et al. Experimental sinusitis in a rhinogenic model. Laryngoscope. 2004; 114:273–8.
181. Kara CO. Animal models of sinusitis: relevance to human disease. Curr Allergy Asthma Rep 2004; 4:496–9.
182. Kerschner JE, Cruz MJ, Beste DJ, et al. Computed tomography vs. magnetic resonance imaging of acute bacterial sinusitis: a rabbit model. Am J Otolaryngol 2000; 21:298–305.
183. Kennedy CA, Jyonouchi H, Kajander KC, et al. Middle ear pathologic changes associated with chronic anaerobic sinusitis in rabbits. Laryngoscope 1999; 109:498–503.
184. Irvin CG. Sinusitis and asthma: an animal model. J Allergy Clin Immunol 1992; 90:521–33.
185. Brugman SM, Larsen GL, Henson PM, et al. Increased lower airway responsiveness associated with sinusitis in a rabbit model. Am Rev Respir Dis 1993; 147:314–20.
186. Drettner B, Johansson P, Kumlien J. Experimental acute sinusitis in rabbit. A study of mucosal blood flow. Acta Otolaryngol 1987; 103:432–4.

187. Johansson P, Kumlien J, Soderlund K, et al. Experimental acute sinusitis in rabbits. Energy metabolism in sinus mucosa and secretion. Acta Otolaryngol 1988; 106:460–7.
188. Stierna P, Soderlund K, Hultman E. Chronic maxillary sinusitis. Energy metabolism in sinus mucosa and secretion. Acta Otolaryngol 1991; 111:135–43.
189. Stierna P, Kumlien J, Carlsoo B. Experimental sinusitis in rabbits induced by aerobic and anaerobic bacteria: models for research in sinusitis. J Otolaryngol 1991; 20:376–8.
190. Norlander T, Fukami M, Westrin KM, et al. Formation of mucosal polyps in the nasal and maxillary sinus cavities by infection. Otolaryngol Head Neck Surg 1993; 109:522–9.
191. Westrin KM, Stierna P, Carlsoo B, et al. Mucosal fine structure in experimental sinusitis. Ann Otol Rhinol Laryngol 1993; 102:639–45.
192. Beste DJ, Capper DT, Shaffer K, et al. Antimicrobial effect on rabbit sinusitis after temporary ostial occlusion. Am J Rhinol 1997; 11:485–9.
193. Kara CO, Cetin CB, Demirkan N, et al. Experimental sinusitis in a rhinogenic model. Laryngoscope 2004; 114:273–8.
194. Cable B, Wassmuth Z, Mann EA. The effect of corticosteroids in the treatment of experimental sinusitis. Am J Rhinol 2000; 14:217–22.
195. Hurley DB, Smith GS, Vogler GA. Leukotriene B4 levels in rabbit maxillary sinusitis: limitations of the current model. Am J Rhinol 2001; 15:47–8.
196. Karasen Rm, Uslu C, Gundogdu C. Effect of WEB 2170 BS, platelet activating factor receptor inhibitor, in the rabbit model of sinusitis. Ann Otol Rhinol Laryngol 2004; 113:477–82.
197. Otori N, Paydas G, Stierna P. The anti-inflammatory effect of fusafungine during experimentally induced rhinosinusitis in the rabbit. Eur Arch Otorhinolaryngol 1998; 255:195–201.
198. Brown CL, Graham SM, Cable BB, et al. Xylitol enhances bacterial killing in the rabbit maxillary sinus. Laryngoscope 2004; 114:2021–4.
199. Bende M, Fukami M, Arfors KE, et al. Effect of oxymetazoline nose drops on acute sinusitis in the rabbit. Ann Otol Rhinol Laryngol 1996; 105:222–5.
200. Suh SH, Chon KM, Min YG, et al. Effects of topical nasal decongestants on histology of nasal respiratory mucosa in rabbits. Acta Otolaryngol 1995; 115:664–71.
201. Scheld WM. Evaluation of quinolones in experimental animal models of infections. Eur J Clin Microbiol Infect Dis 1991; 10:275–90.
202. Verwoerd-Verhoef HL, Verwoerd CD. Surgery of the lateral nasal wall and ethmoid: effects on sinonasal growth: an experimental study in rabbits. Int J Pediatr Otorhinolaryngol 2003; 67:263–9.
203. Benninger MS, Kaczor J, Stone C. Natural ostiotomy vs. inferior antrostomy in the management of sinusitis: an animal model. Otolaryngol Head Neck Surg 1993; 109:1034–42.
204. Perko D, Karin RR. Nasoantral windows: an experimental study in rabbits. Laryngoscope 1992; 102:320–6.
205. Min YG, Lee YM, Lee BJ, et al. The effect of ostial opening on experimental maxillary sinusitis in rabbits. Rhinology 1993; 31:101–5.
206. Beste D, Capper D, Shaffer K, et al. Antimicrobial effect on rabbit sinusitis after temporary ostial occlusion. Am J Rhinol 1997; 11:485–9.
207. Scharf K, Lawson W, Shapiro J, et al. Pressure measurements in the normal and occluded rabbit maxillary sinus. Laryngoscope 1995; 105:570–4.
208. Matsune S, Masahiko E, Ohyama M. Application of YAMIK sinus catheter for patients with paranasal sinusitis with and without nasal allergy. Auris Nasus Larynx 2000; 27:343–7.
209. Roche AK, Koutlas IG, Kajander KC. Labeling of calcitonin gene-related peptide and substance P increases in subnucleus caudalis of rabbit during maxillary sinusitis. Brain Res 1998; 791:283–9.
210. Hinni ML, McCaffrey TV, Kasperbauer JL. Early mucosal changes in experimental sinusitis. Otolaryngol Head Neck Surg 1992; 107:537–48.
211. Dufour X, Kauffmann-Lacroix C, Goujon JM, et al. Experimental model of fungal sinusitis: a pilot study in rabbits. Ann Otol Rhinol Laryngol 2005; 114:167–72.

212. Cetin CB, Kara CO, Colakoglu N, et al. Experimental sinusitis in nasally catheterised rabbits. Rhinology 2002; 40:154–8.
213. Westrin KM, Stierna P, Carlsoo B, et al. Mucosal fine structure in experimental sinusitis. Ann Otol Rhinol Laryngol 1993; 102:639–45.
214. Sabirov A, Kodama S, Sabirova N, et al. Intranasal immunization with outer membrane protein P6 and cholera toxin induces specific sinus mucosal immunity and enhances sinus clearance of nontypeable Haemophilus influenzae. Vaccine 2004; 22:3112–21.
215. Schlosser RJ, Spotnitz WD, Peters EJ, et al. Elevated nitric oxide metabolite levels in chronic sinusitis. Otolaryngol Head Neck Surg 2000; 123:357–62.
216. Kumlien J, Schiratzki H. Blood flow in the rabbit sinus mucosa during experimentally induced chronic sinusitis. Measurement with a diffusible and with a non-diffusible tracer. Acta Otolaryngol 1985; 99:630–6.
217. Kennedy DW. Pathogenesis of chronic rhinosinusitis. Ann Otol Rhinol Laryngol Suppl 2004; 193:6–9.
218. Bomer K, Brichta A, Baroody F, et al. A mouse model of acute bacterial rhinosinusitis. Arch Otolaryngol Head Neck Surg 1998; 124:1227–32.
219. Won YS, Brichta A, Baroody F, et al. Bactrim reduces the inflammatory response in a murine model of acute rhinosinusitis. Rhinology 2000; 38:68–71.
220. Blair C, Nelson M, Thomson K, et al. Allergic inflammation enhances bacterial sinusitis in mice. J Allergy Clin Immunol 2001; 108:424–429.
221. Yu X, Sperling A, Blair C, Thompson K, et al. Antigen stimulation of TH2 cells augments acute bacterial sinusitis in mice. J Allergy Clin Immunol 2004; 114:328–34.
222. Kirtsreesakul V, Blair C, Yu X, et al. Desloratadine partially inhibits the augmented bacterial responses in the sinuses of allergic and infected mice. Clin Exp Allergy 2004; 34:1649–54.
223. Blair C, Naclerio RM, Yu X, et al. Role of type 1 T helper cells in the resolution of acute *Streptococcus pneumoniae* sinusitis: A mouse model. J Infect Dis. 2005; 192:1237–44.
224. Xie M. A comparative experimental study between recombinant active gene 1-deficient mice and C57BL/6 mice model of acute bacterial rhinosinusitis Zhonghua Er Bi Yan Hou Ke Za Zhi 2002; 37:23–6.
225. Lemanske RF Jr. Viral infections and asthma inception. J Allergy Clin Immunol 2004; 114:1023–26.
226. Jacob A, Faddis BT, Chole RA. Chronic bacterial rhinosinusitis: description of a mouse model. Arch Otolaryngol Head Neck Surg 2001; 127(6):657-664.
227. McCool TL, Weiser JN. Limited role of antibody in clearance of *Streptococcus pneumoniae* in a murine model of colonization. Infect Immun 2004; 72, 5807–13.
228. Lipsitch M, Dykes JK, Johnson SE, et al. Competition among *Streptococcus pneumoniae* for intranasal colonization in mouse model. Vaccine 2000; 18:2895–901.
229. Gwaltney JM Jr, Hendley JO, Patrie JT. Symptom severity patterns in experimental common colds and their usefulness in timing onset of illness in natural colds. Clin Infect Dis 2003; 36:714–23.
230. Turner RB, Witek TJ Jr, Riker DK. Comparison of symptom severity in natural and experimentally induced colds. Am J Rhinol 1996; 10:167–172.
231. Turner RB, Bauer R, Woelkart K, et al. An evaluation of Echinacea angustifolia in experimental rhinovirus infections. N Engl J Med 2005; 353:341–8.
232. Buchman CA, Doyle WJ, Pilcher O, et al. Nasal and otologic effects of experimental respiratory syncytial virus infection in adults. Am J Otolaryngol 2002; 23:70–5.
233. Fakhri S, Christodoulopoulos P, Tulic M, et al. Role of microbial toxins in the induction of glucocorticoid receptor beta expression in an explant model of rhinosinusitis. J Otolaryngol 2003; 32:388–93.
234. Fakhri S, Tulic M, Christodoulopoulos P, et al. Microbial superantigens induce glucocorticoid receptor beta and steroid resistance in a nasal explant model. Laryngoscope 2004; 114:887–92.
235. Hauber HP, Daigneault P, Frenkiel S, et al. Niflumic acid and MSI-2216 reduce TNF-alpha-induced mucin expression in human airway mucosa. J Allergy Clin Immunol 2005; 115:266–71.

4 Innate and Acquired Immunity and Epithelial Cell Function in Chronic Rhinosinusitis

R. P. Schleimer
Division of Allergy-Immunology, Northwestern University Feinberg School of Medicine, Chicago, Illinois, U.S.A.

Andrew P. Lane and J. Kim
Department of Otolaryngology–Head and Neck Surgery, Johns Hopkins University, Baltimore, Maryland, U.S.A.

INTRODUCTION

The purpose of this review is to discuss the role of epithelial cells in chronic rhinosinusitis (CRS) from the perspective of their participation in immunity in the upper airways and sinuses and their mediation of components of the inflammatory response. Triggering of CRS is complex and not well understood. Inanimate airborne materials, antigens and pathogenic organisms can all play a role in CRS and influence the function and phenotype of the airway epithelium. Epithelial cells are prominently involved in the defense of the airways from all these external forces and this can come at the cost of inflammation and disease. We have provided an overview of the many processes in which epithelial cells participate, including innate immunity, adaptive immunity, inflammation, and remodeling. While CRS is an inflammatory disease that is mediated by several cell types and impacts several cell types, we believe that the epithelium is uniquely involved both as a target and mediator of this disease.

OVERVIEW OF MUCOSAL IMMUNITY IN THE SINONASAL MICROENVIRONMENT

The nasal cavity is often the first point of contact between the airway mucosa and the external environment. Inspired air contains a wide assortment of microbial and non-microbial elements, some of which have the potential to harm the host. Multiple mechanisms exist at the mucosal surface to defend against such threats. Primary among these is the continuously flowing mucus blanket, which traps particulates in the air and sweeps them towards the nasopharynx. Contained within the mucus are a variety of antimicrobial products, including enzymes, immunoglobulins, opsonins, and defensins. Acute challenge by inspired irritants stimulates additional mucus and tear production and accelerates mucociliary transport. Triggering of sensory C fibers in the nasal cavity also elicits a sneeze reflex that expels entrapped particles from the nose. Through these non-specific, constitutively active pathways, the majority of airborne particles and organisms are harmlessly removed without further activation of the immune system.

At the same time, the mucosa of the sinonasal tract plays an important sentinel role in sampling the contents of the external environment and initiating the appropriate immune response. In many cases, the response is one of tolerance and suppression of adaptive immune system activation. Antigens at the mucosal surface are routinely internalized by dendritic cells (DCs) and processed for antigen presentation to T cells in lymphatic tissue. Antigen-specific T cells move to the sinonasal mucosa to become activated upon re-exposure to the same antigen, in the context of proper costimulation. Under normal conditions, the sinonasal mucosa exists in a state of readiness, capable of directing local, specific immune mechanisms when challenged. The stimulation of adaptive immune processes or the removal of inhibitory signals that restrain them, allows the full force of the immune system to come to bear on threats within the nasal cavity lumen through a cascade of pro-inflammatory and host defense-directed products and the recruitment of potent granulocytes. The interaction between the innate and adaptive immune systems in the nose must be regulated tightly to control the destructive potential of the inflammatory reaction.

At the front line of the mucosal surface are the ciliated respiratory epithelial cells. These cells have been shown over recent years to play more than a simple passive barrier function, but rather to act as complex and active participants in the mucosal immune response. Not only are epithelial cells capable of producing antimicrobial products, but they are also able to directly recognize pathogens through pattern recognition receptors and to express costimulatory molecules necessary for communication with T lymphocytes. At present, the role of the sinonasal epithelial cell in the pathogenesis of CRS is suspected but has not been firmly established. Some existing theories of CRS postulate that the underlying inflammatory mechanism may lead to an abnormal host mucosal immune response to microbial agents present in the nasal airway lumen. Fungi, staphylococcal superantigens, bacterial biofilms, and viral infections have all been suggested as potential triggers (1–6). If this is indeed the case, and CRS represents a dysregulated immune response to one or more of these exogenous agents, it is likely that epithelial cells play critical roles in the initiation or maintenance of the sustained mucosal inflammatory state. Therefore, an understanding of the immune function of the sinonasal epithelial cell in healthy and diseased states may lead to the development of novel treatment strategies for CRS.

INNATE IMMUNITY AND CRS
Review of Innate Immune Effector Systems
Cells

Direct sensing of pathogens in the sinonasal tract occurs via multiple mechanisms. Patrolling macrophages and DCs at or near the mucosal surface interact with microbial and non-microbial elements through cell-surface receptors. Opsonization of such entities with antibody or complement allows efficient binding and internalization by these common phagocytic cells. Polymorphonuclear leukocytes and other inflammatory cells—eosinophils, basophils, and mast cells—also interact with opsonized foreign particles and microbes to activate extracellular release of potent antimicrobial enzymes. Although many of the immune activities of fixed tissue and circulating phagocytes are generally considered to be pathogen-non-specific, the presence of opsonins with specificity for pathogen structures (e.g., mannose, galactofuranose and other carbohydrate-binding proteins such as collectins, pentraxins) and macrophage mannose receptors can provide some specificity. Innate phagocytic immune function, which occurs in coordination with the adaptive immune system, acts to recruit particular effector cell populations to the mucosal surface and produce antigen-specific antibodies. Although they generally do not phagocytize large quantities of microbes, epithelial cells have the ability to detect potential pathogens and respond via secreted products that are described in detail below. Leukocyte cell populations and resident epithelial macrophages also elaborate effector proteins that are secreted extracellularly to inhibit microbial growth.

Non-specific Innate Mucosal Defense Mechanisms
Mucociliary Clearance
One of the primary functions of the nasal cavity is to serve as a filter of inspired air. This is accomplished in part through the narrow physical dimensions of the nasal passages themselves, but mainly by the presence of an adherent blanket of mucus that is perpetually propelled by the ciliary action of epithelial cells. The epithelial lining fluid covering the airways derives its proteins from plasma transudate, mucous and serous cells in submucosal glands, goblet cells, Clara cells, epithelial cells, and other cells within the mucosa (plasma cells, mast cells, phagocytes, and fibroblasts). Airborne particulates that enter the nose become immediately deposited on the mucosal surface and are cleared over a relatively short period of time (7). The primary factors influencing the efficiency of mucociliary clearance include the ciliary beat frequency and the quantity and viscoelastic properties of the mucus. The viscous mucous gel rides over the surface of a more fluid periciliary liquid layer directly above the epithelium. The major constituents of mucus are high-molecular-weight, heavily glycosylated macromolecules that are derived from two distinct mucin genes known as *MUC5AC* and *MUC5B* (8). The viscoelastic properties of the mucus are largely determined by the tangled network of these mucin molecules, which is in turn modulated by the water content, ion concentration, and pH of the mucus. Mucin macromolecules bind and trap inhaled particles with extraordinary avidity owing to the diversity of their carbohydrate side chains. Other mucins such as MUC1 and MUC4 are tethered to the epithelial cell surface and extend out to the airway lumen, allowing indirect interaction of epithelial cells with particles in the environment.

There is a wide variability in the rate of mucociliary clearance in normal subjects and patients with inflammatory sinonasal disease even over the course of a day in an individual subject. Although it is unclear how the rate of mucociliary movement is regulated, the process is postulated to involve tachykinin-mediated neural mechanisms or via cyclic nucleotides released in response to airway luminal stress (9). Increased mucociliary flow in response to airborne irritants is an important non-specific defense mechanism employed by the sinonasal epithelium. The presence of antimicrobial factors to be described below suppresses the growth of microbes trapped within the mucus layer while they are trafficked into the nasopharynx. However, chronic stasis of mucus due to poor mucociliary function gives these organisms an opportunity to overcome secreted defenses and grow exponentially within the sinonasal cavities.

Secreted Antimicrobials
Sinonasal epithelial cells secrete a large array of molecules that are involved in inflammatory and immune processes (10–12). Some of these mediators are involved in the chemoattraction and activation of effector cells of the innate and adaptive immune system, while others act directly to immobilize and kill microorganisms. These endogenous "antibiotics" serve a critical role in immediate host defense against potential pathogens entering the body through nasal breathing. Examples of these molecules include small cationic peptides such as β-defensins,

as well as larger antimicrobial proteins such as lysozyme, lactoferrin, and secretory leukocyte proteinase inhibitor (SLPI) (13–15). The inhibition of microbial growth and direct microbicidal activity provides time to eliminate the threat through the mucociliary apparatus, or to recruit phagocytic cells and develop an adaptive immune response when necessary. Therefore, the pathologic deficiency of the antimicrobial properties of airway secretions may contribute to epithelial colonization by microorganisms in CRS.

A major antibacterial product secreted by nasal epithelial cells is lysozyme, a 14-kDa enzyme directed against glycosidic bonds in the peptidoglycan cell wall of bacteria. In 1922, when Alexander Fleming first described the intrinsic antimicrobial properties of human nasal secretions, he attributed them to lysozyme (16). In addition to the enzymatic lysis of bacterial cell walls, lysozyme can also kill bacteria by a non-enzymatic mechanism (17). While lysozyme is highly effective against many common upper airway gram-positive species, such as streptococci, it appears to kill gram-negative bacteria only when potentiated by cofactors such as lactoferrin, antibody–complement complexes, or ascorbic acid (18). Presumably, these other agents act to disrupt the outer membrane of gram-negative bacteria sufficiently to allow lysozyme access to the sensitive peptidoglycan layer. Lysozyme is produced by monocytes, macrophages, and epithelial cells, and it is a major component of both phagocytic and secretory granules of neutrophils. Despite the multiple sources of lysozyme, it is believed that the airway epithelium and seromucous glands are the major sources of lysozyme in airway secretions. The important role of lysozyme in airway defense is exemplified by transgenic mice overexpressing lysozyme, which demonstrate increased resistance to lung infection with group *B. Streptococcus* or *Pseudomonas aeruginosa* (19).

Next to lysozyme, the most commonly secreted antimicrobial product is lactoferrin, an 80-kDa iron-binding protein that inhibits microbial growth by sequestering iron (20). Lactoferrin is stored and released by serous mucosal glands, and is also a major component of neutrophil granules. It can also be directly microbicidal, an activity that is concentrated in its N-terminal cationic fragment "lactoferricin" (21). Another defensive molecule found in nasal mucus is SLPI, a 12-kDa protein with two separate functional domains. The N-terminal domain has been demonstrated in vitro to have activity against both gram-negative and gram-positive bacteria (22). The C-terminal domain inhibits neutrophil elastase and may also be involved in the intracellular regulation of responses to lipopolysaccharide (LPS) (23). Secretory phospholiphase A_2 (sPLA$_2$) is another secreted product identified from methacholine-induced nasal lavage that has Ca^{2+}-dependent antimicrobial activity against both gram-positive and gram-negative bacteria (24,25).

Defensins and cathelicidins are large families of antimicrobial peptides produced in the sinonasal tract. Human defensins are 3- to 5-kDa peptides with a characteristic three-dimensional fold and six-cysteine/three-disulfide patterns (26). α-defensins are contained in granules of neutrophils and Paneth cells of the intestine. The β-defensins of the upper airways are human beta defensin (HBD)-1, -2, -3, and -4. Whereas HBD-1 is expressed constitutively, expression of HBD-2–4 has been shown to be induced by exposure to pro-inflammatory cytokines or endotoxin. The cathelicidin family of microbicidal peptides has highly heterogeneous C-terminal peptides that are freed and activated by extracellular proteolytic cleavage (27–29). The only known human cathelicidin has been named hCAP18 and FALL-39/LL-37 by different groups that described the gene, the cDNA, and the peptide (29–31). Antimicrobial peptides have a broad-spectrum activity against the surface membranes of gram-positive and gram-negative bacteria as well as against fungi and enveloped viruses. Their activity is synergistic with that of lysozyme and lactoferrin (32). The importance of antimicrobial peptides in vivo is supported by a number of studies in mice. For example, knock-out mice lacking matrix metalloprotease-7 (MMP-7), an enzyme that cleaves and activates antimicrobial peptides, have been shown to have increased susceptibility to enteric pathogens (33). Similarly, transgenic mice lacking either the murine homolog of LL-37 or of β-defensin 1 also have impaired ability to clear bacterial infections (34,35). Conversely, overexpression of LL-37 or defensins appears to augment immune function and provide increased protection against infection.

Recent experiments utilizing epithelial cell lines in vitro have shown that acute-phase proteins such as complement components and serum amyloid A (SAA) are also produced by epithelial cells (36). Expression of these genes can be induced BEAS2B cells (a lung epithelial cell line) by exposure to the double-stranded RNA (dsRNA) analog, polyI:C, a ligand for Toll-like receptor 3 (TLR3) (see below). In vivo, the presence of complement component 3 protein can be demonstrated in both normal and inflamed sinonasal mucosa (37,38). Previously, these proteins have been presumed to be derived from plasma exudation, rather than local production. However, mRNA for all components of the alternative pathway of complement activation are present in mucosal specimens obtained from the ethmoid sinuses of human subjects. Cleavage products of C3 are potent chemoattractants for granulocytes and act to opsonize particulates for removal by phagocytes. In addition, the SAA gene has been shown to be expressed in sinus mucosa, and this expression occurs at a significantly higher level in patients with recalcitrant CRS with polyps when compared with those with treatment-responsive CRS (39). SAA has been shown to bind directly to gram-positive bacteria and is probably an important opsonin. The functional role of acute-phase proteins in the pathogenesis of CRS has not yet been demonstrated.

PATTERN RECOGNITION RECEPTORS

Toll-like receptors are a family of evolutionarily ancient proteins involved in the recognition of conserved motifs associated with pathogens (40–42). TLRs were originally identified by their similarity to *Drosophila* Toll, a protein implicated in dorsoventral patterning in embryogenesis, which also was shown to induce nuclear factor kappa-B (NF-κB) activation when stimulated by fungal antigens. There are 11 known mammalian TLRs, all characterized by the presence of an extracellular domain with leucine-rich repeats and an intracellular signaling domain similar to that of the interleukin-1 (IL-1) receptor family [Toll/IL-1 receptor (TIR) domain]. Factors important in the signal transduction pathway of TLRs include MyD88, IL-1 receptor-associated kinase (IRAK), tumor necrosis factor (TNF)-receptor associated factor-6 (TRAF-6), mitogen-activated protein kinases (MAPK), and NF-κB. Although the function of each of the TLRs has not been fully elucidated, the individual TLR proteins appear to recognize distinct pathogen-associated molecular patterns (PAMPs), such as zymosan, lipopeptides, endotoxin, flagellin, dsRNA, or bacterial DNA. There is increasing evidence that TLRs mediate the well-known activation of epithelial cells by microorganisms and their products.

Situated at the interface between the external environment and the mucosal surface, it is not surprising that epithelial cells of the respiratory, digestive, and urogenital tract express TLRs. Activation of TLRs at the mucosal surface allows primary defensive immune mechanisms to be initiated locally, while initiating communication of the presence of pathogens to the adaptive immune system. It is important to recognize that these mucosal surfaces are normally colonized with microbes, and that encounters with potential pathogens are commonplace. This is to be contrasted with TLRs expressed by epithelial cells in sterile body compartments or on internal mucosal surfaces that are not directly exposed to the external environment. In the nasal cavity, where microbial interaction is frequent, there is likely to be negative regulation of TLR activation and development of tolerance to normal upper airway flora. This process has not yet been demonstrated in the sinonasal tract, but is known to occur in the intestinal epithelium. There are multiple negative regulators of the TLR signal transduction pathway that are active in epithelial cells, including SIGRR, Tollip, splice variants of MyD88 or IRAK, and A20. It has been established that epithelial cells develop tolerance to LPS after multiple stimulations, and that cross-inhibition of other TLR occurs as well. It is possible that TLRs can discriminate structural differences in pathogen-associated ligands, thus permitting differentiation between commensal and pathogenic microbes. For example, TLR4-mediated cytokine production is decreased when LPS is derived from normal commensal intestinal bacteria when compared with pathogenic strains. Recent studies indicate that TLR signaling can be involved in immune tolerance as well as inflammatory responses.

SIGNALING MOLECULES

Nucleotide-binding oligomerization proteins (Nods) are a family of cytosolic pattern recognition proteins that activate NF-κB and caspase pathways. Nod proteins are phylogenetically ancient and are related to the disease resistance genes of plants. The best-studied members of the Nod family are Nod1 and Nod2, which recognize peptidoglycans (PGN) of bacteria. Mutations in the Nod2 gene have been linked to increased susceptibility to Crohn's disease. Nod1 seems to be most specific to gram-negative bacterial PGN, whereas Nod2 acts as a general sensor for all PGN molecules. It is hypothesized that dysfunction of the bacterial-sensing capabilities of Nod proteins may undermine local immune defenses and allow bacterial infection to occur. Similar to TLRs, Nods are believed to be involved in the coupling of the innate and adaptive immune responses to pathogens. Activation of Nods requires that the bacterial PGN be delivered to the cytosol, either by direct invasion or through phagosomes. The signaling pathways utilized by Nods and TLRs differ, with Nod1 and Nod2 utilizing a common downstream molecule, Rip2, which is independent of MyD88.

Lessons from Deficiencies in Humans and Mice

Many of the agents that have been shown to be ligands for TLRs were identified in knock-out mice deficient for the individual receptors. In other experiments, mice lacking TLR signaling molecules or other innate immune components have been bred to study the in vivo functions of these genes. In humans, there are known to be common loss-of-function polymorphisms of the TLR5 gene, involved in the recognition of bacterial flagellin. A stop codon polymorphism present in approximately 10% of the population has been shown to result in production of a dominant negative receptor. Individuals with this genotype have an increased susceptibility to pneumonia caused by the flagellated *Legionella* bacteria (43).

However, there does not appear to be any defect in the immune response to another flagellated bacterial species, *Salmonella enterica*, which is the pathogen causing typhoid fever (44). The lack of a consistent disease phenotype associated with TLR5 deficiency suggests that the immune function of TLR5 may be largely redundant. Reduced function polymorphisms in TLR4 have been linked to increases in the risk of gram-negative infections and respiratory syncytial virus (RSV); polymorphisms in TLR2 have been linked to increased infections with tuberculosis and staphylococcal infections (for review see Ref. 45). Genetic analyses have revealed that human TLR11 is a pseudogene, although the murine counterpart is not, and therefore there is no disease phenotype of human TLR11 deficiency (46).

Inherited disorders of Toll-like receptor signaling pathways exist in humans and are associated with primary immunodeficiency syndromes. Certain mutations of the NF-κB essential modulator (NEMO) and of IκBα are associated with anhidrotic ectodermal dysplasia with immunodeficiency (EDA-ID). EDA-ID is characterized by a number of developmental anomalies as well as an array of infectious diseases. Autosomal recessive mutations in IRAK4 also result in immunological defects that are more restricted. In such patients, there is a susceptibility to pyogenic bacterial infections, as well as a reduced response to TIR agonists.

Knock-out mice have been bred to study the effect of deletion of most of the TLR genes. Disruption of the TLR1 and TLR2 genes leads to a loss of response to triacylated lipopeptides and peptidoglycans, respectively, demonstrating these ligand–receptor relationships. TLR2 forms heterodimers with other TLRs to create receptors specific for different lipopeptides. Discrimination of mycoplasmal macrophage-activating lipopeptide-2-kDa (MALP-2) requires the presence of TLR6, and knock-out mice lacking TLR6 cannot recognize MALP-2 even with a functional TLR2 receptor (47). TLR3−/− mice lose responsiveness to poly(I:C), a synthetic analog of viral dsRNA, while TLR4−/− mice are resistant to systemic endotoxin. Knock-out mice lacking TLR4 also demonstrate impaired DC function, with decreased expression of the costimulatory molecule CD86. The lack of CD86 costimulation reduces the ability of DCs to activate (Th2) T lymphocytes upon presentation of non-pathogenic antigens. Although TLR2 and TLR4 have been implicated in innate mycobacterial recognition in vitro, knock-out mice lacking TLR2, TLR4, and TLR6 do not have increased susceptibility to infection with *Mycoplasma bovis*. However, deficiency of TLR7 leads to reduced immune responses to vesicular stomatitis virus. Absence of TLR9 confers resistance to CpG DNA.

Knock-out mice with deficiencies in TLR signaling molecules also have phenotypes that shed light on the immune system functions of innate pattern recognition receptors. MyD88−/− mice have abrogated NF-κB responses to TLR2 and TLR9 ligands, but TLR4 is capable of signaling via an MyD88-independent pathway. MyD88 deficiency in knock-out mice is associated with impaired clearance of *Chlamydia pneumoniae* infection. Knock-out mice lacking Nod2 have defective macrophage responses to the muramyl dipeptide motif of peptidoglycans. Deficiency of Nod2 leads to increased Th1 cytokine production, secondary to loss of the negative regulation by Nod2 of TLR2-mediated NF-κB activation (48).

Evidence that Innate Immune Effector Systems Are Involved in CRS
Cells
Chronic rhinosinusitis is an inflammatory disorder involving the mucosa of the nose and paranasal sinuses. The definition of CRS is based on a series of clinical

parameters and symptoms persisting for more than 12 consecutive weeks. Although infection is not always present, CRS is frequently complicated by viral, fungal, or bacterial infections. Objective findings by sinonasal endoscopy and radiologic imaging support the diagnosis but were only recently incorporated in the definition (6). The manner in which CRS has been defined has led to a large degree of heterogeneity in the underlying pathophysiology and associated histologic features.

Chronic rhinosinusitis is broadly classified into two categories—one with nasal polyps (CRS with NP) and one without (CRS without NP). The histologic patterns of inflammation in these two entities overlap, but they differ principally with respect to the unique characteristics of nasal polyps. In CRS with NP, the predominant inflammatory cells are eosinophils and lymphocytes. Nasal polyps include dense concentrations of eosinophils in a stroma that may be variably dense or loosely edematous. The eosinophils extend through the thickened basement membrane and may infiltrate into the epithelium and out to the nasal cavity lumen. The epithelium tends to be hypertrophic, and there may be metaplastic changes present. The eosinophils are activated and degranulating either within the tissue or at the mucosal surface. Investigators at the Mayo Clinic have demonstrated the clustering of degranulating eosinophils in the nasal mucus surrounding fungal elements. Certain forms of CRS with NP, such as Churg-Strauss disease and aspirin sensitivity triad disease, are especially associated with profound tissue eosinophilia. Eosinophilic CRS also tends to be associated with asthma and elevated eosinophil counts in peripheral blood. The two notable exceptions to the relationship between nasal polyps and eosinophils are cystic fibrosis (CF) and antrochoanal polyps (conditions that should not be classified as CRS with NP). In both these disorders, the polyps lack eosinophilic infiltrates. Although the polyps in CF tend to be inflammatory and multiple, antrochoanal polyps are not heavily infiltrated by leukocytic cells and occur singly.

In contrast to CRS with NP, CRS without NP tends to be characterized by the presence of substantial numbers of neutrophils, macrophages, and lymphocytes, rather than eosinophils. That being said, there is a broad spectrum of eosinophilic sinonasal inflammatory disease that extends into the CRS without NP category. For example, eosinophils may be present in the sinonasal mucosa, to varying degrees, due to underlying allergic rhinosinusitis, even in the absence of CRS. CRS without NP is frequently associated with anatomic obstruction of sinus outflow and colonization of entrapped mucus with microbes. The microbial species that infect the sinuses frequently enter along with inspired air and are present in normal hosts as well. Anatomic or functional defects in mucociliary clearance undermine the orderly and harmless transit of potential pathogens through the nasal passages. The histologic appearance of non-eosinophilic CRS without NP is most notable for the presence of tissue edema, neutrophilic inflammatory infiltrate, and thickening of the basement membrane and epithelial layer. As CRS without NP is also a heterogeneous disorder, there may be other underlying conditions, such as auto-immune vasculitis or granulomatous disease, which have additional histologic features.

Signaling Molecules
The adaptive immune signaling molecules associated with CRS are largely related to the type of inflammation present. In eosinophilic varieties of CRS, the predominant types of cytokines present are Th2-related. Chemokines with eosinophilic

chemoattractive properties are also highly expressed in these cases. Despite the Th2 bias, many studies have demonstrated a mixed profile of Th1 and Th2 cytokines in eosinophilic CRS, including CRS with NP. In contrast, non-eosinophilic varieties of CRS have a Th1 cytokine profile only.

The expression of innate immune signaling molecules in CRS has not been extensively studied. TLR1–TLR10 are expressed in sinonasal tissue and on isolated nasal epithelial cells. Studies using real-time polymerase chain reaction (PCR) suggest that there may be differences in the level of expression of TLRs in CRS when compared with control subjects. Unfortunately, significant differences in housekeeping gene expression between control and CRS tissues hamper normalization of mRNA levels and confound interpretation. That said, recent experiments appear to show an increase in TLR2 gene expression in CRS when mRNA levels are normalized to 18S ribosomal RNA (39). Normalization to other housekeeping genes, however, demonstrates reduced expression in CRS of a number of other TLR genes. Separate groups have reported increased or decreased levels of TLR2 mRNA in sinusitis (49–51). Further studies will be required to resolve these discrepant findings, as well as to determine whether such alterations in TLR gene expression are involved in the pathogenesis of the disease.

Effector Molecules
The innate immune effector molecules expressed in CRS have not been examined in great detail. Those that have been identified are also present in normal sinonasal tissue. The local expression of complement components and SAA has been demonstrated in control and CRS tissue specimens. Real-time PCR has not revealed a significant alteration in the expression of complement C3 or SAA in CRS mucosa. On the other hand, the aforementioned mRNA normalization issues may be masking significant differences between control and CRS tissues. Analysis of treatment-responsive and recalcitrant CRS groups demonstrates increased expression of SAA mRNA in recalcitrant eosinophilic CRS (38,39). Alterations in the expression of defensins have been suggested in CRS.

Innate Immune Inflammation vs. Host Defense
An important function of the sinonasal mucosa is to protect the lower respiratory tract and the host from inhaled pathogens and potentially harmful particulates. A complex set of innate and adaptive immune pathways are active at the mucosal surface both constitutively and in response to specific challenges. Hypofunction of these critical processes may lead to infection and endanger the health of the host. On the other hand, overactivity or dysregulation of these same mucosal immune mechanisms could lead to damaging persistent inflammation. Disruption of normal mucosal functions caused by ongoing inflammation eventually leads to impaired immune capabilities and possible infectious injury to the host.

In eosinophilic CRS, a Th2-dominated inflammatory cascade exists in the absence of an identifiable trigger. Although it has been suggested that a microbial element (e.g., fungi or toxin-producing staphylococci) may be the underlying target of the immune system in CRS, no consistent agent has been identified to this point. Moreover, the suggested microbial triggers are fairly ubiquitous, existing in both healthy individuals as well as in CRS patients. For this reason, theories of CRS pathogenesis have invoked the concept that it is the abnormal host response to the trigger, rather than the trigger itself, that is ultimately responsible for the disease process. To address this hypothesis further, it is necessary to understand the manner in which the sinonasal mucosa interacts with the external environment. At present, mucosal immunity of the sinonasal tract is incompletely understood. Much is known about the adaptive immune mediators and effectors that participate in CRS, but the roles of recently discovered innate immune genes and their products are only now beginning to be explored.

ADAPTIVE IMMUNITY AND CRS

T cells play a central role in orchestrating the adaptive immune response of the airways. The majority of T cells express the alpha–beta T-cell antigen receptor (TCR) and undergo TCR rearrangement in the thymus during development. There are approximately 10^6 combinations of rearrangements possible for TCRs. This provides an enormous array of diversity and specificity in defining T cell-antigen interactions. Such rearrangements result in mature T cells that recognize antigens in the context of self-major histocompatibility complex (MHC) antigens. Once the CD4+ T cell is released into circulation from the thymus, it is considered naïve until it comes in contact with a specific antigen. One major class of T cells, CD4+ T cells, or T helper cells, recognize antigen presented by class II MHC, a marker found primarily on antigen-presenting cells (APC). The second subset of T cells, CD8+ T cells, or cytotoxic T cells (Tc), recognize antigen presented by class I MHC molecules, are typically activated by pathogens such as viruses, and function to enhance airway inflammation in allergic disease.

Signaling Mechanisms: Antigen Presentation and Costimulation

Optimal activation of T cells requires engagement of the TCR with antigen peptide in the context of MHC class II molecules. The "second signal" is provided by engagement of a costimulatory receptor on the T-cell surface by a costimulator on the APC. Engagement of the TCR in the absence of costimulation may result in T-cell anergy. Costimulatory interactions between the B7 family ligands expressed on APCs and their receptors on T cells play important roles in the growth, differentiation and death of T cells (52–56). The best-described costimulatory receptor on T cells is CD28. Engagement of the T-cell costimulatory receptor CD28 by its ligands B7-1 (CD80) and B7-2 (CD86) promotes the activation and survival of T cells in part by activation of Jun kinase (JNK), which is required for the induction of cytokine gene transcription (57). Physical interactions between T cells and APC are facilitated by adhesion molecules (e.g., intercellular adhesion molecule (ICAM-1) and β2 integrins) located on both the T cell and the APC. Co-ligation of TCR and costimulatory receptor CD28 within the immunologic synapse results in a sustained state of T-cell activation (58). In contrast, T-cell responses can be inhibited by the engagement of CTLA-4, a homolog of CD28 on T cells that delivers a negative signal and has been proposed to be an important mediator of T-cell tolerance (55,59–62).

Costimulatory Molecules

Counter-ligands for both CD28 and CTLA4 are B7-1 and B7-2, which have been found to be expressed on professional APCs of lymphoid origin, including B cells, monocytes, and DCs (63). Studies in the recent two decades have led to the identification of a sizeable family of costimulatory molecules related to B7-1 and B7-2. These homologs of the original B7-1 and -2 molecules are B7-H1, B7-H2, B7-H3, B7-H4, and B7-DC. A summary of terms and interactions of costimulatory molecules is provided in Table 1. B7-H2 has been shown to be expressed on the cell surface of B cells and macrophages and serves as a ligand for the inducible costimulatory molecule receptor (ICOS) expressed on antigen-primed T cells (64,65). This engagement results in the activation of T-helper memory cells with bias toward Th2 cytokine production and increased expression of cell-surface chemokine receptors (66–71). B7-H3 is a costimulatory ligand expressed in non-lymphoid tissue, whose expression can be induced on lymphoid DCs and monocytes by inflammatory cytokines (72). Its complementary receptor on T cells is not known. Engagement results in proliferation of CD4+ and CD8+ T cells, induction of cytotoxic T cells, and bias toward Th1 cytokine production. Thus, B7-H3 may play a role in Th1 cell differentiation and in primary cytotoxic T-cell activation. B7-H1 (PD-L1) and B7-DC (PD-L2) have been identified in both lymphoid and several non-lymphoid tissues, as well as in several tumor cell lines and are putative inhibitory costimulatory ligands (73). Interaction of these ligands with the counter-receptor PD-1 can result in inhibition of T- and B-cell responses (74,75). These observations have led to the suggestion that tumors may escape immuno-surveillance by attenuation of T-cell responses upon PD-1 engagement. More recently, new findings suggest that there may exist a new paradigm for PD-1-mediated immune regulation. Yamakazi et al. recently reported finding PD-1 on activated B cells and B7-H1 on activated T cells (76). This suggested that the engagement of PD-1 on B cells by B7-H1 on T cells may constitute a novel mechanism of T-cell-mediated B-cell suppression. B7-DC engagement on DCs was found to costimulate T-cell proliferation more efficiently than B7-1 and induce secretion of interferon-γ (IFNγ), but not IL-4 or IL-10, from isolated naïve T cells, suggesting that signaling through PD-1 by B7-H1 and B7-DC may sometimes be stimulatory (76,77). The importance of costimulatory molecules in immunity and inflammatory disease is illustrated by the profound effects of inhibitors of these molecules in human clinical trials (78,79). More recently, B7-H4 has been identified (80,81). Engagement of B7-H4 by its receptor BTLA results in inhibition of T-cell growth, cytokine secretion, and development of cytotoxicity (80,81). B7-H4 mRNA expression was widely observed in human tissues, but constitutive cell-surface expression was not found in most tissues including leukocytes. However, expression of B7-H4 can be induced on T cells, B cells, monocytes, and DCs by in vitro stimulation with IFNγ, LPS, phytohemaglutinin (PHA), PMA, or ionomycin for 72 hours (81). A positive costimulatory signal results in high IL-2 production by the engaged T-cell. This subsequently promotes T-cell proliferation and maturation to

TABLE 1 B7 Family Ligands and Their Receptors

Ligand	HLDA workshop designation	Receptor	Function
B7-1	CD80	CD28	Stimulatory
		CTLA-4 (CD125)	Inhibitory
B7-2	CD86	CD28	Stimulatory
		CTLA-4 (CD125)	Inhibitory
B7-H1 (PD-L1)	CD274	PD-1 (CD279)	Inhibitory
B7-H2 (ICOS-L)	CD275	ICOS (CD278)	Stimulatory
B7-H3	CD276	?	Stimulatory
B7-H4		BTLA (CD272)	Inhibitory
B7-DC (PD-L2)	CD273	PD-1 (CD279)	Inhibitory

become an effector T cell. Once T-cell activation has been initiated, the T cell expresses yet another additional costimulatory molecule CD40L, which can bind to CD40 on APCs to further promote its own activation. When the activated T cell finally transforms into an effector T cell, it can respond to antigen with much greater speed than its naïve counterpart, without the need for costimulation, to produce high levels of appropriate cytokines and chemokines. After the Th1/Th2 dichotomy of commitment is established for an effector T cell, the response remains stable and reflects terminal differentiation (82). This suggests that an established pool of memory CD4+ T cells exists throughout the host's life. In allergic disease and asthma, memory CD4+ Th2 cells are thought to be central to the pathophysiology of the disease.

Evidence that Adaptive Immune Effector Systems Are Involved in CRS
Proinflammatory Roles
Proinflammatory cytokines have been implicated in the pathophysiology of CRS which can variably present as an infectious or hyperplastic response. Correlations have been noted between temporal patterns of insurance claims for upper respiratory viral infections (URI) and for CRS (83). Additionally, 45% of sinus brushings from patients with acute rhinosinusitis showed the presence of virus, as detected by real-time PCR, while only 3% of a corresponding control group were virus-positive (84). Despite the strong links between URI and acute rhinosinusitis, the direct role of viruses in the development of CRS has not been firmly established. Viral infections trigger the production of inflammatory cytokines that produce tissue edema, anatomic obstruction, hypoxia, ciliary dysfunction, and mucous stasis. Infection of epithelial cells in vitro with rhinovirus, influenza virus or RSV induces the production of cytokines, including IL-8, IL-6, IL-11, granulocyte macropage-colony stimulating factor (GM-CSF), and regulated upon activation normal T-cell expressed and secreted (RANTES) (85–92). Increased concentrations of many of these cytokines have also been detected in nasal secretions in case of experimentally induced, or naturally acquired colds (93,94).

Increased levels of both eosinophils and neutrophils have been noted in sinus mucosa and lavages from subjects with CRS (95,96). Expression of IL-8, a chemoattractant for neutrophils and lymphocytes, is increased in CRS compared to either allergic rhinitic or normal subjects (95–97). The immunopathologic profile of CRS associated with nasal polyps is characterized by a high degree of tissue eosinophilia, presence of IL-5-producing lymphocytes, expression of C–C chemokines by epithelial cells, expression of proinflammatory cytokines, and expression of the adhesion molecule vascular adhesion molecule-1 (VCAM-1), regardless of atopic status (98). There is an abundance of mRNA for cytokines which promote the recruitment, activation, and survival of eosinophils, such as TNFα, GM-CSF, IL-3, IL-5, and IL-13 (99–101). Additionally, RANTES and eotaxin were found to be strongly expressed by the epithelial cells of nasal polyps (102–104).

Host Defense Roles
Recent studies have implicated the role of innate immune effector molecules in the pathogenesis of CRS by virtue of their presence, in either increased or decreased amounts. Studies suggest that NO may play a vital role in the local host defense mechanisms in the upper airways (105). Evidence favors the paranasal sinuses, and not the nasal cavity per se, as a major airway source of NO. Immunohistochemical and in situ hybridization studies showed dense staining for NOS in sinus

epithelium versus only weak staining in nasal epithelium (106). Interestingly, NO levels were significantly decreased in various forms of rhinosinusitis. Although the study was limited, Lindberg et al. found that patients with CRS displayed greater than 50% decreased nasal NO levels compared to normal, allergic rhinitis, and URI subjects (107). Patients with acute rhinosinusitis showed decreased nasal NO which returned to normal values after antibiotic therapy (108). In diseases displaying severe forms of rhinosinusitis, such as CF and primary ciliary dyskinesia (PCD), reductions in exhaled nasal NO of 70% and 98% were measured, respectively (109,110). NO has also been shown to affect ciliary function. In the study by Lindberg et al. (107), two of the 12 patients with CRS with the greatest reduction in NO levels had an absence of mucociliary transport measured by the saccharine test. A paucity of beating cilia and ultrastructural changes typical of acquired ciliary dysfunction, including lack of dynein arms and derangements of microtubules were also observed (107). Other studies support the hypothesis that NO is important for maintenance of ciliary function. Ciliary beat frequency was decreased in ex vivo studies of sinus mucosa (111) and in primary airway epithelial cell cultures (112) after application of the iNOS inhibitor N^G-nitro-L-arginine methyl ester (L-NAME).

The role of innate antimicrobials in CRS pathogenesis is less clear. Innate antimicrobials such as human beta defensins 1 and 2 were detected more frequently in human polyp tissue (13) and inflamed maxillary sinus tissue (113) than in control nasal turbinate tissue, whereas others have found these molecules to be decreased in nasal polyps relative to control inferior turbinate tissue (114). Messenger RNA for cathelicidin LL-37, another antimicrobial peptide, was found to be increased in the nasal polyps of patients with CRS (115). In contrast, the antimicrobial protein lysozyme was decreased in patients with recurrent sinusitis and perennial allergic rhinitis (116).

Role of the Epithelium in Adaptive Immune Responses
Recruitment/Activation of Cells

It has become clear that the epithelial cell is not just a passive barrier, but responds to pathogens and other stimuli by generating a broad range of cellular products that can play a major role in regulating airway inflammation and physiology (117,118). The ability of the epithelium to secrete proinflammatory cytokines and chemokines for recruitment of both granulocytes and leukocytes establishes a key role for this structural barrier cell in participating in the adaptive response of the airways. The distribution of T cells in human nasal mucosa has been examined and compared to that of intestinal mucosa (119). Most of the T cells seen in nasal tissue are localized to the epithelium and immediate submucosa of the lamina propria. CD8+ T cells were twice as abundant as CD4+ T cells in the epithelium. Conversely, there was only a slight predominance of CD4+ T cells in the lamina propria. Almost 80% of intraepithelial T cells express the $\alpha_E\beta_7$ integrin adhesion molecule (CD103). Additionally, ICAM-1 is expressed on nasal epithelial cells, and is likely to serve as a ligand for leukocyte function-associated molecule 1 (LFA-1) expressed by T cells. Most of the nasal T cells in the epithelium and lamina propria have been found to express TCR subtype α/β, and not TCR γ/δ (119,120), although increased numbers of TCR-γ/δ+ T cells have been observed in patients with chronic allergic rhinitis (121). Large numbers of CD45RO+, CD45RA-, CD8+ and CD4+ memory T cells are found in polyps and biopsy specimens from CRS patients (122–124). These cells displayed TCR-$\alpha\beta$, CD3, and CD28 at lower levels than in matched peripheral blood T cells. Nasal polyp T cells were also found to express T-cell activation molecules CD69, HLA-DR and CD54, and secrete cytokines. Unlike peripheral blood T cells, $\alpha_E\beta_7$ integrin (CD103), a potential ligand for epithelial E-cadherin, was highly expressed in nasal polyp T cells, suggesting that this molecule may help retain T cells in the mucosa (122). Nasal polyp T cells displayed CD95 (Fas) but did not undergo apoptosis after cross-linking with monoclonal anti-CD95. Taken together, these results suggest that nasal polyps contain large numbers of activated memory T cells.

Costimulation/T-Cell Effects

Growing evidence suggests that airway epithelial cells interact with T cells in multiple and distinct pathways to modulate immune responses. T-cell infiltration of the epithelium and submucosa are striking features of CRS (122), providing evidence for a direct physical interaction between T cells and epithelial cells in the disease. Epithelial cells also express other cell-surface molecules typically associated with T-cell interactions, including HLA-DR, Fas and Fas ligand, and CD40. Studies in our laboratory and others suggest that epithelial cells may present antigen and/or regulate T-cell activation. We recently reported that human airway epithelial cells, both in vivo and in vitro, display significant constitutive cell-surface expression of costimulatory ligands, B7-H1, B7-H2, B7-H3, and B7-DC, and thus display the requisite machinery required for T-cell activation (125). We have found that inflammatory stimuli, such as cytokines (126,127), rhinovirus and TLR ligand dsRNA (128) can induce expression of B7-H1 and B7-DC. Expression of B7-H1 and B7-DC was selectively induced by stimulation of either BEAS2B or primary nasal epithelial cells (PNEC) in culture with IFNγ or dsRNA (128). Interestingly, presence of sinus disease appeared to correlate with costimulatory molecule expression patterns (126,127). Immunohistochemical staining of human sinonasal surgical tissue confirmed the presence of B7-H1, B7-H2, and B7-H3 in the epithelial cell layer, especially in samples of patients diagnosed with Samter's Triad, a severe form of CRS. Additionally, real-time PCR analysis of sinonasal tissue revealed elevated levels of B7-H1 and B7-DC in CRS patients compared to controls.

Immunomodulation

Published reports in the literature have demonstrated the functional activation of T cells by airway epithelial cells in vitro (129–132). Functional analysis in our laboratories demonstrated that monoclonal antibody blockade of B7-H1 or B7-DC enhanced IFNγ expression by purified T cells in co-culture with BEAS2B cells, suggesting that these two B7 homologs inhibit T-cell responses at the mucosal surface (126). Additionally, others have demonstrated that BEAS2B bronchial epithelial cells stimulated the proliferation of allogeneic mixtures of T and B lymphocytes when the BEAS2B cells were cultured with IFNγ (132). T-cell proliferation was inhibited by treating cultured primary nasal epithelial cells (NEC) with addition of anti-class II monoclonal antibody (VG2.2) (129). IFNγ was shown to induce antigen trafficking and uptake of immune complexes in NEC and BEAS2B cell lines (131). Additional evidence supports the notion of direct activation of T cells by airway epithelial cells: (1) epithelial cells express high levels of HLA-DR (119); (2) T cells and epithelial cells are in direct contact within the nasal airways; and (3) epithelial cells express functional TLRs, an established characteristic of APCs (133–138). The precise details of how epithelial expression of B7 homologs may play a role in regulation of T cells is unclear. However, the notion that epithelial cells present antigen to activated memory T cells in the airways provides a mechanism whereby T cells can receive feedback regarding the continued presence of antigen in the airways.

Epithelial cells have been shown to prominently express CD95 (Fas) and CD95L (FasL) (139–145). Fas (CD95) is a 45-kDa type I transmembrane protein belonging to the TNF receptor family that triggers apoptosis (146). Since both epithelial cells and T cells can express both Fas and FasL, it has been proposed that each of these cell types can regulate the survival of the other depending on their respective state of activation and expression. Epithelial cells have also been found to interact with T cells via the CD40/CD40L pathway to modulate immune responses (147). Crosslinking of CD40 on epithelial cells has been shown to induce profound activation associated with chemokine production (148–150). T cells bearing CD40L may activate epithelial cells via direct physical interactions with CD40. Engagement of CD40 on APCs by CD40L on T cells can enhance the release of T-cell-activating cytokines by the APC. CD40/CD40L interactions between cutaneous epithelial cells and T cells have been shown to play a role in IL-8 secretion, expression of CD54 and Bcl-x, growth inhibition, and cell death (151–153). Finally, the ability of T-cell-derived cytokines such as IFNγ, IL-4, and IL-13 to activate epithelial responses, including chemokine expression, mucous glycoproteins, and other mediators of allergic inflammation is well established (154).

EPITHELIUM AS A CENTRAL CELL IN AIRWAY INFLAMMATION

The sections above delineate the roles of airway epithelium in innate and adaptive immune responses. These responses, while protective of the airways, often initiate the cardinal signs of inflammation, including vascular dilation and leak, swelling, pain, and loss of function. Epithelial cells, by virtue of their location, large numbers, and ability to be activated by diverse stimuli, can stimulate all of these processes. In some cases, the epithelium is an initiating cell, as may occur following the direct activation of TLR in epithelium by exposure to a potential pathogen. In other cases, the epithelial response comes secondary to stimulation by infiltrating immune or inflammatory cells such as T cells or DCs. Of particular relevance to allergic inflammation (i.e., characterized by increased numbers of eosinophils, basophils and Th2 cells) is the profound response of epithelial cells to Th2-derived cytokines such as IL-4 and IL-13. Knock-out analysis and gene promoter studies indicate that STAT6 is a central regulator of the expression by epithelial cells and other cell types of numerous genes involved in the allergic inflammatory process. STAT6 activation occurs when the Th2 cytokines IL-4 or IL-13 bind to type I or type II IL-4 receptors and activate members of the Janus kinase (JAK) family which phosphorylate and activate STAT6 (155). Homodimerization of two phosphorylated STAT6 monomers and translocation to the nucleus are necessary for the binding of this transcription factor to the STAT6 consensus sequence (156) and initiation of STAT6-dependent gene expression. A recent analysis of whole-lung extracts from antigen-exposed STAT6 knock-out mice revealed that expression of a host of chemokine genes including chemoattractants of eosinophils and basophils was absent and that the animals did not manifest allergic inflammation in standard challenge models (157). The promoters of these chemokine genes (e.g., eotaxins, monocyte chemotactic proteins (MCPs)) contain STAT6 consensus sequence sites, and those that have been studied have been found to require STAT6 for activation by IL-4 and IL-13. It has been demonstrated that genetic restoration of STAT6 solely in airway epithelial cells of STAT6−/− mice was sufficient to restore both IL-13-induced airway hyperresponsiveness and mucus production (158). Interestingly, restoration of epithelial STAT6 was not sufficient to restore leukocyte infiltration, possibly because endothelial STAT6 may be required for proper expression of adhesion molecules necessary for the response, such as VCAM-1 (159). Profound epithelial activation also occurs secondary to exposure to the TH1 cytokine IFNγ and to the inflammatory cytokine TNFα. Activation of epithelial cells by both immune and type I interferons is mediated to a great extent via other members of the JAK-STAT family (e.g., JAK1, JAK2, and STAT1) and via IRF signaling. Interestingly, the coexistence of both Th1 and Th2 cells and cytokines has been shown to lead to severe inflammation in mouse models of asthma (160). Since both Th2 and Th1 cytokines are detected in CRS, it is likely that crosstalk between these inflammatory responses also worsens inflammation in the upper airways and sinuses in CRS. Both Th1- and Th2-type cytokines can trigger the expression of the various classes of inflammatory cytokines and enzymes shown in the lower half of Figure 1. As discussed above, the nature of the chemokines and the consequent makeup of the infiltrating leukocytes (e.g., neutrophils vs. eosinophils) depends on the relative abundance of Th1 and Th2 cells and their cytokine products. It has recently been suggested that polypoid CRS and non-polypoid CRS reflect a preponderance of Th2 and Th1 inflammation, respectively.

Some of the epithelial responses that have been discussed elsewhere in this review and are potentially important in both innate immunity and CRS are indicated in Figure 1. When the airways encounter bacteria, fungi or viruses, pathogen recognition structures including TLR, CD14/LBP and Nod proteins can trigger signaling pathways involved in both immunity and inflammation. When infection exceeds the capacity of the local cells and mediators for containment and/or elimination of an organism in a tissue site, a systemic host response can ensue. This response involves release of numerous acute-phase proteins from the liver in response to pathogen products (e.g., endotoxin) and cytokines (e.g., IL-1β,

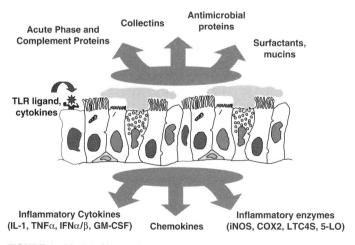

FIGURE 1   Model of innate immune response and epithelium.

TNFα, and IL-6 generated locally and acting systemically). The liver produces complement, collectins, and pentraxins along with numerous other classes of acute-phase molecules that can regulate inflammation, clotting and cardiovascular function and contribute to host defense (161,162). Evidence is accumulating to suggest that a local version of this response occurs in the airways. We and others have demonstrated that both immortalized and primary airway epithelial cells taken from patients express mRNA for TLR1–10 and that several of these receptors are functionally active (36,163). Preliminary results from our laboratory, and a few published studies, indicate that many acute-phase proteins, including complement proteins, pentraxins, and collectins can be produced by epithelial cells after activation with TLR ligands and cytokines. For example, a recent study showed that C-reactive protein (CRP) is highly expressed by airway epithelium and that CRP is found at levels in sputum and nasal lavage high enough to kill bacteria (164). Further studies are needed to determine the relative importance of local acute-phase responses in host defense in the airways. In the liver, the acute-phase response is mediated to a great extent by activation of proteins of the CCAAT-enhancer-binding protein family (C/EBP) (165,166). Epithelial cells have been reported to express C/EBP proteins (167,168), and we have recently determined that the expression of mRNA and protein for C/EBPβ and C/EBPδ is increased by stimulation with glucocorticoids, especially in combination with the TLR3 ligand dsRNA. We have also obtained evidence that there is a role of C/EBP proteins in the response of epithelial cells to TLR ligands, cytokines and glucocorticoids (Zhang, Schleimer et al., unpublished observations).

The interface between innate and adaptive responses may partially hinge on interactions between epithelial cells and DCs (see 1 and 2 in Fig. 2). Recent studies have shown that DCs form a network among epithelial cells and project processes between epithelial cells into the airways that enable them to sample the intraluminal airway contents (169,170). The rapid activation of DC and epithelial cells by TLR ligands may trigger a local host defense response by the epithelium that takes the form of the release of antimicrobial products and the triggering of processes that recruit both innate and adaptive immune cells (see 1 and 2 in Fig. 2).

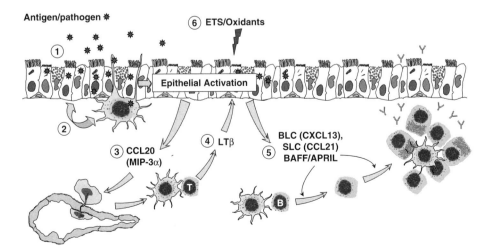

FIGURE 2 Model of adaptive immune response and epithelium. See text for details.

Prominent recruitment of DC occurs in inflamed airways and is now known to be an important event in the initiation of an adaptive immune response as well as in non-specific airway inflammation (171). Among the chemotactic factors for DC, macropage inflammatory protein (MIP-3α) (CCL20) is particularly potent and effective (see 3 in Fig. 2) (172). It is notable therefore, that the most powerful inducers of these chemokines include TLR3 activation and activation with either type I interferons (IFNα or IFNβ) or immune interferon (IFNγ) (36,173). Interestingly, particulate matter and proteolytic allergens (e.g., Der p l) also induce CCL20 expression by epithelial cells, possibly explaining some of the interactions between irritants and allergens (173,174). Recruitment of DC to the airways is likely to be essential in the adaptive B-, T- and NK-cell-mediated immune responses that are important in defense against infection and in inflammation of the airways and sinuses. Studies in animal asthma models suggest that DC activation is essential for airway disease (175,176). Infiltrating DC almost certainly play a key role in the activation of inflammatory T cells and antigen-specific B cells in the airways.

As discussed above and displayed in Figure 2, epithelial cells are likely to be involved in the coordination of the adaptive immune response in the airways. This can occur through regulation of TCR via B7 homologs, fas, CD40, etc. Epithelial cells are also likely to play a role in the formation of lymphoid structures in the airways. Epithelial cells respond to lymphotoxin-beta derived from T cells (see 4 in Fig. 2). Studies of mice genetically manipulated to be deficient in cysteinyl leukotrienes β (LTβ) or its receptors have demonstrated a lack of lymph nodes, implicating LTβ in the formation of secondary lymphoid tissue (177,178). Studies of the gastrointestinal epithelium have shown that LTβ is a potent stimulator of the expression of MIP-3α, the DC-attracting chemokine (179). One role that LTβ may play in CRS is thus the activation of airway epithelium to produce chemoattractants. Receptors for LTβ have been shown to be expressed by airway epithelial cells, although relatively little is known about the effects of LTβ on airway epithelial responses (179,180). In the gut, LTβ is known to be essential in the formation of Peyer's patches, lymphoid aggregates that are important in antigen-specific responses (181,182). Isolated lymphoid follicles (ILF) are recently recognized tertiary lymphoid structures that form at mucosal surfaces. While formation of ILF is also dependent on LTβ, antigen stimulation is not necessary for the event (183–185). Formation of both Peyer's patches and ILF is thought to involve the release of B-cell-attracting chemokines such as BLC induced by LTβ in epithelium (Fig. 2) (178,185). BAFF and APRIL are cytokines that induce proliferation, immunoglobulin isotype switch recombination and differentiation of B lymphocytes to become plasma cells and secrete immunoglobulin. Recent studies indicate that these cytokines are produced by airway epithelial cells (Kato, Schleimer et al., unpublished observations). This response is of significant potential importance in both immunity and inflammation in the airways, a site where IgA-and IgE-isotype immunoglobulins are abundantly produced. Interestingly, BAFF and APRIL are probably also involved along with lymphotoxin in the formation of isolated lymphoid follicles (see 5 in Fig. 2) (183,186,187).

The interface between innate and adaptive immune responses may be influenced by exposure to several environmental pollutants, including ozone, diesel exhaust and tobacco smoke, all recognized to be risk factors for airway inflammatory disease (see 6 in Fig. 2). Exposure of the airways to oxidants from the environment or generated in response to irritants can activate inflammatory pathways that promote allergic sensitization and elicitation of antigen-specific responses. For example, residual oil fly ash has been shown to be a potent activator of epithelial cell expression of the DC chemoattractant, MIP-3α, which is likely to increase the antigen-processing and immune-activation functions of DC (173). Diesel exhaust extract is well known for its ability to promote Th2 responses, B-cell immunoglobulin class-switching and allergic inflammation in the airways (188,189). Similarly, tobacco smoke is an important and ubiquitous environmental stimulus that increases the prevalence of asthma and produces airway inflammation that can exacerbate allergic disease (190,191).

While substantial remodeling of the airways occurs in CRS, there are no established animal models of most of the processes involved and little is known about the pathogenesis. Prominent features include the formation of polyps and hyperplasia of mucous glandular structures. Interestingly, polyp formation is often associated with aspirin sensitivity, and elevations of leukotriene C4 synthase (192). It is postulated that dysregulation of arachidonic acid metabolism may therefore play some role. The relationship between edema and polyp formation is not clear, as edema can occur without the formation of polyps. As in asthma, thickening of the sub-basement membrane is often associated with CRS. Consequently, Th2 cytokines are implicated in this process along with activation of the expression of fibrogenic cytokines including transforming growth factor-beta (TGF-β). Increases in the number and activity of mucus-secreting cells occur and are suspected to involve Th2 cytokines and the activation of STAT6 as discussed above.

SUMMARY

We have outlined the myriad of roles, both proven and suspected, of epithelial cells in airway inflammation in general and CRS in particular. There is little doubt that these remarkable cells are essential for host defense, tissue responses to injury and threats, and inflammation that cause disease. We believe that many of these responses are likely to be amenable to the development of new therapies for CRS. As we acquire more information on the signaling processes that drive the protective responses in epithelial cells, we will improve our chances of developing approaches to enhance these responses without triggering deleterious inflammatory responses. Enhanced clearance of fungi and bacteria by local immune responses would likely be beneficial in reducing disease. As we better understand the signals that epithelial cells give and get from DCs, B and T lymphocytes, new opportunities for productive intervention will arise.

REFERENCES

1. Shin SH, Ponikau JU, Sherris DA, et al. Chronic rhinosinusitis: an enhanced immune response to ubiquitous airborne fungi. J Allergy Clin Immunol 2004; 114:1369–75.
2. Bernstein JM, Kansal R. Superantigen hypothesis for the early development of chronic hyperplastic sinusitis with massive nasal polyposis. Curr Opin Otolaryngol Head Neck Surg 2005; 13:39–44.
3. Bachert C, van Zele T, Gevaert P, De Schrijver L, Van Cauwenberge P. Superantigens and nasal polyps. Curr Allergy Asthma Rep 2003; 3:523–31.
4. Ramadan HH, Sanclement JA, Thomas JG. Chronic rhinosinusitis and biofilms. Otolaryngol Head Neck Surg 2005; 132:414–7.
5. Perloff JR, Palmer JN. Evidence of bacterial biofilms on frontal recess stents in patients with chronic rhinosinusitis. Am J Rhinol 2004; 18:377–80.

6. Meltzer EO, Hamilos DL, Hadley JA et al. Rhinosinusitis: establishing definitions for clinical research and patient care. Otolaryngol Head Neck Surg 2004; 131:S1–62.

7. Wanner A, Salathe M, O'Riordan TG. Mucociliary clearance in the airways. Am J Respir Crit Care Med 1996; 154:1868–902.

8. Knowles MR, Boucher RC. Mucus clearance as a primary innate defense mechanism for mammalian airways. J Clin Invest 2002; 109:571–7.

9. Quinlan MF, Salman SD, Swift DL, Wagner HN Jr, Proctor DF. Measurement of mucociliary function in man. Am Rev Respir Dis 1969; 99:13–23.

10. Travis SM, Singh PK, Welsh MJ. Antimicrobial peptides and proteins in the innate defense of the airway surface. Curr Opin Immunol 2001; 13:89–95.

11. Cole AM, Dewan P, Ganz T. Innate antimicrobial activity of nasal secretions. Infect Immun 1999; 67:3267–75.

12. Kaliner MA. Human nasal respiratory secretions and host defense. Am Rev Respir Dis 1991; 144:S52–6.

13. Lee SH, Kim JE, Lim HH, Lee HM, Choi JO. Antimicrobial defensin peptides of the human nasal mucosa. Ann Otol Rhinol Laryngol 2002; 111:135–41.

14. Raphael GD, Jeney EV, Baraniuk JN, Kim I, Meredith SD, Kaliner MA. Pathophysiology of rhinitis. Lactoferrin and lysozyme in nasal secretions. J Clin Invest 1989; 84:1528–35.

15. Lee CH, Igarashi Y, Hohman RJ, Kaulbach H, White MV, Kaliner MA. Distribution of secretory leukoprotease inhibitor in the human nasal airway. Am Rev Respir Dis 1993; 147:710–6.

16. Fleming A. On a remarkable bacteriolytic element found in tissues and secretions. Proc R Soc Lond B Biol Sci 1922; 93:306–17.

17. During K, Porsch P, Mahn A, Brinkmann O, Gieffers W. The non-enzymatic microbicidal activity of lysozymes. FEBS Lett 1999; 449:93–100.

18. Ellison RT 3rd, Giehl TJ. Killing of gram-negative bacteria by lactoferrin and lysozyme. J Clin Invest 1991; 88:1080–91.

19. Akinbi HT, Epaud R, Bhatt H, Weaver TE. Bacterial killing is enhanced by expression of lysozyme in the lungs of transgenic mice. J Immunol 2000; 165:5760–6.

20. Arnold RR, Cole MF, McGhee JR. A bactericidal effect for human lactoferrin. Science 1977; 197:263–5.

21. Kuwata H, Yip TT, Yip CL, Tomita M, Hutchens TW. Bactericidal domain of lactoferrin: detection, quantitation, and characterization of lactoferricin in serum by SELDI affinity mass spectrometry. Biochem Biophys Res Commun 1998; 245:764–73.

22. Hiemstra PS, Maassen RJ, Stolk J, Heinzel-Wieland R, Steffens GJ, Dijkman JH. Antibacterial activity of antileukoprotease. Infect Immun 1996; 64:4520–4.

23. Zhu J, Nathan C, Ding A. Suppression of macrophage responses to bacterial lipopolysaccharide by a non-secretory form of secretory leukocyte protease inhibitor. Biochim Biophys Acta 1999; 1451:219–23.

24. Stadel JM, Hoyle K, Naclerio RM, Roshak A, Chilton FH. Characterization of phospholipase A2 from human nasal lavage. Am J Respir Cell Mol Biol 1994; 11:108–13.

25. Aho HJ, Grenman R, Sipila J, Peuravuori H, Hartikainen J, Nevalainen TJ. Group II phospholipase A2 in nasal fluid, mucosa and paranasal sinuses. Acta Otolaryngol 1997; 117:860–3.

26. Lehrer RI, Lichtenstein AK, Ganz T. Defensins: antimicrobial and cytotoxic peptides of mammalian cells. Annu Rev Immunol 1993; 11:105–28.

27. Zanetti M, Gennaro R, Romeo D. Cathelicidins: a novel protein family with a common proregion and a variable C-terminal antimicrobial domain. FEBS Lett 1995; 374:1–5.

28. Zanetti M. Cathelicidins, multifunctional peptides of the innate immunity. J Leukoc Biol 2004; 75:39–48.

29. Sorensen OE, Follin P, Johnsen AH et al. Human cathelicidin, hCAP-18, is processed to the antimicrobial peptide LL-37 by extracellular cleavage with proteinase 3. Blood 2001; 97:3951–9.

30. Gudmundsson GH, Agerberth B, Odeberg J, Bergman T, Olsson B, Salcedo R. The human gene FALL39 and processing of the cathelin precursor to the antibacterial peptide LL-37 in granulocytes. Eur J Biochem 1996; 238:325–32.

31. Larrick JW, Hirata M, Balint RF, Lee J, Zhong J, Wright SC. Human CAP18: a novel antimicrobial lipopolysaccharide-binding protein. Infect Immun 1995; 63:1291–7.

32. Bals R, Weiner DJ, Moscioni AD, Meegalla RL, Wilson JM. Augmentation of innate host defense by expression of a cathelicidin antimicrobial peptide. Infect Immun 1999; 67:6084–9.

33. Wilson CL, Ouellette AJ, Satchell DP, et al. Regulation of intestinal alpha-defensin activation by the metalloproteinase matrilysin in innate host defense. Science 1999; 286:113–7.

34. Moser C, Weiner DJ, Lysenko E, Bals R, Weiser JN, Wilson JM. beta-Defensin 1 contributes to pulmonary innate immunity in mice. Infect Immun 2002; 70:3068–72.

35. Iimura M, Gallo RL, Hase K, Miyamoto Y, Eckmann L, Kagnoff MF. Cathelicidin mediates innate intestinal defense against colonization with epithelial adherent bacterial pathogens. J Immunol 2005; 174:4901–7.

36. Sha Q, Truong-Tran AQ, Plitt JR, Beck LA, Schleimer RP. Activation of airway epithelial cells by toll-like receptor agonists. Am J Respir Cell Mol Biol 2004; 31:358–64.

37. Vandermeer J, Sha Q, Lane AP, Schleimer RP. Innate immunity of the sinonasal cavity: expression of messenger RNA for complement cascade components and toll-like receptors. Arch Otolaryngol Head Neck Surg 2004; 130:1374–80.

38. Lane A, VanderMeer J, Sha Q, et al. Toll-like receptors, complement factors, and acute phase proteins are expressed by the sinonasal epithelium in chronic rhinosinusitis. 2004; (in press).

39. Lane AP, Truong-Tran QA, Schleimer RP. Altered expression of genes associated with innate immunity and inflammation in recalcitrant rhinosinusitis with polyps. Am J Rhinology 2006; 20(2):138–144.

40. Medzhitov R. Toll-like receptors and innate immunity. Nat Rev 2001; 1:135–45.

41. Beutler B. Inferences, questions and possibilities in Toll-like receptor signalling. Nature 2004; 430:257–63.

42. Akira S. Toll-like receptors and innate immunity. Adv Immunol 2001; 78:1–56.

43. Hawn TR, Verbon A, Lettinga KD, et al. A common dominant TLR5 stop codon polymorphism abolishes flagellin signaling and is associated with susceptibility to legionnaires' disease. J Exp Med 2003; 198:1563–72.

44. Dunstan SJ, Hawn TR, Hue NT, et al. Host susceptibility and clinical outcomes in toll-like receptor 5-deficient patients with typhoid fever in Vietnam. J Infect Dis 2005; 191:1068–71.

45. Cook DN, Pisetsky DS, Schwartz DA. Toll-like receptors in the pathogenesis of human disease. Nat Immunol 2004; 5:975–9.

46. Roach JC, Glusman G, Rowen L, et al. The evolution of vertebrate Toll-like receptors. Proc Natl Acad Sci U S A 2005.

47. Takeuchi O, Kawai T, Muhlradt PF, et al. Discrimination of bacterial lipoproteins by Toll-like receptor 6. Int Immunol 2001; 13:933–40.

48. Watanabe T, Kitani A, Murray PJ, Strober W. NOD2 is a negative regulator of Toll-like receptor 2-mediated T helper type 1 responses. Nat Immunol 2004; 5:800–8.

49. Dong Z, Yang Z, Wang C. Expression of TLR2 and TLR4 messenger RNA in the epithelial cells of the nasal airway. Am J Rhinol 2005; 19:236–9.

50. Claeys, S, de Belder T., Holtappels G, et al. Human beta-defensins and toll-like receptors in the upper airway. Allergy 2003; 58:748–53.

51. Pitzurra L, Bellocchio S, Nocentini A, et al. Antifungal immune reactivity in nasal polyposis. Infect Immun 2004; 72:7275–81.

52. Fraser JD, Irving BA, Crabtree GR, Weiss A. Regulation of interleukin-2 gene enhancer activity by the T cell accessory molecule CD28. Science 1991; 251:313–6.

53. Harding FA, McArthur JG, Gross JA, Raulet DH, Allison JP. CD28-mediated signallingr co-stimulates murine T cells and prevents induction of anergy in T-cell clones. Nature 1992; 356:607–9.

54. June, CH, Ledbetter JA, Gillespie MM, Lindsten T, Thompson CB. T-cell proliferation involving the CD28 pathway is associated with cyclosporine-resistant interleukin 2 gene expression. Mol Cell Biol 1987; 7:4472–81.

55. Chambers CA, Allison JP. Co-stimulation in T cell responses. Curr Opin Immunol 1997;9:396–404.
56. Gause, WC, Mitro V, Via C, Linsley P, Urban JF Jr, Greenwald RJ. Do effector and memory T helper cells also need B7 ligand costimulatory signals? J Immunol 1997; 159:1055–8.
57. Su B, Jacinto E, Hibi M, Kallunki T, Karin M, Ben-Neriah Y. JNK is involved in signal integration during costimulation of T lymphocytes. Cell 1994; 77:727–36.
58. Wulfing C, Davis MM. A receptor/cytoskeletal movement triggered by costimulation during T cell activation. Science 1998; 282:2266–9.
59. Bugeon L, Dallman MJ. Costimulation of T cells. Am J Respir Crit Care Med 2000; 162:S164–8.
60. Walunas TL, Lenschow DJ, Bakker CY, et al. CTLA-4 can function as a negative regulator of T cell activation. Immunity 1994; 1:405–13.
61. Krummel MF, Allison JP. CD28 and CTLA-4 have opposing effects on the response of T cells to stimulation. J Exp Med 1995; 182:459–65.
62. Walunas TL, Bakker CY, Bluestone JA. CTLA-4 ligation blocks CD28-dependent T cell activation. J Exp Med 1996; 183:2541–50.
63. Carreno BM, Collins M. The B7 family of ligands and its receptors: new pathways for costimulation and inhibition of immune responses. Annu Rev Immunol 2002; 20:29–53.
64. Tamatani T, Tezuka K, Hanzawa-Higuchi N. AILIM/ICOS: a novel lymphocyte adhesion molecule. Int Immunol 2000; 12:51–5.
65. Beier KC, Hutloff A, Dittrich AM, et al. Induction, binding specificity and function of human ICOS. Eur J Immunol 2000; 30:3707–17.
66. Hutloff A, Dittrich AM, Beier KC, et al. ICOS is an inducible T-cell co-stimulator structurally and functionally related to CD28. Nature 1999; 397:263–66.
67. Wang S, Zhu G, Chapoval AI, et al. Costimulation of T cells by B7-H2, a B7-like molecule that binds ICOS. Blood 2000; 96:2808–13.
68. Yoshinaga SK, Zhang M, Pistillo J, et al. Characterization of a new human B7-related protein: B7RP-1 is the ligand to the co-stimulatory protein ICOS. Int Immunol 2000; 12:1439–47.
69. Coyle AJ, Lehar S, Lloyd C, et al. The CD28-related molecule ICOS is required for effective T cell-dependent immune responses. Immunity 2000; 13:95–105.
70. McAdam AJ, Chang TT, Lumelsky AE, et al. Mouse inducible costimulatory molecule (ICOS) expression is enhanced by CD28 costimulation and regulates differentiation of CD4+ T cells. J Immunol 2000; 165:5035–40.
71. McAdam AJ, Greenwald RJ, Levin MA, et al. ICOS is critical for CD40-mediated antibody class switching. Nature 2001; 409:102–5.
72. Chapoval AI, Ni J, Lau JS, et al. B7-H3: a costimulatory molecule for T cell activation and IFN-gamma production. Nat Immunol 2001; 2:269–74.
73. Latchman Y, Wood CR, Chernova T, et al. PD-L2 is a second ligand for PD-1 and inhibits T cell activation. Nat Immunol 2001; 2:261–8.
74. Nishimura H, Honjo T. PD-1: an inhibitory immunoreceptor involved in peripheral tolerance. Trends Immunol 2001; 22:265–8.
75. Freeman GJ, Long AJ, Iwai Y, et al. Engagement of the PD-1 immunoinhibitory receptor by a novel B7 family member leads to negative regulation of lymphocyte activation. J Exp Med 2000; 192:1027–34.
76. Yamazaki T, Akiba H, Iwai H, et al. Expression of programmed death 1 ligands by murine T cells and APC. J Immunol 2002; 169:5538–45.
77. Tseng SY, Otsuji M, Gorski K, et al. B7-DC, a new dendritic cell molecule with potent costimulatory properties for T cells. J Exp Med 2001; 193:839–46.
78. Vincenti F. What's in the pipeline? New immunosuppressive drugs in transplantation. Am J Transplant 2002; 2:898–903.
79. Halloran PF. Immunosuppressive agents in clinical trials in transplantation. Am J Med Sci 1997; 313:283–8.
80. Carreno BM, Collins M. BTLA: a new inhibitory receptor with a B7-like ligand. Trends Immunol 2003; 24:524–7.

81. Choi IH, Zhu G, Sica GL, et al. Genomic organization and expression analysis of b7-h4, an immune inhibitory molecule of the b7 family. J Immunol 2003; 171:4650–4.
82. Swain SL. Generation and in vivo persistence of polarized Th1 and Th2 memory cells. Immunity 1994; 1:543–52.
83. Jones J, Gable C, Floor M, et al. Prior upper respiratory infection and allergic rhinitis: relationship to chronic sinusitis. In Int Conf Sinus Disease 1993.
84. Pitkaranta A, Arruda E, Malmberg H, Hayden FG. Detection of rhinovirus in sinus brushings of patients with acute community-acquired sinusitis by reverse transcription-PCR. J Clin Microbiol 1997; 35:1791–3.
85. Subauste MC, Jacoby DB, Richards SM, Proud D. Infection of a human respiratory epithelial cell line with rhinovirus. Induction of cytokine release and modulation of susceptibility to infection by cytokine exposure. J Clin Invest 1995; 96:549–57.
86. Einarsson O, Geba GP, Zhu Z, et al. Interleukin-11: stimulation in vivo and in vitro by respiratory viruses and induction of airways hyperresponsiveness. J Clin Invest 1996; 97:915–24.
87. Zhu Z, Tang W, Ray A, et al. Rhinovirus stimulation of interleukin-6 in vivo and in vitro. Evidence for nuclear factor kappa B-dependent transcriptional activation. J Clin Invest 1996; 97:421–30.
88. Becker S, Koren HS, Henke DC. Interleukin-8 expression in normal nasal epithelium and its modulation by infection with respiratory syncytial virus and cytokines tumor necrosis factor, interleukin-1, and interleukin-6. Am J Respir Cell Mol Biol 1993; 8:20–7.
89. Becker S, Reed W, Henderson FW, Noah TL. RSV infection of human airway epithelial cells causes production of the beta-chemokine RANTES. Am J Physiol 1997; 272:L512–20.
90. Saito T, Deskin RW, Casola A, et al. Respiratory syncytial virus induces selective production of the chemokine RANTES by upper airway epithelial cells. J Infect Dis 1997; 175:497–504.
91. Choi AM, Jacoby DB. Influenza virus A infection induces interleukin-8 gene expression in human airway epithelial cells. FEBS Lett 1992; 309:327–9.
92. Matsukura S, Kokubu F, Noda H, Tokunaga H, Adachi M. Expression of IL-6, IL-8, and RANTES on human bronchial epithelial cells, NCI-H292, induced by influenza virus A. J Allergy Clin Immunol 1996; 98:1080–7.
93. Noah TL, Henderson FW, Wortman IA, et al. Nasal cytokine production in viral acute upper respiratory infection of childhood. J Infect Dis 1995; 171:584–92.
94. Grunberg K, Timmers MC, Smits HH, de Klerk EP, Dick EC, Spaan WJ, Hiemstra PS, Sterk PJ. Effect of experimental rhinovirus 16 colds on airway hyperresponsiveness to histamine and interleukin-8 in nasal lavage in asthmatic subjects in vivo. Clin Exp Allergy 1997; 27:36–45.
95. Takeuchi K, Yuta A, Sakakura Y. Interleukin-8 gene expression in chronic sinusitis. Am J Otolaryngol 1995; 16:98–102.
96. Suzuki H, Takahashi Y, Wataya H, et al. Mechanism of neutrophil recruitment induced by IL-8 in chronic sinusitis. J Allergy Clin Immunol 1996; 98:659–70.
97. Rhyoo C, Sanders SP, Leopold DA, Proud D. Sinus mucosal IL-8 gene expression in chronic rhinosinusitis. J Allergy Clin Immunol 1999; 103:395–400.
98. Hamilos DL. Noninfectious sinusitis. ACI International 2001; 13:27–32.
99. Hamilos DL, Leung DY, Wood R, et al. Evidence for distinct cytokine expression in allergic versus nonallergic chronic sinusitis. J Allergy Clin Immunol 1995; 96:537–44.
100. Broide DH, Stachnick G, Castaneda D, Nayar J, Sriramarao P. Inhibition of eosinophilic inflammation in allergen-challenged TNF receptor p55/p75—and TNF receptor p55-deficient mice. Am J Respir Cell Mol Biol 2001; 24:304–11.
101. Hamilos DL, Leung DY, Wood R, et al. Chronic hyperplastic sinusitis: association of tissue eosinophilia with mRNA expression of granulocyte-macrophage colony-stimulating factor and interleukin-3. J Allergy Clin Immunol 1993; 92:39–48.
102. Hamilos DL, Leung DY, Wood R, et al. Eosinophil infiltration in nonallergic chronic hyperplastic sinusitis with nasal polyposis (CHS/NP) is associated with endothelial

VCAM-1 upregulation and expression of TNF-alpha. Am J Respir Cell Mol Biol 1996; 15:443–50.

103. Minshall EM, Cameron L, Lavigne F, et al. Eotaxin mRNA and protein expression in chronic sinusitis and allergen- induced nasal responses in seasonal allergic rhinitis. Am J Respir Cell Mol Biol 1997; 17:683–90.

104. Stellato C, Beck LA, Gorgone GA, et al. Expression of the chemokine RANTES by a human bronchial epithelial cell line. Modulation by cytokines and glucocorticoids. J Immunol 1995; 155:410–8.

105. Fang FC. Perspectives series: host/pathogen interactions. Mechanisms of nitric oxide-related antimicrobial activity. J Clin Invest 1997; 99:2818–25.

106. Lundberg JO, Farkas-Szallasi T, Weitzberg E, et al. High nitric oxide production in human paranasal sinuses. Nat Med 1995; 1:370–3.

107. Lindberg S, Cervin A, Runer T. Nitric oxide (NO) production in the upper airways is decreased in chronic sinusitis. Acta Otolaryngol 1997; 117:113–7.

108. Baraldi, E, Azzolin NM, Biban P, Zacchello F. Effect of antibiotic therapy on nasal nitric oxide concentration in children with acute sinusitis. Am J Respir Crit Care Med 1997; 155:1680–3.

109. Lundberg JO, Nordvall SL, Weitzberg E, Kollberg H, Alving K. Exhaled nitric oxide in paediatric asthma and cystic fibrosis. Arch Dis Child 1996; 75:323–6.

110. Lundberg JO, Weitzberg E, Nordvall SL, Kuylenstierna R, Lundberg JM, Alving K. Primarily nasal origin of exhaled nitric oxide and absence in Kartagener's syndrome. Eur Respir J 1994; 7:1501–4.

111. Kim JW, Min YG, Rhee CS, et al. Regulation of mucociliary motility by nitric oxide and expression of nitric oxide synthase in the human sinus epithelial cells. Laryngoscope 2001; 111:246–50.

112. Jain B, Rubinstein I, Robbins RA, Leise KL, Sisson JH. Modulation of airway epithelial cell ciliary beat frequency by nitric oxide. Biochem Biophys Res Commun 1993; 191:83–8.

113. Carothers DG, Graham SM, Jia HP, Ackermann MR, Tack BF, McCray PB Jr. Production of beta-defensin antimicrobial peptides by maxillary sinus mucosa. Am J Rhinol 2001; 15:175–9.

114. Meyer JE, Harder J, Gorogh T, Schroder JM, Maune S. hBD-2 gene expression in nasal mucosa. Laryngorhinootologie 2000; 79:400–3.

115. Chen PH, Fang SY. The expression of human antimicrobial peptide LL-37 in the human nasal mucosa. Am J Rhinol 2004; 18:381–5.

116. Kalfa VC, Spector SL, Ganz T, Cole AM. Lysozyme levels in the nasal secretions of patients with perennial allergic rhinitis and recurrent sinusitis. Ann Allergy Asthma Immunol 2004; 93:288–92.

117. Polito AJ, Proud D. Epithelia cells as regulators of airway inflammation. J Allergy Clin Immunol 1998; 102:714–8.

118. Schwiebert LM, Stellato C, Schleimer RP. The epithelium as a target of glucocorticoid action in the treatment of asthma. Am J Respir Crit Care Med 1996; 154:S16–19; discussion S19–20.

119. Jahnsen FL, Farstad IN, Aanesen JP, Brandtzaeg P. Phenotypic distribution of T cells in human nasal mucosa differs from that in the gut. Am J Respir Cell Mol Biol 1998; 18:392–401.

120. Goto E, Kohrogi H, Hirata N, et al. Human bronchial intraepithelial T lymphocytes as a distinct T-cell subset: their long-term survival in SCID-Hu chimeras. Am J Respir Cell Mol Biol 2000; 22:405–11.

121. Pawankar RU, Okuda M, Suzuki K, Okumura K, Ra C. Phenotypic and molecular characteristics of nasal mucosal gamma delta T cells in allergic and infectious rhinitis. Am J Respir Crit Care Med 1996; 153:1655–65.

122. Sanchez-Segura A, Brieva JA, Rodriguez C. T lymphocytes that infiltrate nasal polyps have a specialized phenotype and produce a mixed TH1/TH2 pattern of cytokines. J Allergy Clin Immunol 1998; 102:953–60.

123. Berger G, Kattan A, Bernheim J, Ophir D. Polypoid mucosa with eosinophilia and glandular hyperplasia in chronic sinusitis: a histopathological and immunohistochemical study. Laryngoscope 2002; 112:738–45.

124. Grevers G, Klemens A, Menauer F, Sturm C. Involvement of inferior turbinate mucosa in chronic sinusitis—localization of T-cell subset. Allergy 2000; 55:1155–62.

125. Kurosawa S, Myers AC, Chen L, et al. Expression of the costimulatory molecule B7-H2 (inducible costimulator ligand) by human airway epithelial cells. Am J Respir Cell Mol Biol 2003; 28:563–73.

126. Kim J, Myers AC, Chen L, et al. Constitutive and inducible expression of b7 family of ligands by human airway epithelial cells. Am J Respir Cell Mol Biol 2005; 33:280–9.

127. Kim J, Plitt J, Myers A, Schleimer RP. Expression of B7 homolog costimulatory molecules in airway epithelial cells. FASEB J 2003; 17:C14.

128. Kim J, Sanders SP, Plitt J, Pardoll D, Chen L, Schleimer RP. Modulation of expression of B7 homologs by human rhinovirus and double-stranded RNA in airway epithelial cells in vitro and in vivo. J Allergy Clin Immunol 2003; 113:S247.

129. Kalb TH, Chuang MT, Marom Z, Mayer L. Evidence for accessory cell function by class II MHC antigen-expressing airway epithelial cells. Am J Respir Cell Mol Biol 1991; 4:320–9.

130. Kalb TH, Yio XY, Mayer L. Human airway epithelial cells stimulate T-lymphocyte lck and fyn tyrosine kinase. Am J Respir Cell Mol Biol 1997; 17:561–70.

131. Salik E, Tyorkin M, Mohan S, et al. Antigen trafficking and accessory cell function in respiratory epithelial cells. Am J Respir Cell Mol Biol 1999; 21:365–79.

132. Tanaka H, Maeda K, Nakamura Y, Azuma M, Yanagawa H, Sone S. CD40 and IFN-gamma dependent T cell activation by human bronchial epithelial cells. J Med Invest 2001; 48:109–17.

133. Wang X, Moser C, Louboutin JP, et al. Toll-like receptor 4 mediates innate immune responses to Haemophilus influenzae infection in mouse lung. J Immunol 2002; 168:810–5.

134. Bocker U, Yezerskyy O, Feick P, et al. Responsiveness of intestinal epithelial cell lines to lipopolysaccharide is correlated with Toll-like receptor 4 but not Toll-like receptor 2 or CD14 expression. Int J Colorectal Dis 2003; 18:25–32.

135. Putnins EE, Sanaie AR, Wu Q, Firth JD. Induction of keratinocyte growth factor 1 Expression by lipopolysaccharide is regulated by CD-14 and toll-like receptors 2 and 4. Infect Immun 2002; 70:6541–8.

136. Imasato A, Desbois-Mouthon C, Han J, et al. Inhibition of p38 MAPK by glucocorticoids via induction of MAPK phosphatase-1 enhances nontypeable Haemophilus influenzae-induced expression of toll-like receptor 2. J Biol Chem 2002; 277:47444–50.

137. Schulz C, Farkas L, Wolf K, Kratzel K, Eissner G, Pfeifer M. Differences in LPS-induced activation of bronchial epithelial cells (BEAS-2B) and type II-like pneumocytes (A-549). Scand J Immunol 2002; 56:294–302.

138. Song PI, Park YM, Abraham T, et al. Human keratinocytes express functional CD14 and toll-like receptor 4. J Invest Dermatol 2002; 119:424–32.

139. Rezai KA, Semnani RT, Farrokh-Siar L, et al. Human fetal retinal pigment epithelial cells induce apoptosis in allogenic T-cells in a Fas ligand and PGE2 independent pathway. Curr Eye Res 1999; 18:430–9.

140. Hamann KJ, Dorscheid DR, Ko FD, et al. Expression of Fas (CD95) and FasL (CD95L) in human airway epithelium. Am J Respir Cell Mol Biol 1998; 19:537–42.

141. Jorgensen A, Wiencke AK, la Cour M, et al. Human retinal pigment epithelial cell-induced apoptosis in activated T cells. Invest Ophthalmol Vis Sci 1998; 39:1590–9.

142. Zhang J, Miranda K, Ma BY, Fine A. Molecular characterization of the mouse Fas ligand promoter in airway epithelial cells. Biochim Biophys Acta 2000; 1490:291–301.

143. Dorscheid DR, Wojcik KR, Yule K, White SR. Role of cell surface glycosylation in mediating repair of human airway epithelial cell monolayers. Am J Physiol Lung Cell Mol Physiol 2001; 281:L982–92.

144. Gochuico BR, Miranda KM, Hessel EM, et al. Airway epithelial Fas ligand expression: potential role in modulating bronchial inflammation. Am J Physiol 1998; 274:L444–9.

145. Wen LP, Madani K, Fahrni JA, Duncan SR, Rosen GD. Dexamethasone inhibits lung epithelial cell apoptosis induced by IFN-gamma and Fas. Am J Physiol 1997; 273:L921–9.

146. De Maria R, Testi R. Fas-FasL interactions: a common pathogenetic mechanism in organ-specific autoimmunity. Immunol Today 1998; 19:121–5.
147. van Kooten C, Banchereau J. CD40-CD40 ligand. J Leukoc Biol 2000; 67:2–17.
148. Propst SM, Estell K, Schwiebert LM. CD40-mediated activation of NF-kappa B in airway epithelial cells. J Biol Chem 2002; 277:37054–63.
149. Propst SM, Denson R, Rothstein E, Estell K, Schwiebert LM. Proinflammatory and Th2-derived cytokines modulate CD40-mediated expression of inflammatory mediators in airway epithelia: implications for the role of epithelial CD40 in airway inflammation. J Immunol 2000; 165:2214–21.
150. Atsuta J, Sterbinsky SA, Plitt J, Schwiebert LM, Bochner BS, Schleimer RP. Phenotyping and cytokine regulation of the BEAS-2B human bronchial epithelial cell: demonstration of inducible expression of the adhesion molecules VCAM-1 and ICAM-1. Am J Respir Cell Mol Biol 1997; 17:571–82.
151. Companjen AR, van der Wel LI, Boon L, Prens EP, Laman JD. CD40 ligation-induced cytokine production in human skin explants is partly mediated via IL-1. Int Immunol 2002; 14:669–76.
152. Jolles S, Christensen J, Holman M, Klaus GB, Ager A. Systemic treatment with anti-CD40 antibody stimulates Langerhans cell migration from the skin. Clin Exp Immunol 2002; 129:519–26.
153. Denfeld RW, Hollenbaugh D, Fehrenbach A, et al. CD40 is functionally expressed on human keratinocytes. Eur J Immunol 1996; 26:2329–34.
154. Nickel R, Beck LA, Stellato C, Schleimer RP. Chemokines and allergic disease. J Allergy Clin Immunol 1999; 104:723–42.
155. Hou J, Schindler U, Henzel WJ, Ho TC, Brasseur M, McKnight SL. An interleukin-4-induced transcription factor: IL-4 stat. Science 1994; 265:1701–6.
156. Mikita T, Campbell D, Wu P, Williamson K, Schindler U. Requirements for interleukin-4-induced gene expression and functional characterization of Stat6. Mol Cell Biol 1996; 16:5811–.
157. Zhang S, Lukacs NW, Lawless VA, Kunkel SL, Kaplan MH. Cutting edge: differential expression of chemokines in Th1 and Th2 cells is dependent on Stat6 but not Stat4. J Immunol 2000; 165:10–4.
158. Kuperman DA, Huang X, Koth LL, et al. Direct effects of interleukin-13 on epithelial cells cause airway hyperreactivity and mucus overproduction in asthma. Nat Med 2002; 8:885–9.
159. Palmer-Crocker RL, Hughes CCW, Pober JS. IL-4 and IL-13 activate the JAK2 tyrosine kinase and Stat6 in cultured human vascular endothelial cells through a common pathway that does not involve the g_c chain. J Clin Invest 1996; 98:604–9.
160. Hansen G, Berry G, DeKruyff RH, Umetsu DT. Allergen-specific Th1 cells fail to counterbalance Th2 cell-induced airway hyperreactivity but cause severe airway inflammation. J Clin Invest 1999; 103:175–83.
161. Ceciliani F, Giordano A, Spagnolo V. The systemic reaction during inflammation: the acute-phase proteins. Protein Pept Lett 2002; 9:211–23.
162. Desiderio S, Yoo JY. A genome-wide analysis of the acute-phase response and its regulation by Stat3beta. Ann N Y Acad Sci 2003; 987:280–4.
163. Diamond G, Legarda D, Ryan LK. The innate immune response of the respiratory epithelium. Immunol Rev 2000; 173:27–38.
164. Gould JM, Weiser JN. Expression of C-reactive protein in the human respiratory tract. Infect Immun 2001; 69:1747–54.
165. Baumann H, Morella KK, Campos SP, Cao Z, Jahreis GP. Role of CAAT-enhancer binding protein isoforms in the cytokine regulation of acute-phase plasma protein genes. J Biol Chem 1992; 267:19744–51.
166. Baumann H, Jahreis GP, Morella KK, et al. Transcriptional regulation through cytokine and glucocorticoid response elements of rat acute phase plasma protein genes by C/EBP and JunB. J Biol Chem 1991; 266:20390–9.
167. Jamaluddin M, Garofalo R, Ogra PL, Brasier AR. Inducible translational regulation of the NF-IL6 transcription factor by respiratory syncytial virus infection in pulmonary epithelial cells. J Virol 1996; 70:1554–63.

168. Land SC, Darakhshan F. Thymulin evokes IL-6-C/EBPbeta regenerative repair and TNF-alpha silencing during endotoxin exposure in fetal lung explants. Am J Physiol Lung Cell Mol Physiol 2004; 286:L473–87.
169. Lambrecht BN. Allergen uptake and presentation by dendritic cells. Curr Opin Allergy Clin Immunol 2001; 1:51–9.
170. Niess JH, Brand S, Gu X, et al. CX3CR1-mediated dendritic cell access to the intestinal lumen and bacterial clearance. Science 2005; 307:254–8.
171. Lambrecht BN, Hammad H. Taking our breath away: dendritic cells in the pathogenesis of asthma. Nat Rev Immunol 2003; 3:994–1003.
172. Dieu MC, Vanbervliet B, Vicari A, et al. Selective recruitment of immature and mature dendritic cells by distinct chemokines expressed in different anatomic sites. J Exp Med 1998; 188:373–86.
173. Reibman J, Hsu Y, Chen LC, Bleck B, Gordon T. Airway epithelial cells release MIP-3alpha/CCL20 in response to cytokines and ambient particulate matter. Am J Respir Cell Mol Biol 2003; 28:648–54.
174. Pichavant M, Charbonnier AS, Taront S, et al. Asthmatic bronchial epithelium activated by the proteolytic allergen Der p 1 increases selective dendritic cell recruitment. J Allergy Clin Immunol 2005; 115:771–8.
175. Lambrecht BN. Dendritic cells and the regulation of the allergic immune response. Allergy 2005; 60:271–82.
176. Lambrecht BN, Hammad H. The other cells in asthma: dendritic cell and epithelial cell crosstalk. Curr Opin Pulm Med 2003; 9:34–41.
177. De Togni P, Goellner J, Ruddle NH, et al. Abnormal development of peripheral lymphoid organs in mice deficient in lymphotoxin. Science 1994; 264:703–7.
178. Ware CF. Network communications: lymphotoxins, LIGHT, and TNF. Annu Rev Immunol 2005; 23:787–819.
179. Rumbo M, Sierro F, Debard N, Kraehenbuhl JP, Finke D. Lymphotoxin beta receptor signaling induces the chemokine CCL20 in intestinal epithelium. Gastroenterology 2004; 127:213–23.
180. Boussaud V, Soler P, Moreau J, Goodwin RG, Hance AJ. Expression of three members of the TNF-R family of receptors (4-1BB, lymphotoxin-beta receptor, and Fas) in human lung. Eur Respir J 1998; 12:926–31.
181. Drayton DL, Ying X, Lee J, Lesslauer W, Ruddle NH. Ectopic LT alpha beta directs lymphoid organ neogenesis with concomitant expression of peripheral node addressin and a HEV-restricted sulfotransferase. J Exp Med 2003; 197:1153–63.
182. Dohi T, Rennert PD, Fujihashi K, et al. Elimination of colonic patches with lymphotoxin beta receptor-Ig prevents Th2 cell-type colitis. J Immunol 2001; 167:2781–90.
183. Lorenz RG, Chaplin DD, McDonald KG, McDonough JS, Newberry RD. Isolated lymphoid follicle formation is inducible and dependent upon lymphotoxin-sufficient B lymphocytes, lymphotoxin beta receptor, and TNF receptor I function. J Immunol 2003; 170:5475–82.
184. McDonald KG, McDonough JS, Newberry RD. Adaptive immune responses are dispensable for isolated lymphoid follicle formation: antigen-naive, lymphotoxin-sufficient B lymphocytes drive the formation of mature isolated lymphoid follicles. J Immunol 2005; 174:5720–8.
185. Corbett M, Kraehenbuhl JP. Lung immunity: necessity is the mother of induction. Nat Med 2004; 10:904–5.
186. Magliozzi R, Columba-Cabezas S, Serafini B, Aloisi F. Intracerebral expression of CXCL13 and BAFF is accompanied by formation of lymphoid follicle-like structures in the meninges of mice with relapsing experimental autoimmune encephalomyelitis. J Neuroimmunol 2004; 148:11–23.
187. Rahman ZS, Manser T. B cells expressing Bcl-2 and a signaling-impaired BAFF-specific receptor fail to mature and are deficient in the formation of lymphoid follicles and germinal centers. J Immunol 2004; 173:6179–88.
188. Diaz-Sanchez D, Dotson AR, Takenaka H, Saxon A. Diesel exhaust particles induce local IgE production in vivo and alter the pattern of IgE messenger RNA isoforms. J Clin Invest 1994; 94:1417–25.

189. Diaz-Sanchez D, Tsien A, Fleming J, Saxon A. Combined diesel exhaust particulate and ragweed allergen challenge markedly enhances human in vivo nasal ragweed-specific IgE and skews cytokine production to a T helper cell 2-type pattern. J Immunol 1997; 158:2406–13.
190. Meyers DA, Postma DS, Stine OC, et al. Genome screen for asthma and bronchial hyperresponsiveness: interactions with passive smoke exposure. J Allergy Clin Immunol 2005; 115:1169–75.
191. Choudhry S, Avila PC, Nazario S, et al. CD14 tobacco gene-environment interaction modifies asthma severity and immunoglobulin E levels in Latinos with asthma. Am J Respir Crit Care Med 2005; 172:173–82.
192. Steinke JW, Bradley D, Arango P, et al. Cysteinyl leukotriene expression in chronic hyperplastic sinusitis-nasal polyposis: importance to eosinophilia and asthma. J Allergy Clin Immunol 2003; 111:342–9.

5 Role of Inflammatory T Cells and Eosinophils in Chronic Rhinosinusitis

Susan Foley and Qutayba Hamid

Meakins-Christie Laboratories, McGill University, Montreal, Quebec, Canada

INTRODUCTION

The last 10 years have witnessed new insights into the inflammatory mechanisms of chronic rhinosinusitis (CRS). Investigation of the inflammatory roles of cytokines and chemokines has shed considerable light on the pathogenesis of this disease. T lymphocytes and activated eosinophils are prominent within the sinus mucosa of patients with CRS, especially in atopic patients. Distinct cytokine and inflammatory cell profiles have been found in atopic and non-atopic patients, suggesting that different pathophysiologies may be present in these two subgroups of patients. Recruitment and activation of the inflammatory cell infiltrate has largely been attributed to the effects of T-helper (Th2) cytokines [namely interleukin (IL)-4, IL-5, IL-13, and granulocyte monocyte-colony stimulating factor (GM-CSF)], and the eosinophil-associated chemokines, eotaxin, and monocyte chemotactic proteins (MCPs). This review focuses on the roles of inflammatory T cells and eosinophils in CRS, and discusses recent developments regarding the inflammatory processes in this complex disease.

Chronic rhinosinusitis exists with or without nasal polyposis and is a complex, multifactorial process (1). An inflammatory disease of the nasal and paranasal sinus mucosa, it is classified as allergic or non-allergic, depending on the presence or absence of atopy. In the United States, CRS represents one of the most common chronic diseases in adults with an estimated prevalence of 16.8% (32 million patients) (2). Nasal polyps are found on clinical examination in about 20% of patients with CRS.

The immunopathologic mechanisms underlying the development of CRS in allergic patients are largely related to the effects of Th2 cytokines and their corresponding receptors. In contrast, a combination of Th1 and Th2 cytokines seems to orchestrate the inflammatory response in non-allergic CRS patients. Similar observations have been made in CRS with and without nasal polyposis (3,4). Despite these distinct mechanisms, the common outcome in CRS, in both atopic and non-atopic patients is an intense eosinophilic infiltration.

Compared with healthy control subjects, the sinus mucosa of patients with allergic CRS is characterized by a higher number of eosinophils, T cells, and B cells (Fig. 1) (3,5). Kamil et al. (4) observed that there is heterogeneity in the inflammatory process in different sinus compartments. In patients with allergic CRS, the ethmoid sinus exhibits a more severe inflammatory response than the maxillary, evident by an increased CD4 helper/CD8 suppressor ratio as well as raised eosinophil and mast cell numbers. Tissues of patients with non-allergic CRS also demonstrate high numbers of eosinophils but have lower numbers of T cells and a different cytokine profile (discussed below).

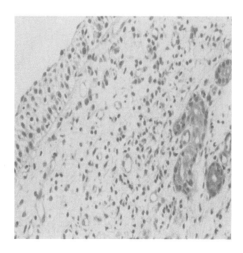

FIGURE 1 (*See color insert.*) H&E staining showing inflammatory T cells and eosinophils in nasal mucosa in CRS.

The reported incidence of asthma within the CRS population nears 50% (6), supporting a clinical link between these two conditions. Eosinophilic inflammation is a key common link between these two diseases.

ROLE OF LYMPHOCYTES IN CRS

T and B lymphocytes are prominent in the sinus mucosa of patients with allergic CRS compared with normal control subjects. Activated T lymphocytes and plasma cells are found in regions surrounding mucosal glandular cells and to a lesser extent in the subepithelial area. The profile of locally-expressed cytokines in sinus mucosa in CRS suggests that T lymphocytes play a major role in disease pathogenesis.

Biopsy tissues of nasal mucosa obtained from subjects with allergic rhinitis 24 hours after allergen challenge (outside the pollen season) demonstrate a marked increase in the number of CD4+ T lymphocytes (Fig. 2) (7). Furthermore, use of in situ hybridization with antisense complementary riboprobes designed to detect cytokine messenger RNA (mRNA), has shown increased numbers of Th2-type cytokines IL-4, IL-5, IL-13, and GM-CSF mRNA+ cells (8,9) (Fig. 3). In contrast, the Th1-type cytokines interferon (IFN)-γ and IL-12 are not increased. T cells are a major source of Th2 cytokine expression within the nasal mucosa, seen 24 hours after allergen exposure. Co-localization studies have demonstrated that the majority of IL-4, IL-5, and IL-13 mRNA+ cells (approximately 70–80%) were T cells (8,10,11). In CRS patients with associated allergies (allergic CRS), a similar pattern of Th2 cytokine mRNA expression has been found in sinus tissues, suggesting that chronic "late-phase" allergic inflammation occur in the sinus tissues (4,12).

A relatively modest increase in CD3+ T lymphocytes has been found in nasal polyp tissue in patients with "chronic hyperplastic sinusitis/nasal polyposis", a condition now referred to as "Chronic rhinosinussitis with nasal polyps (CRS with NP)". The increase in T lymphocytes is seen primarily in CRS with NP patients with associated allergies. A substantial proportion of these patients are non-allergic on the basis of allergy skin testing, and in these patients the numbers of T lymphocytes are similar to that in control uninflamed nasal turbinate tissue (3,5). The cytokine profile found in patients with CRS with NP depends on the presence or absence of allergy (3) (see below).

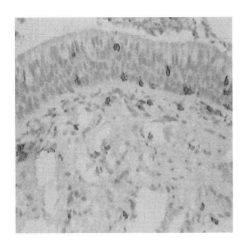

FIGURE 2 (*See color insert.*) Immunostaining with CD4 antibody showing infiltration of the nasal mucosa and epithelium with T cells.

Cytokines Produced by T Cells

Interleukin-4, a Th2 cytokine, has been shown to induce naïve T cells to commence production of other Th2 cytokines (13). It also induces isotype switching of B cells in favor of IgE, and facilitates eosinophil infiltration by enhancing endothelial migration of eosinophils and lymphocytes (not neutrophils) through interaction with the integrin molecule very late activation antigen-4 (VLA-4). A recent study by Bradley et al. (14) reported that patients with CRS/NP demonstrated increased transcription of transforming growth factor-beta (TGF-β) in response to IL-4 treatment, suggesting that IL-4 may also play a role in mediating stromal proliferation in the formation of nasal polyposis. T cells are likely the major source of IL-4 in CRS. Increased mRNA expression for IL-4 has been found in allergic CRS (both Chronic rhinosinussitis without nasal polyps (CRS without NP) and CRS with NP) (3,12,15).

Although local production of IL-4 appears to be a feature of CRS (and CRS with NP) with associated allergies, IL-5 appears to be less distinguishing.

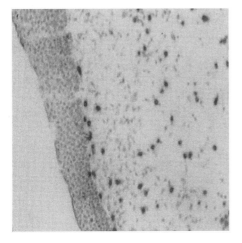

FIGURE 3 (*See color insert.*) In-situ hybridization showing Th2-type cytokines produced by T cells.

An increase in local production of IL-5 was also found in non-allergic subjects with CRS with NP, and the IL-5 producing cells were found to be primarily T lymphocytes (16). Therefore, T cells are the principal source of IL-5 production in both allergic and non-allergic patients with CRS. IL-5 plays a critical role in the activation and differentiation of eosinophils (17). IL-4 and IL-5 act through hetero-dimeric receptors composed of a ligand-specific alpha subunit and a signal-transducing beta subunit, respectively. Upregulation of receptors for IL-4 and IL-5 has been demonstrated in the mucosa of subjects with allergic CRS (15). Wright et al. (16) demonstrated that IL-4(R) and IL-5(R) mRNA expression was increased in the lamina propria of subjects with CRS, particularly in those with associated allergies. IL-5R expression is a fundamental property of eosinophil/basophil pro-genitor cells and mature eosinophils (18). A study by Simon et al. demonstrated that IL-5 was the principal eosinophil survival-enhancing cytokine in nasal polyp tissue (19).

Interleukin-13, a cytokine with functional similarities to IL-4, is elevated in the sinus mucosa of both allergic and non-allergic subjects with CRS (12). In both allergic and non-allergic CRS/NP, there is also increased tissue density of cells expressing GM-CSF and IL-13 mRNA (20). IL-13 has activities critical to the development of the asthma phenotype in experimental animals. These activities include production of muc5ac, goblet cell metaplasia, and epithelial production of pro-eosinophilic chemokines, including eotaxin, eotaxin-2, MCP-1-2-3-5, macro-phage inflammatory protein (MIP-1α) and MIP-1β (21). GM-CSF promotes eosino-phil survival in mucosal tissue (22).

Interleukin-3, possibly produced by activated T cells, mast cells, and eosino-phils in the sinus mucosa, may have multiple important effects in CRS (5,23). It may indirectly contribute to fibrosis and the on-going mucosal thickening that ultimately results in obstruction of the sinus ostia, specifically the ostiomeatal complex (23,24).

Expression of IFN-γ mRNA was found to be increased in the tissues of patients with non-allergic nasal polyps (CRS with NP) (5). In this study, an inverse relationship was observed between the expression of IL-4 and IFN-γ. A similar finding of increased local production of IFN-γ was also reported in non-allergic CRS without NP (25). IFN-γ has many proinflammatory effects, including the ability to stimulate intercellular adhesion molecule (ICAM-1) and regulated upon activation, normal T-cell expressed and secreted (RANTES) expression in airway epithelial cells (26,27). The expression of IFN-γ in association with IL-5 and IL-13 constitutes the characteristic "mixed Th1/Th2 phenotype" profile of non-allergic CRS with NP and CRS without NP (6).

Interleukin-12, a Th1-associated cytokine, is thought to play a suppressive role in allergic responses. Wright et al. (28) demonstrated a decreased expression of IL-12 (p40) mRNA in sinus biopsy specimens from both allergic and non-allergic patients with CRS. Furthermore, IL-12R (β2) was decreased in allergic CRS, possibly due to the upregulation of IL-4 which has inhibitory effects on Th1 cytokines (29). However, the role of IL-12 in CRS pathogenesis remains relatively poorly understood.

Molet et al. (30) recently examined the role of a relatively new T-cell cytokine, IL-17, in the remodeling process that takes place in CRS with NP. This cytokine is produced primarily, but not exclusively, by CD4+ and CD8+ T lymphocytes (31,32), Increased expression of IL-17 was demonstrated in subjects with CRS with NP compared to normal control nasal turbinate tissue (30). Correlating with the presence of CD4+ and CD8+ T lymphocytes, 43.3% of the detected IL-17+ inflammatory cells were T lymphocytes. These findings suggest that IL-17 may contribute, at least partly, to the structural abnormalities such as stromal fibrosis and basement membrane thickening that characterize NP.

Cytokines mediate their effects by binding to membrane-associated receptors on inflammatory cells. The upregulation of IL-4, IL-5, and GM-CSF in CRS is paralleled by an increase in the expression of their receptors on inflammatory cells. Expression of GM-CSF receptors has been found to be increased predominantly in patients with non-allergic CRS. Conversely, IL-12 receptors were found to be decreased in those with allergic CRS, in accordance with a downregulation of IL-12 (a Th1-associated cytokine) (29).

B Cells

A resident population of B cells can be found within the nasal and sinus mucosa (33,34). IgE production has long been ascribed to B cells within secondary lymphoid tissue, bone marrow, and blood, however, certain patients exhibit IgE in nasal secretions but not in serum (35) or salivary secretions (36). Furthermore, it has been demonstrated that IgE protein, ε-mRNA, and DNA switch circles, generated as a consequence of isotype switching to IgE, are present in nasal lavage of allergic rhinitis patients following allergen challenge supporting the concept of local IgE isotype switching (37,38).

Interleukin-4, IL-13, and costimulation via CD40 target the ε promoter (Iε for germline transcription, giving rise to germline transcripts (39–41). These transcripts are considered necessary for the recombination of DNA so that genes coding for ε-mRNA (Cε) may be placed in favorable positions for transcription (42). The factors required for inducing isotype switching of resident B cells to IgE, IL-4, IL-13, and CD40L (8,39,43,44) are expressed within nasal sinus tissue in individuals with allergic rhinitis and CRS (8,10,12,45). With the use of antisense riboprobes, increased numbers of Iε and Cε RNA+ cells, in the absence of a change in B-cell numbers have been observed within allergic nasal mucosa after allergen challenge (37,38) as well as within the ethmoid sinus mucosa of allergic patients with CRS (34). This indicates that resident B cells undergo ε germline transcription, a process necessary for DNA rearrangement and isotype switching, within the mucosal tissue.

EOSINOPHILS IN CRS

An elevation in the number of inflammatory cells in the tissues, particularly eosinophils, is a feature common to allergic diseases. Eosinophils arise predominantly in the bone marrow from CD34+ pluripotent progenitor cells in the presence of IL-3, IL-5, and GM-CSF (47–50). IL-5 is critical to their development, influencing mainly terminal differentiation of CD34/CD33+ progenitor cells (50). They are the only human leukocytes that express membrane-bound receptors specific to IL-5, demonstrating the importance of this cytokine in the development of eosinophilia (51,52).

The presence of eosinophils within mucosal tissue of allergic airways disease is believed to be due to de novo infiltration of mature cells from the bone marrow. Recent studies, however, by Cameron et al., using an explant system of human allergic nasal mucosa, provide strong evidence that a sub-population of eosinophils

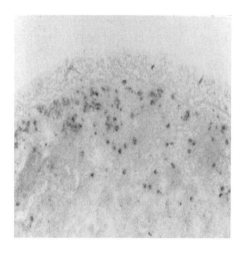

FIGURE 4 (*See color insert.*) MBP staining of eosinophils in the mucosa and epithelium in nasal tissue in CRS.

may undergo local differentiation within the mucosa itself. Following ex-vivo stimulation with specific allergen or recombinant human (rh) IL-5, more major basic protein (MBP)-immunoreactive and IL-5mRNA+ cells, along with fewer CD34/IL-5Rα cells, were found in nasal mucosal tissues (53). The process was found to be highly IL-5-dependent, implying that it might be regulated in vivo by endogenous production of sIL-5Rα. Since the alpha subunit of the IL-5 receptor (IL-5Rα) is almost exclusively expressed by eosinophils, the co-localization of CD34 immunoreactivity with IL-5Rα is considered to be a marker for precursor eosinophils (CD34/IL-5Rα+) (54). Such precursors have been found in nasal polyps, and in the presence of locally produced IL-5 likely differentiate into mature eosinophils (18). Similarly, eosinophil precursors and IL-5 mRNA have been identified by Robinson et al. in the lungs of asthmatic patients (55), indicating that a similar process of local differentiation of eosinophils may occur within the asthmatic lung.

Eosinophils are major effectors in allergic tissue reactions. They have the capacity to synthesize and store cytokines, particularly of the Th2-type, which may lead to increased cell survival within tissues (56). IL-4 and IL-5 production by eosinophils may amplify local allergic inflammation. Eosinophils are also a potent source of leukotriene C_4 (LTC_4) (57), and increased levels of cysteinyl leukotrienes have been found in eosinophilic nasal polyps (58). Increased levels of eosinophil-derived proteins such as MBP and eosinophil cationic protein (ECP) are also present within the sinus mucosa in allergic rhinitis (Fig. 4). These proteins have been shown to cause degranulation of other inflammatory cells and to promote epithelial cell damage (59–61). Hamilos et al. (5) found tissue eosinophilia to be a prominent feature of both allergic and non-allergic CRS/NP, correlating in both groups with the density of GM-CSF and IL-3 mRNA+ cells.

Recruitment and Activation of Eosinophils

A variety of factors, including chemokines such as eotaxin, are responsible for the infiltration of eosinophils into the nasal tissue in CRS. Eotaxin is an eosinophil-specific C–C chemokine that has been shown to increase after allergen challenge in allergic rhinitis (62,63) and to be present in the sinus mucosa of both allergic and non-allergic CRS (63,64) (Fig. 5). Eotaxin is a potent eosinophil chemoattractant,

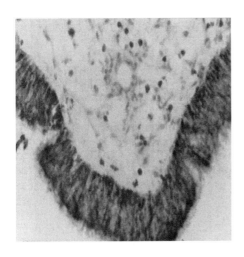

FIGURE 5   (*See color insert.*) Eotaxin immunostaining in the epithelium in CRS.

inducing eosinophil migration in vivo (64) and is increased in patients with both
allergic and non-allergic rhinosinusitis (63,65).

Other CC–chemokines, such as RANTES and MCP-3, have also been implicated in the recruitment of eosinophils to the inflamed nasal mucosa in patients
with CRS with NP. Bartels et al. (65) found elevated expression of eotaxin- and
RANTES-mRNA, but not of MCP-3-mRNA, in non-atopic and atopic nasal polyps,
compared to normal nasal mucosa. Lee et al. (66) recently demonstrated that,
compared with controls, the expression of RANTES is increased in vivo within
allergic and non-allergic nasal polyp tissue, and that such increase is correlated
with eosinophil infiltration. However, the importance of RANTES in the recruitment of eosinophils within nasal polyps has been questioned, as Bachert et al. (67)
found no difference in protein levels between nasal polyps and control tissues.
It is possible that the main involvement of RANTES lies in the localization of
eosinophils within polyp regions (68).

In CRS, the selective recruitment of eosinophils might occur through upregulation of endothelial vascular adhesion molecule-1 (VCAM-1). This adhesion
molecule facilitates the selective transendothelial migration of eosinophils and
lymphocytes (not neutrophils) through interaction with its counterligand, VLA
antigen-4. VCAM-1 can be activated on endothelial cells by cytokines, particularly
IL-4, IL-13, and tumor necrosis factor (TNFα) (20,69). TNFα is known to increase
transendothelial migration of eosinophils through the induction of ICAM-1,
VCAM-1, and E-selectin (70). Hamilos et al. (20) found evidence that upregulation
of VCAM-1 and elaboration of RANTES may contribute to the marked accumulation of eosinophils in non-allergic CRS with NP. Furthermore, a correlation was
found between TNFα expression and local upregulation of VCAM-1, suggesting a
critical role for TNFα in this process.

An increase in endothelial expression of P-selectin was also found in nasal
polyps (71). P-selectin, which is induced on human endothelial cells by IL-4
and IL-13 (72), may also play a role in eosinophil recruitment into nasal polyp
tissue (73).

Interleukin-3, IL-5, and GM-CSF are critically involved in the activation and
survival of human eosinophils (74,75). In CRS, as in other forms of allergic tissue

inflammation, IL-5 mediates the activation and selective migration of eosinophils from the peripheral circulation into the tissues (76,77). As previously mentioned, local IL-5 production is critical for eosinophil survival in nasal polyps (19). The density of mRNA expression for GM-CSF (a cytokine that is produced by both Th1 and Th2 cells and eosinophils) also correlated well with the level of eosinophilia observed in CRS with NP, suggesting that GM-CSF may also play a role in the local differentiation, activation, and prolonged survival of eosinophils (79).

EG2, a marker that solely stains secreted ECP, has been proposed as a specific marker for activated eosinophils (78,79). The number and ratio of activated and non-activated eosinophils within tissues have been shown to be reduced in association with systemic or topical corticosteroid treatment, suggesting that these measures may serve as an indicator of the level of chronic inflammation in nasal polyposis (79).

The activation of eosinophils and the subsequent release of their cytotoxic mediators, such as MBP, ECP, and eosinophil peroxidase (EPO), have been associated with many pathologic features, namely, epithelial desquamation, subepithelial fibrosis, and airway hyperresponsiveness (80,81) that characterize allergic inflammation. Eosinophils are known to directly damage the epithelium of the upper, as well as the lower respiratory tract (59). The toxic products produced by eosinophilic granule constituents also induce ciliostasis and lysis of epithelial cells (82). Eosinophil granules also contain vasoactive substances, chemotactic mediators, including leukotriene C_4 (LTC_4) and platelet-activating factor (PAF). Specific granule proteins and the lipid mediators LTC_4 and PAF are thought to be responsible for the observed swelling and hyperresponsiveness of the nasal mucosa (83). Furthermore, eosinophils are known to stimulate collagen synthesis (84). Eosinophils also produce multiple cytokines, notably IL-4, IL-5, GM-CSF, TNF-α, IL-12, and TGF-β among others.

There are several histologic markers for eosinophils. BMK13 and EG1 constitute pan-eosinophilic markers; the former is known to detect MBP, and the latter is used to detect secreted or stored ECP. Activated eosinophils have greater toxicity, and appear hypodense in light microscopy, as they contain less MBP, and possess smaller granules. Their chemotactic response to PAF and their oxygen demand are higher than in resting eosinophils (78). Another antibody, EG2, stains only secreted ECP and has been proposed as a specific marker for detecting eosinophil activation. Activated, degranulated, and EG2-positive eosinophils are seen to predominate in polyp stroma, and participate in the development and maintenance of mature polyp disease (75,79,85). The majority of eosinophils in nasal polyps stain for both MBP and EG2 and are sensitive to suppression by topical fluticasone (71).

Among the inflammatory cells, eosinophils (MBP+ or EG2) predominate, found in 80–90% of nasal polyps. Appenroth et al. (79) found that the relative number of activated versus non-activated eosinophils was a reliable indicator of the level of inflammatory activity in chronic polyposis. In contrast, CRS patients without nasal polyps have fewer resting and activated eosinophils.

T CELL AND EOSINOPHIL INTERACTION

The development of CRS represents a complex, multi-step process characterized by inflammation of the nasal and sinus mucosa. There is dynamic interplay between inflammatory cells, cytokines, inflammatory mediators, and microbial products. In allergic patients, the immunopathology of CRS has many similarities to that of allergic rhinitis, as well as in the late-phase response to antigen challenge. IgE-dependent mast cell activation and the release of inflammatory mediators ultimately lead to the recruitment and activation of various leukocytes, including mast cells, eosinophils, and T lymphocytes. Such events are mediated by a strong Th2-type cytokine profile, whereby IL-4 and IL-5 are crucially implicated in the processes leading up to the eosinophilia characteristic of CRS. IL-5, though mainly produced by Th2 cytokines, is also produced by eosinophils, and is crucial for their survival.

In non-allergic patients, the pathologic events leading to eosinophilic inflammation are less clear. Recent studies, however, have suggested that colonizing fungi induce antigen-specific T-lymphocyte activation, leading to local production of a "mixed Th1/Th2 phenotype" of IL-5, IL-13, and IFN-γ that promotes the local accumulation and survival of eosinophils. Alternatively, at least in the case of nasal polyposis, the pathogenesis may involve a localized Th2 response to colonizing *Staphylococcus aureus*. The evidence underlying these recent hypotheses are reviewed elsewhere in this monograph (see Chapters 10 and 11).

REFERENCES

1. Ponikau JU, Sherris DA, Kephart GM, et al. Features of airway remodeling and eosinophilic inflammation in chronic rhinosinusitis: is the histopathology similar to asthma? J Allergy Clin Immunol 2003; 112:877–82.
2. Blackwell DL, Collins JG, Coles R. Summary health statistics for U.S. adults: National Health Interview Survey. Vital Health Stat 1997; 10:2002:1–109.
3. Hamilos DL, Leung DY, Wood R, et al. Evidence for distinct cytokine expression in allergic versus nonallergic chronic sinusitis. J Allergy Clin Immunol 1995; 96:537–44.
4. Kamil A, Ghaffar O, Lavigne F, et al. Comparison of inflammatory cell profile and Th2 cytokine expression in the ethmoid sinuses, maxillary sinuses, and turbinates of atopic subjects with chronic sinusitis. Otolaryngol Head Neck Surg 1998; 118:804–9.
5. Hamilos DL, Leung DY, Wood R, et al. Chronic hyperplastic sinusitis: association of tissue eosinophilia with mRNA expression of granulocyte-macrophage colony-stimulating factor and interleukin-3. J Allergy Clin Immunol 1993; 92:39–48.
6. Hamilos DL. Chronic sinusitis. J Allergy Clin Immunol 2000; 106:213–27.
7. Varney VA, Jacobson MR, Sudderick RM, et al. Immunohistology of the nasal mucosa following allergen-induced rhinitis. Identification of activated T lymphocytes, eosinophils, and neutrophils. Am Rev Respir Dis 1992; 146:170–6.
8. Ghaffar O, Laberge S, Jacobson MR, et al. IL-13 mRNA and immunoreactivity in allergen-induced rhinitis: comparison with IL-4 expression and modulation by topical glucocorticoid therapy. Am J Respir Cell Mol Biol 1997; 17:17–24.
9. Durham SR, Ying S, Varney VA, et al. Cytokine messenger RNA expression for IL-3, IL-4, IL-5, and granulocyte/macrophage-colony-stimulating factor in the nasal mucosa after local allergen provocation: relationship to tissue eosinophilia. J Immunol 1992; 148:2390–4.
10. Ying S, Durham SR, Barkans J, et al. T cells are the principal source of interleukin-5 mRNA in allergen-induced rhinitis. Am J Respir Cell Mol Biol 1993; 9:356–60.
11. Ying S, Durham SR, Jacobson MR, et al. T lymphocytes and mast cells express messenger RNA for interleukin-4 in the nasal mucosa in allergen-induced rhinitis. Immunology 1994; 82:200–6.
12. al Ghamdi K, Ghaffar O, Small P, et al. IL-4 and IL-13 expression in chronic sinusitis: relationship with cellular infiltrate and effect of topical corticosteroid treatment. J Otolaryngol 1997; 26:160–6.
13. Sornasse T, Larenas PV, Davis KA, et al. Differentiation and stability of T helper 1 and 2 cells derived from naive human neonatal CD4+ T cells, analyzed at the single-cell level. J Exp Med 1996; 184:473–83.

14. Bradley DT, Kountakis SE. Role of interleukins and transforming growth factor-beta in chronic rhinosinusitis and nasal polyposis. Laryngoscope 2005; 115:684–6.
15. Wright ED, Frenkiel S, Al-Ghamdi K, et al. Interleukin-4, interleukin-5, and granulo-cyte-macrophage colony-stimulating factor receptor expression in chronic sinusitis and response to topical steroids. Otolaryngol Head Neck Surg 1998; 118:490–5.
16. Hamilos DL, Leung DY, Huston DP, Kamil A, Wood R, Hamid Q. GM-CSF, IL-5 and RANTES immunoreactivity and mRNA expression in chronic hyperplastic sinusitis with nasal polyposis (NP). Clin Exp Allergy 1998; 28:1145–52.
17. Lopez AF, Sanderson CJ, Gamble JR, et al. Recombinant human interleukin 5 is a selective activator of human eosinophil function. J Exp Med 1988; 167:219–24.
18. Kim YK, Uno M, Hamilos DL, et al. Immunolocalization of CD34 in nasal polyposis. Effect of topical corticosteroids. Am J Respir Cell Mol Biol 1999; 20:388–97.
19. Simon HU, Yousefi S, Schranz C, Schapowal A, Bachert C, Blaser K. Direct demonstra-tion of delayed eosinophil apoptosis as a mechanism causing tissue eosinophilia. J Immunol 1997; 158:3902–8.
20. Hamilos DL, Leung DY, Wood R, et al. Eosinophil infiltration in nonallergic chronic hyperplastic sinusitis with nasal polyposis (CHS/NP) is associated with endothelial VCAM-1 upregulation and expression of TNF-alpha. Am J Respir Cell Mol Biol 1996; 15:443–50.
21. Elias JA, Lee CG, Zheng T, et al. Interleukin-13 and Leukotrienes: An Intersection of Pathogenetic Schema. Am J Respir Cell Mol Biol 2003; 28:401–4.
22. Owen WF Jr, Rothenberg ME, Silberstein DS, et al. Regulation of human eosinophil viability, density, and function by granulocyte/macrophage colony-stimulating factor in the presence of 3T3 fibroblasts. J Exp Med 1987; 166:129–41.
23. Rudack C, Bachert C. Cytokines and chemokines in paranasal sinus diseases. Laryn-gorhinootologie 1999; 78:481–90.
24. Persson CG, Erjefalt JS, Andersson M, et al. Epithelium, microcirculation, and eosinophils–new aspects of the allergic airway in vivo. Allergy 1997; 52:241–55.
25. Jyonouchi H, Sun S, Rimell FL. Cytokine production by sinus lavage, bronchial lavage, and blood mononuclear cells in chronic rhinosinusitis with or without atopy. Arch Otolaryngol Head Neck Surg 2000; 126: 522–8.
26. Look DC, Rapp SR, Keller BT, Holtzman MJ. Selective induction of intercellular adhesion molecule-1 by interferon-gamma in human airway epithelial cells. Am J Physiol 1992; 263(1 Pt 1):L79–87.
27. Taguchi M, Sampath D, Koga T, Castro M, Look DC, Nakajima S, Holtzman MJ. Patterns for RANTES secretion and intercellular adhesion molecule 1 expression mediate transepithelial T cell traffic based on analyses in vitro and in vivo. J Exp Med 1998; 187:1927–40.
28. Wright ED, Christodoulopoulos P, Frenkiel S, et al. Expression of interleukin (IL)-12 (p40) and IL-12 (beta 2) receptors in allergic rhinitis and chronic sinusitis. Clin Exp Allergy 1999; 29:1320–5.
29. Szabo SJ, Jacobson NG, Dighe AS, et al. Developmental commitment to the Th2 lineage by extinction of IL-12 signaling. Immunity 1995; 2:665–75.
30. Molet SM, Hamid QA, Hamilos DL. IL-11 and IL-17 expression in nasal polyps: relationship to collagen deposition and suppression by intranasal fluticasone propio-nate. Laryngoscope 2003; 113:1803–12.
31. Shin HC, Benbernou N, Fekkar H, et al. Regulation of IL-17, IFN-gamma and IL-10 in human CD8(+) T cells by cyclic AMP-dependent signal transduction pathway. Cyto-kine 1998; 10:841–50.
32. Fossiez F, Djossou O, Chomarat P, et al. T cell interleukin-17 induces stromal cells to produce proinflammatory and hematopoietic cytokines. J Exp Med 1996; 183:2593–603.
33. Davidsson A, Karlsson MG, Hellquist HB. Allergen-induced changes of B-cell pheno-types in patients with allergic rhinitis. Rhinology 1994; 32:184–90.
34. Ghaffar O, Durham SR, Al-Ghamdi K, et al. Expression of IgE heavy chain transcripts in the sinus mucosa of atopic and nonatopic patients with chronic sinusitis. Am J Respir Cell Mol Biol 1998; 18:706–11.
35. Huggins KG, Brostoff J. Local production of specific IgE antibodies in allergic-rhinitis patients with negative skin tests. Lancet 1975; 2:148–50.

36. Platts-Mills TA. Local production of IgG, IgA and IgE antibodies in grass pollen hay fever. J Immunol 1979; 122:2218–25.
37. Durham SR, Gould HJ, Thienes CP, et al. Expression of epsilon germ-line gene transcripts and mRNA for the epsilon heavy chain of IgE in nasal B cells and the effects of topical corticosteroid. Eur J Immunol 1997; 27:2899–906.
38. Cameron LA, Durham SR, Jacobson MR, et al. Expression of IL-4, Cepsilon RNA, and Iepsilon RNA in the nasal mucosa of patients with seasonal rhinitis: effect of topical corticosteroids. J Allergy Clin Immunol 1998; 101:330–6.
39. Punnonen J, Cocks BG, de Vries JE. IL-4 induces germ-line IgE heavy chain gene transcription in human fetal pre-B cells. Evidence for differential expression of functional IL-4 and IL-13 receptors during B cell ontogeny. J Immunol 1995; 155:4248–54.
40. Iciek LA, Delphin SA, Stavnezer J. CD40 cross-linking induces Ig epsilon germline transcripts in B cells via activation of NF-kappaB: synergy with IL-4 induction. J Immunol 1997; 158:4769–79.
41. Warren WD, Berton MT. Induction of germ-line gamma 1 and epsilon Ig gene expression in murine B cells. IL-4 and the CD40 ligand-CD40 interaction provide distinct but synergistic signals. J Immunol 1995; 155:5637–46.
42. Lorenz M, Jung S, Radbruch A. Switch transcripts in immunoglobulin class switching. Science 1995; 267:1825–8.
43. Gauchat JF, Lebman DA, Coffman RL, et al. Structure and expression of germline epsilon transcripts in human B cells induced by interleukin 4 to switch to IgE production. J Exp Med 1990; 172:463–73.
44. Xu J, Foy TM, Laman JD, Elliott EA, et al. Mice deficient for the CD40 ligand. Immunity 1994; 1:423–31.
45. Pawankar R, Okuda M, Yssel H, et al. Nasal mast cells in perennial allergic rhinitics exhibit increased expression of the Fc epsilonRI, CD40L, IL-4, and IL-13, and can induce IgE synthesis in B cells. J Clin Invest 1997; 99:1492–9.
46. Denburg JA, Telizyn S, Messner H, et al. Heterogeneity of human peripheral blood eosinophil-type colonies: evidence for a common basophil-eosinophil progenitor. Blood 1985; 66:312–8.
47. Clutterbuck EJ, Hirst EM, Sanderson CJ. Human interleukin-5 (IL-5) regulates the production of eosinophils in human bone marrow cultures: comparison and interaction with IL-1, IL-3, IL-6, and GMCSF. Blood 1989; 73:1504–12.
48. Shalit M, Sekhsaria S, Malech HL. Modulation of growth and differentiation of eosinophils from human peripheral blood CD34+ cells by IL5 and other growth factors. Cell Immunol 1995; 160:50–7.
49. Gibson PG, Dolovich J, Girgis-Gabardo A, et al. The inflammatory response in asthma exacerbation: changes in circulating eosinophils, basophils and their progenitors. Clin Exp Allergy 1990; 20:661–8.
50. Ema H, Suda T, Nagayoshi K, et al. Target cells for granulocyte colony-stimulating factor, interleukin-3, and interleukin-5 in differentiation pathways of neutrophils and eosinophils. Blood 1990; 76:1956–61.
51. Migita M, Yamaguchi N, Mita S, et al. Characterization of the human IL-5 receptors on eosinophils. Cell Immunol 1991; 133:484–97.
52. Egan RW, Umland SP, Cuss FM, et al. Biology of interleukin-5 and its relevance to allergic disease. Allergy 1996; 51:71–81.
53. Cameron L, Christodoulopoulos P, Lavigne F, et al. Evidence for local eosinophil differentiation within allergic nasal mucosa: inhibition with soluble IL-5 receptor. J Immunol 2000; 164:1538–45.
54. Sehmi R, Wood LJ, Watson R, et al. Allergen-induced increases in IL-5 receptor alpha-subunit expression on bone marrow-derived CD34+ cells from asthmatic subjects. A novel marker of progenitor cell commitment towards eosinophilic differentiation. J Clin Invest 1997; 100:2466–75.
55. Robinson DS, Damia R, Zeibecoglou K, et al. CD34(+)/interleukin-5Ralpha messenger RNA+ cells in the bronchial mucosa in asthma: potential airway eosinophil progenitors. Am J Respir Cell Mol Biol 1999; 20:9–13.
56. Kay AB, Barata L, Meng Q, et al. Eosinophils and eosinophil-associated cytokines in allergic inflammation. Int Arch Allergy Immunol 1997; 113:196–9.

57. Holgate ST, Bradding P, Sampson AP. Leukotriene antagonists and synthesis inhibitors: new directions in asthma therapy. J Allergy Clin Immunol 1996; 98:1–13.

58. Steinke JW, Bradley D, Arango P, Crouse CD, Frierson H, Kountakis SE, Kraft M, Borish L. Cysteinyl leukotriene expression in chronic hyperplastic sinusitis-nasal polyposis: importance to eosinophilia and asthma. J Allergy Clin Immunol. 2003; 111:342–9.

59. Hisamatsu K, Ganbo T, Nakazawa T, et al. Cytotoxicity of human eosinophil granule major basic protein to human nasal sinus mucosa in vitro. J Allergy Clin Immunol 1990; 86:52–63.

60. Moy JN, Gleich GJ, Thomas LL. Noncytotoxic activation of neutrophils by eosinophil granule major basic protein. Effect on superoxide anion generation and lysosomal enzyme release. J Immunol 1990; 145:2626–32.

61. Oddera S, Silvestri M, Balbo A, et al. Airway eosinophilic inflammation, epithelial damage, and bronchial hyperresponsiveness in patients with mild-moderate, stable asthma. Allergy 1996; 51:100–7.

62. Griffiths-Johnson DA, Collins PD, Rossi AG, et al. The chemokine, eotaxin, activates guinea-pig eosinophils in vitro and causes their accumulation into the lung in vivo. Biochem Biophys Res Commun 1993; 197:1167–72.

63. Minshall EM, Cameron L, Lavigne F, et al. Eotaxin mRNA and protein expression in chronic sinusitis and allergen-induced nasal responses in seasonal allergic rhinitis. Am J Respir Cell Mol Biol 1997; 17:683–90.

64. Lukacs NW, Strieter RM, Kunkel SL. Leukocyte infiltration in allergic airway inflammation. Am J Respir Cell Mol Biol 1995; 13:1–6.

65. Bartels J, Maune S, Meyer JE, et al. Increased eotaxin-mRNA expression in non-atopic and atopic nasal polyps: comparison to RANTES and MCP-3 expression. Rhinology 1997; 35:171–4.

66. Lee CH, Lee KS, Rhee CS, et al. Distribution of rantes and interleukin-5 in allergic nasal mucosa and nasal polyps. Ann Otol Rhinol Laryngol 1999; 108:594–8.

67. Bachert C, Wagenmann M, Rudack C, et al. The role of cytokines in infectious sinusitis and nasal polyposis. Allergy 1998; 53:2–13.

68. Min YG, Lee KS. The role of cytokines in rhinosinusitis. J Korean Med Sci 2000; 15:255–9.

69. Christodoulopoulos P, Cameron L, Durham S, et al. Molecular pathology of allergic disease. II: Upper airway disease. J Allergy Clin Immunol 2000; 105:211–23.

70. Tonnel AB, Gosset P, Molet S, et al. Interactions between endothelial cells and effector cells in allergic inflammation. Ann N Y Acad Sci 1996; 796:9–20.

71. Hamilos DL, Thawley SE, Kramper MA, Kamil A, Hamid QA. Effect of intranasal fluticasone on cellular infiltration, endothelial adhesion molecule expression, and proinflammatory cytokine mRNA in nasal polyp disease. J Allergy Clin Immunol 1999; 103(1 Pt 1):79–87.

72. Woltmann G, McNulty CA, Dewson G, Symon FA, Wardlaw AJ. Interleukin-13 induces PSGL-1/P-selectin-dependent adhesion of eosinophils, but not neutrophils, to human umbilical vein endothelial cells under flow. Blood 2000; 95:3146–52.

73. Symon FA, Walsh GM, Watson SR, Wardlaw AJ. Eosinophil adhesion to nasal polyp endothelium is P-selectin-dependent. J Exp Med 1994; 180:371–6.

74. Simon HU. Dysregulated apoptosis in chronic eosinophilic diseases–new therapeutic strategies for allergies and bronchial asthma. Pneumologie 1996; 50:790–6.

75. Bachert C, Wagenmann M, Hauser U, et al. IL-5 synthesis is upregulated in human nasal polyp tissue. J Allergy Clin Immunol 1997; 99:837–42.

76. Terada N, Konno A, Natori T, et al. Interleukin-5 preferentially recruits eosinophils from vessels in nasal mucosa. Acta Otolaryngol Suppl 1993; 506:57–60.

77. Walsh GM, Wardlaw AJ, Hartnell A, et al. Interleukin-5 enhances the in vitro adhesion of human eosinophils, but not neutrophils, in a leucocyte integrin (CD11/18)-dependent manner. Int Arch Allergy Appl Immunol 1991; 94:174–8.

78. Stoop AE, van der Heijden HA, Biewenga J, et al. Eosinophils in nasal polyps and nasal mucosa: an immunohistochemical study. J Allergy Clin Immunol 1993; 91:616–22.

79. Appenroth E, Gunkel AR, Muller H, et al. Activated and non-activated eosinophils in patients with chronic rhinosinusitis. Acta Otolaryngol 1998; 118:240–2.

80. Terada N, Konno A, Togawa K. Biochemical properties of eosinophils and their preferential accumulation mechanism in nasal allergy. J Allergy Clin Immunol 1994; 94:629–42.
81. Ohno I, Lea RG, Flanders KC, et al. Eosinophils in chronically inflamed human upper airway tissues express transforming growth factor beta 1 gene (TGF beta 1). J Clin Invest 1992; 89:1662–8.
82. Danzig M, Cuss F. Inhibition of interleukin-5 with a monoclonal antibody attenuates allergic inflammation. Allergy 1997; 52:787–94.
83. Konno A, Terada N, Ito E, et al. The reaction of nasal mucosa to platelet-activating factor and leukotrienes in nasal allergy. ORL Toyko 1988; 7(Suppl.): 241–2.
84. Jankowski R. Eosinophils in the pathophysiology of nasal polyposis. Acta Otolaryngol 1996; 116:160–3.
85. Yoshimi R, Takamura H, Takasaki K, et al. Immunohistological study of eosinophilic infiltration of nasal polyps in aspirin-induced asthma. Nippon Jibiinkoka Gakkai Kaiho 1993; 96:1922–5.

6 Role of Mast Cells and Basophils in Chronic Rhinosinusitis

Ruby Pawankar, Kun Hee Lee, Manabu Nonaka, and Ryuta Takizawa
Department of Otolaryngology, Nippon Medical School, Tokyo, Japan

INTRODUCTION

Chronic rhinosinusitis (CRS) is a multifactorial chronic inflammatory disease of the upper airways occurring with or without nasal polyps (NP) that is characterized histologically by the infiltration of inflammatory cells, eosinophils, neutrophils, mast cells, and T cells. Mast cells and basophils are inflammatory cells that are known to play a key role not only in IgE-mediated diseases but also in non-IgE-mediated eosinophilic respiratory inflammatory diseases. Mast cells and basophils are increased in nasal and sinus mucosa in chronic rhinosinusitis with and without nasal polyps (CRS with NP and CRS without NP). Basophils are mostly distributed in the surface layer, whereas mast cells are localized in the epithelium as well as the stroma of NP. Furthermore, the majority of degranulated mast cells are localized to the deep stroma of NP. Mast cells in CRS are an important source of a variety of multifunctional cytokines, and mast cells interact with other effector cells and structural cells to induce and upregulate (i.e., amplify) inflammation in CRS. While the properties of mast cells in CRS with NP have been characterized, less is known of the characteristics and role of basophils in CRS. The present review will therefore focus primarily on the studies of mast cells in CRS with NP.

Chronic rhinosinusitis with and without nasal polyps (CRS with and without NP) is a multifactorial chronic inflammatory disease often associated with asthma and other respiratory diseases such as cystic fibrosis, primary ciliary dyskinesia, and aspirin sensitivity. In the general population the overall prevalence of CRS with NP ranges from 1% to 4% (1). It is more common in adults than in children under 10 years except when associated with cystic fibrosis. The incidence of NP is higher in non-atopic asthmatics and rhinitics than in atopic rhinitics and asthmatics and is particularly high (60%) in individuals with aspirin sensitivity. However, a higher incidence of recurrence of NP has been observed in patients who are either atopic or aspirin sensitive.

While a variety of inflammatory cells such as eosinophils, mast cells (MCs), T cells, neutrophils, and structural cells such as epithelial cells and fibroblasts contribute to the inflammatory process in CRS, the present review will focus on the roles of MCs in CRS with NP.

CELLULAR COMPOSITION AND CYTOKINE PROFILE OF NASAL POLYPS

In the majority of NP eosinophils comprise more than 60% of the cell population. The exceptions are cystic fibrosis polyps and a subset of NP termed the *chronic inflammatory type* that contains predominantly neutrophils and lymphocytes. There is also an increase in activated T cells (CD45RO$^+$) with CD8$^+$ T cells predominating over CD4$^+$

T cells (2). MCs and plasma cells are also increased in comparison with normal nasal mucosa (3–6). Varga et al. also reported an increase in the number of activated T cells, MCs, and eosinophils in aspirin-sensitive NP (7).

Besides increased inflammatory cell infiltration a variety of pro-inflammatory cytokines and chemokines have also been found to be increased in NP. These contribute to the chronic eosinophilic inflammation by regulating the migration, survival, and activation of eosinophils. Among the cytokines, tumor necrosis factor-α (TNF-α and Interleukin-4 (IL-4)/IL-13 upregulate vascular cell adhesion molecule-1 (VCAM-1) expression and facilitate eosinophil migration into the tissue, and granulocyte macropage-colony stimulating factor (GM-CSF) and IL-5 prolong eosinophil survival (by reducing apoptosis) and promote eosinophil activation (8,9). Similarly, the potent eosinophil chemoattractant chemokines regulated upon activation, normal T-cell expressed and secreted (RANTES) and eotaxin are increased in NP, particularly in the epithelium (10,11). In addition to promoting eosinophil infiltration into NP tissue, eotaxin can also act locally within the polyp by contributing to tissue damage (12).

Interleukin-8, which is a known neutrophil chemoattractant, is also increased in NP compared to normal nasal mucosa. Furthermore, pro-inflammatory cytokines such as IL-1β and TNF-α are produced, and these contribute to the upregulation of adhesion molecules within the polyp, particularly intercellular ashesion molecule (ICAM-1) and VCAM-1, that promote the migration of T cells and leukocytes into the polyp.

Transforming growth factor-β (TGF-β) is another cytokine important to NP pathogenesis. TGF-β induces fibroblast proliferation, and the increased stromal fibrosis seen in NP may be due to the increased expression of TGF-β (13,14). Recent studies have shown that TGF-β upregulates the function of fibroblasts by enhancing the IL-4 and LPS (bacterial product)-induced production of eotaxin from these cells (15). As eosinophils are also an important source of TGF-β it can be hypothesized that eosinophils can enhance their own migration into the polyp tissue by regulating the function of fibroblasts. Vascular endothelial growth factor (VEGF), which is important for inducing angiogenesis and edema, is also increased in NP, and its expression is further upregulated by TGF-α (16).

A variety of cells, including epithelial cells, fibroblasts, T cells, and MCs, are indeed potent sources of cytokines and chemokines, including IL-1, TNF-α, IL-8, GM-CSF, IL-5, RANTES, eotaxin, and thymus- and activation-regulated chemokine (TARC). As such, these cells can orchestrate eosinophil/neutrophil and Th2 cell migration into the polyp tissue (17,18). In addition cell–cell interaction can further upregulate the production of these cytokines/chemokines. For instance, histamine and tryptase from MCs can upregulate RANTES production in epithelial cells and IL-4/IL-13 from MCs and T cells in synergy with TNF-α can upregulate TARC production from epithelial cells/fibroblasts (19). Finally, eosinophils themselves are an important source of a variety of these cytokines/chemokines (IL-5, GM-CSF, TNF-α and TGF-β) and are thus capable of increasing their own survival, activation, and migration in an autocrine manner. The result of these multiple pathways of cytokine and chemokine secretion is a complex set of interactions that is difficult to understand with respect to its capacity to regulate NP inflammation. Eosinophils also elaborate a variety of toxic proteins such as major basic protein (MBP) and eosinophil cationic protein (ECP) that can induce epithelial damage.

Besides cytokines and chemokines, other mediators such as histamine are also markedly increased in NP, exceeding levels of 4000 ng/mL. Increased levels of tryptase, histamine, and ECP have been reported in polyp tissue and the nasal lavages from patients with NP as compared with those without NP (20). In addition, increased levels of immunoglobulins IgA, IgE, IgG, and IgM in polyp fluid and tissue have been reported. In aspirin-intolerant asthmatics, an increased release of cysteinyl leukotrienes and reduced release of prostaglandin E$_2$ (PGE$_2$) from NP tissue and peripheral blood cells has also been reported and contributes to the clinical expression of disease in both the lungs and the sinuses (21).

Matrix metalloproteinases (MMP) play an important role in tissue degradation and may therefore be involved in the pathogenesis of NP. In fact, a significant amount of constitutive MMP-1 mRNA has been reported in NP fibroblasts and this expression was found to be upregulated by cytokines (22). Moreover, the cells expressing MMP-1 and tissue inhibitor of metalloproteinase protein-1 (TIMP-1) mRNAs were detected around areas with loose stroma, suggestive of rapid extracellular matrix (ECM) degradation. Our studies also showed an increased expression of MMP-9 in NP and this may again contribute to the ECM degradation (R. Pawankar et al., unpublished observations).

MAST CELL PHENOTYPES

Human MCs originate from CD34$^+$ hematopoeitic progenitors and undergo maturation in tissue microenvironments under the influence of specific factors such as stem cell factor (SCF). Phenotypically distinct subsets of MCs have been described in rodents based on their staining characteristics, T cell-dependency, and functions, namely connective tissue mast cells (CTMCs), and mucosal mast cells (MMCs) (23–27). Similarly, in humans two types of MCs have been recognized based on their content of neutral proteases, namely TC-type mast cells (MCTCs) which contain tryptase together with chymase, cathepsin-G-like protease, MCs carboxypeptidase A3, and T-type mast cells (MCTs) which contain tryptase, but lack the other neutral proteases present in MCTCs (28).

In humans and many other mammalian species, the numbers of MCs in normal tissues exhibit considerable variation according to the anatomic site. Moreover, the numbers of MCs vary in association with the underlying inflammatory or immunologic condition (29–32). In atopic diseases such as allergic rhinitis and asthma, MCs are known to accumulate within the epithelial compartment of the target organ (33,34). The number of MCs in NP is markedly greater than that in the nasal mucosa of patients with allergic rhinitis (3).

CHARACTERISTICS AND ROLES OF MAST CELLS IN NASAL POLYPS
Allergen/IgE-Mediated Mechanisms of Mast Cell Activation

Mast cells are known to play a key role in IgE-mediated diseases but are also involved in non-IgE-mediated inflammatory diseases. MCs can be detected in the epithelium as well as in the stroma of NP as also seen in the nasal mucosa of allergic rhinitics. In contrast to what is seen in allergic nasal mucosa, in NP the majority of degranulated MCs in NP are localized to the deep stroma suggesting that MCs are not likely to be activated by inhalant allergens. Moreover, while MCs in allergic rhinitis selectively express Th2-type cytokines as opposed to those in infective rhinitis (34), MCs in NP from both atopic and non-atopic patients express Th2-type cytokines IL-5 and IL-13 as well as IL-6 (4). MCs mediators, such as histamine and tryptase, and Th2 cytokines (IL-4 and IL-13) are capable of upregulating the release of RANTES/GM-CSF/SCF/TARC from NP epithelial cells/fibroblasts indicating a vicious cycle that keeps the eosinophilic inflammation ongoing (19). In fact, increased levels of tryptase and ECP were detected in recurrent NP when compared with fresh untreated NP (R. Pawankar et al., unpublished data). Furthermore, a good correlation has been detected between the levels of ECP and tryptase. These findings are further supported by the observations of Di Lorenzo et al. who show that the levels of tryptase and ECP in nasal lavages of patients with NP correlated with symptom scores (20). Furthermore, histamine from MCs can also upregulate the production of fibronectin and chymase, and MCs tryptase can upregulate the production of MMP-9 (R. Pawankar et al., unpublished observations).

In atopic patients, NP mast cells exhibit increased expression of FcεRI, and this is associated with an increased mediator release. IgE is known to upregulate FcεRI in MCs and basophils (4). Thus MCs may play a role in the increased incidence of recurrence of NP in atopic patients via the MCs–IgE–FcεRI receptor cascade.

Certain bacterial and viral products activate FcεRI through novel mechanisms. Bacterial superantigens (protein A from *Staphylococcus aureus* and protein L from *Peptostreptococcus magnus*) and the endogenous virally-induced superallergen, protein Fv, activate Fcε receptor I (FcεRI+) cells by interacting with IgE to release proinflammatory mediators and cytokines in vitro and, in some settings, in vivo (35–37). Whether these mechanisms contribute to MCs mediator release in NP is unknown, they do however, offer an attractive explanation for MCs degranulation in non-allergic patients. Alternatively, Bachert et al. described the presence of specific IgE to staphylococcal enterotoxins A and B in NP and found that the levels of these IgE correlated with the eosinophilic infiltration (38). They demonstrated multiclonal IgE, including specific IgE to staphylococcal enterotoxin A (SEA) and staphylococcal enterotoxin B (SEB), in 50% of bilateral eosinophilic NPs. Increased numbers of IgE-positive MCs have been reported in the sinus mucosa of patients with CRS irrespective of their atopic status (39). These studies provide another potential explanation for MCs participation in nonallergic NP, namely local production of IgE in the absence of systemic IgE production.

Toll-like receptors (TLRs) are a family of pattern recognition receptors that are crucial for cellular responses to a variety of microbial agents (see Chapter 4). Certain TLRs have been identified on mouse bone marrow-derived MCs (TLR2, TLR4, and TLR6) and on human umbilical cord blood-derived MCs (TLR1, TLR2, and TLR6) (40). Malaviya et al. showed that MCs have a pivotal role in innate host immune responses to gram-negative bacteria through the release of TNF-α (41). In another study, LPS and peptidoglycan induced significant release of not only TNF-α, but also IL-5, IL-10, and IL-13 by human MCs and this was mediated through interactions with TLR4 or TLR2, respectively (42). In addition, activation of MCs via TLR induced an increased release of leukotrienes suggesting such a possible mechanism for the overproduction of leukotrienes in patients with NP and aspirin sensitivity. We recently demonstrated that NP mast cells express TLR2 and TLR4 (unpublished observations). Thus, activation of MCs via the TLR may be another mechanism by which MCs contribute to the immune and inflammatory events in CRS with NP independent of conventional allergy.

Potential Role for Mast Cells in Nasal Polyp Growth and Remodeling

It is likely that MCs contribute to NP growth and the remodeling process (Fig. 1). MCs are an important source of TGF-β in NP. TGF-β promotes collagen synthesis and expression of VEGF by NP fibroblasts. VEGF is important for angiogenesis

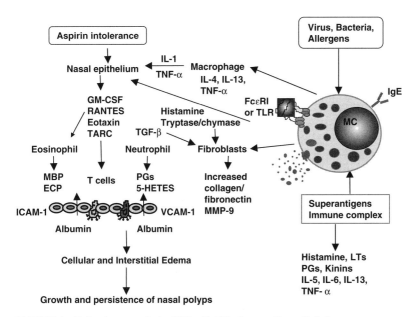

FIGURE 1   Role of mast cells in CRS with NP. *Source*: From Ref. 4.

and edema. TGF-β also promotes eosinophilic inflammation by enhancing the IL-4 and LPS-induced production of eotaxin (43,44).

There is evidence for remodeling in NP with increase in basement membrane thickening and tissue degradation. MMPs are known to play a role in cell migration, edema and ECM degradation. Our recent studies have shown an increase in MMP-9 in NP with relatively low levels of TIMP-1 and 2 (45). Moreover, the levels of MMP-9 were in good correlation with the levels of ECP and tryptase (45). Furthermore, MCs themselves expressed MMP-9, and MCs tryptase and chymase could upregulate the production of MMP-9 from NP epithelial cells suggesting an important role for MCs in ECM degradation in NP. In support of these findings, recent studies indicate that MCs chymase plays a critical role in processing of pro-MMP-9 and pro-MMP-2 to their active forms (46).

ASSOCIATION WITH ASTHMA AND ASPIRIN SENSITIVITY

The association of nasal polyposis with asthma is well recognized with a prevalence ranging from 7% to 20% (1). The association of nasal polyposis, bronchial asthma, and aspirin sensitivity has also been well recognized. Usually, such a triad starts off with rhinitis associated with profuse rhinorrhea, followed by severe nasal congestion, development of nasal polyposis, bronchial asthma, and finally aspirin sensitivity.

Macroscopically NP in aspirin-sensitive patients do not differ from those of NP in aspirin tolerant patients. They generally arise as bilateral and multiple outgrowths of the nasal mucosa from the ethmoid sinus, the middle turbinate, or the maxillary sinus. The precise etiology of aspirin–sensitive NP is unclear but there is evidence that impairment of prostanoid metabolism might be involved. Prostanoids are synthesized by two cyclooxygenase (Cox) enzymes, one constitutive (Cox-1) and another inducible (Cox-2). Cox-1 mRNA was found to be spontaneously upregulated in cultured nasal mucosa but not in NP. A spontaneous but delayed upregulation of Cox-2 mRNA was also found in NP (24 hours) compared with that seen in nasal mucosa (6 hours). After cytokine stimulation (Interferon-γ, IL-1β, and TNF-α), the induction of Cox-2 mRNA and protein was also faster in explants of normal nasal mucosa (1 hour) than in NP (4 hours). These data demonstrate abnormal regulation of Cox-1 and Cox-2 in NP from aspirin-intolerant patients, reinforcing the concept that impaired prostanoid metabolism might be important in the pathogenesis of NP (47). Consistent with these results, Kowalski et al. have demonstrated that epithelial cells from acetyl salicylic acid (ASA)-sensitive NP have a significant abnormality in basal and ASA-induced generation of eicosanoids (48). Although the precise mechanism of MCs activation in NP from ASA patients is not well defined, increased numbers of MCs and eosinophils in NP are well documented (49). These cells may be responsible for the excessive generation of cysteinyl leukotrienes seen in ASA-sensitive NP, and this coupled with impaired generation of prostanoids may contribute to the persistent inflammation in this condition. Consistent with this is the observation that aspirin challenge provokes an acute rise in tryptase levels in serum coincident with aspirin-induced bronchospasm (50).

ASSESSING THE INDIVIDUAL CONTRIBUTION OF MAST CELLS AND BASOPHILS TO NP PATHOGENESIS

Studies in MCs-deficient mice and in certain knockout strains, such as MCs chymase-deficient mouse have allowed for a better assessment of the individual contribution of MCs to disease pathogenesis in experimental animals (46). Given the limitations of current pharmacologic agents, it is not possible to selectively isolate the contribution of MCs or basophils in human diseases. Such studies may eventually be possible using specific inhibitors, such as those of human stem cell factor, a key growth and differentiation factor for human MCs.

SUMMARY

Mast cells and basophils contribute to induction and/or maintenance of eosinophilic inflammation by a variety of mechanisms, including IgE-dependent and IgE-independent processes. The latter include a variety of stimuli that have only recently been elucidated, including mechanisms triggered by bacteria, virus, fungi, complement, or autoantibodies. MCs, and basophils contribute to inflammation both directly through the release of inflammatory mediators, cytokines and growth factors and indirectly through the activation of structural cells. Accumulating evidence places MCs (and most probably basophils) in a position of importance in the pathogenesis of CRS, particularly in the pathogenesis and progression of NP (Fig. 1). Mechanisms other than conventional IgE-dependent activation of MCs are intriguing as potential mechanisms of eosinophilic inflammation in non-allergic CRS/NP. Although it is not possible using current pharmacologic approaches to completely isolate the effects of MCs or basophils in CRS and NP pathogenesis, it seems most likely that such approaches will eventually be available. It might be expected that one or both of these cells will be shown to play important roles, particularly considering their potential for activation by IgE and non-IgE mechanisms, their production of a broad array of inflammatory mediators, cytokines and growth factors, and their unique assortment of proteases.

REFERENCES

1. Settipane GA, Chafee FH. Nasal polyps. Am J Rhinol 1987; 1:119–26.
2. Sanchez-Segura A, Brieva JA, Rodriguez C. T lymphocytes that infiltrate nasal polyps have a specialized phenotype and produce a mixed TH1/TH2 pattern of cytokines. J Allergy Clin Immunol 1998; 102(6 Pt 1):953–60.
3. Seki H, Otsuka H, Pawankar R. Studies on the function of mast cells infiltrating nasal polyps. J Otolaryngol 1992; 95:1012–21.
4. Pawankar R. Nasal polyposis: an update. Curr Opin Allergy Clin Immunol 2003; 3:1–6.
5. Passali D, Bellussi L, Hassan HA, et al. Consensus Conference on Nasal Polyposis. Acta Otorhinolaryngol Ital 2004; 24(2 Suppl. 77):3–61.
6. Meltzer EO, Hamilos DL, Hadley JA, et al. Rhinosinusitis: establishing definitions for clinical research and patient care. J Allergy Clin Immunol 2004; 114(6 Suppl.):155–212.
7. Varga EM, Jacobson MR, Masayuma K, et al. Inflammatory cell populations and cytokine mRNA expression in the nasal mucosa in aspirin-sensitive rhinitis. Intense inflammation of the nasal mucosa characterized by T-lymphocytes, eosinophils and mast cells with predominance of macrophages and IL-5 mRNA was observed in aspirin-sensitive rhinitis. Eur Respir J 1999; 14:610–15.
8. Bachert C, Wagenmann M, Hauser U, Rudack C. IL-5 synthesis is upregulated in human nasal polyp tissue J Allergy Clin Immunol 1997; 99:837–42.
9. Ohno I, Lea R, Finotto S, Dolovich J. Granulocyte/macropage colony stimulating factor (GM-CSF) gene expression by eosinophils in nasal polyps. Am J Resp Cell Mol Biol 1991; 4:11–17.
10. Hamilos DL, Leung DY, Huston DP, Kamil A, Wood R, Hamid Q. GM-CSF, IL-5 and RANTES immunoreactivity and mRNA expression in chronic hyperplastic sinusitis with nasal polyposis (NP). Clin Exp Allergy 1998; 28:1145–52.
11. Nonaka M, Pawankar R, Saji F, Yagi T. Eotaxin expression in nasal polyp fibroblasts. Acta Otolaryngol 1999; 119:314–8.
12. Honda K, Chihara J. Eosinophil activation by eotaxin–eotaxin primes the production of reactive oxygen species from eosinophils. Allergy 1999; 54:1262–9.
13. Elovic C, Wong D, Weller P. Expression of transforming growth factors and β-1 mRNA and product by eosinophils in nasal polyps. J Allergy Clin Immunol 1994; 93:864–9.
14. Chang CH, Chai CY, Ho KY, et al. Expression of transforming growth factor-beta 1 and alpha-smooth muscle actin of myofibroblast in the pathogenesis of nasal polyps. J Med Sci 2001; 17:133–8.
15. Nonaka M, Pawankar R, Fukumoto A, Yagi T. Synergistic induction of eotaxin in fibroblasts by IL-4 and LPS: modulation by TGF-β. J Allergy Clin Immunol 2002; 109: S38 (abstract).
16. Coste A, Brugel L, Maitre B, et al. Inflammatory cells as well as epithelial cells in nasal polyps express vascular endothelial growth factor. Eur Respir J 2000; 5:367–72.
17. Xing Z, Jordana M, Braciak T, Ohtoshi T, Gauldie J. Lipopolysaccharide induces expression of granulocyte/macrophage colony-stimulating factor, interleukin-8, and interleukin-6 in human nasal, but not lung, fibroblasts: evidence for heterogeneity within the respiratory tract. Am J Respir Cell Mol Biol 1993; 9:255–63.
18. Nonaka M, Pawankar R, Saji F, Yagi T. Distinct expression of RANTES and GM-CSF by lipopolysaccharide in human nasal fibroblasts but not in other airway fibroblasts. Int Arch Allergy Immunol 1999; 119:314–21.
19. Pawankar R. Mast cells in rhinitis. In: Watanabe T, Timmerman H, Yanai K, eds. Histamine Research in the New Millennium. Amsterdam: Elsevier Science, 2001: 369–74.
20. Di Lorenzo G, Drago A, Esposito Pellitteri M, et al. Measurement of inflammatory mediators of mast cells and eosinophils in native nasal lavage fluid in nasal polyposis. Int Arch Allergy Immunol 2001; 125:164–75.
21. Schmid M, Gode U, Schafer D, Wigand ME. Arachidonic acid metabolism in nasal tissue and peripheral blood cells in aspirin intolerant asthmatics. Acta Otolaryngol. 1999; 119:277–80.
22. Liu CM, Hong CY, Shun CT, et al. Matrix metalloproteinase-1 and tissue inhibitor of metalloproteinase-1 gene expressions and their differential regulation by

proinflammatory cytokines and prostaglandin in nasal polyp fibroblasts. Ann Otol Rhinol Laryngol 2001; 110:1129–36.

23. Enerbäck L. Mast cells in rat gastrointestinal mucosa: dye-binding and metachromatic properties. Acta Pathol Microbiol Scand 1966; 66:303.

24. Mayerhofer G. Fixation and staining of granules in mucosal mast cells and intraepithelial lymphocytes in the rat jejunum, with special reference to the relationship between the acid glycosaminoglycans in the two cell types. Histochem J 1980; 12:513.

25. Miller HRP, Walshaw R. Immune reactions in mucus membranes. Am J Pathol 1978; 69:195.

26. Befus AD, Pearce FL, Gauldie J, Horsewood P, Bienenstock J: Mucosal mast cells. I. Isolation and functional characteristics of rat intestinal mast cells. J Immunol 1982; 128:2475.

27. Pearce FL, Befus AD, Gauldie J, Bienenstock J. Mucosal mast cells. II. Effects of antiallergic compounds on histamine secretion by isolated intestinal mast cells. J Immunol 1982; 128:2481.

28. Irani AMA, Schecter NM, Craig SS, DeBlois G, Schwartz LB. Two types of human mast cells that have distinct neutral protease compositions. Proc Natl Acad Sci USA 1986; 83:4464–9.

29. Galli SJ. New insights into the riddle of the mast cells. Lab Invest 1990; 62:5–33.

30. Kitamura Y. Heterogeneity of mast cells and phenotypic changes between subpopulations. Annu Rev Immunol 1989; 7:59–76.

31. Church K, Benyon RC, Rees PH, et al. Functional heterogeneity of human mast cells. In: Galli SJ, Austen KF, eds. Mast Cell and Basophil Differentiation and Function in Health and Disease. New York, NY: Raven Press, 1989:161–172.

32. Bienenstock, J, Befus AD, Denburg JA. Mast cell heterogeneity. In: Befus AD, Bienenstock J, Denburg JA, eds. Mast Cell Differentiation and Heterogeneity. New York, NY: Raven Press; 1986:391–403.

33. Enerback L, Pipkorn U, Olofsson A. Intraepithelial migration of mucosal mast cells in hay fever. Int Arch Allergy Appl Immunol 1986; 80:44.

34. Pawankar R, Ra C. Heterogeneity of mast cells and T cells in the nasal mucosa. J Allergy Clin Immunol, 1996; 98:249.

35. Genovese A, Bouvet JP, Florio G, Lamparter-Schummert B, Bjorck L, Marone G. Bacterial immunoglobulin superantigen proteins A and L activate human heart mast cells by interacting with Immunoglobulin E. Infect Immun 2000; 68:5517–24.

36. Genovese A, Borgia G, Bjorck L, et al. Immunoglobulin superantigen protein L induces IL-4 and IL-13 secretion from human Fc epsilon RI+ cells through interaction with the kappa light chains of IgE. J Immunol 2003; 170:1854–61.

37. Patella V, Giuliano A, Bouvet JP, Marone G. Endogenous superallergen protein Fv induces IL-4 secretion from human Fc epsilon RI+ cells through interaction with the VH3 region of IgE. J Immunol 1998; 161:5647–55.

38. Bachert C, Gevaert P, Holtappels G, Johansson SG, van Cauwenberge P. Total and specific IgE in nasal polyps is related to local eosinophilic inflammation. J Allergy Clin Immunol 2001; 107:607–14.

39. Loesel LS. Immunopathologic study of chronic sinusitis: a proposal for atopic and non-atopic IgE-activated mast cell allergic inflammation. Ann Otol Rhinol Laryngol 2001; 110(5Pt 1):447–52.

40. Marshall JS, McCurdy JD, Olynych T. Toll-like receptor-mediated activation of mast cells: implications for allergic disease? Int Arch Allergy Immunol 2003; 132:87–97.

41. Malaviya R, Georges A. Regulation of mast cell-mediated innate immunity during early response to bacterial infection. Clin Rev Allergy Immunol 2002; 22:189–204.

42. Varadaradjalou S, Feger F, Thieblemont N, et al. Toll-like receptor 2 (TLR2) and TLR4 differentially activate human mast cells. Eur J Immunol 2003; 33:899–906.

43. Nonaka M, Pawankar R, Fukumoto A, Yagi T. Synergistic induction of eotaxin in fibroblasts by IL-4 and LPS: modulation by TGF-β. J Allergy Clin Immunol 2002; 109:S38.

44. Nonaka M, Pawankar R, Fukumoto A, Ogihara N, Sakanushi A, Yagi T. Induction of eotaxin production by interleukin-4, interleukin-13 and lipopolysaccharide by nasal fibroblasts. Clin Exp Allergy 2004; 34:804–11.

45. Pawankar R, Watanabe S, Nonaka M, Ozu C, Aida M, Yagi T. Differential expression of matrix metalloproteinase 2 and 9 in the allergic nasal mucosa and nasal polyps. J Allergy Clin Immunol 2004; 113:S332.
46. Tchougounova E, Lundequist A, Fajardo I, Winberg JO, Abrink M, Pejler G. A key role for mast cell chymase in the activation of pro-matrix metalloprotease-9 and pro-matrix metalloprotease-2. J Biol Chem 2005; 280:9291–6.
47. Mullol J, Fernandez-Morata JC, Roca-Ferrer J, et al. Cyclooxygenase 1 and cyclooxygenase 2 expression is abnormally regulated in human nasal polyps. J Allergy Clin Immunol 2002; 109:824–10.
48. Kowalski ML, Pawliczak R, Wozniak J, et al. Differential metabolism of arachidonic acid in nasal polyp epithelial cells cultured from aspirin-sensitive and aspirin-tolerant patients. Am J Respir Crit Care Med 2000; 161(2 Pt 1):391–8.
49. Kowalski ML, Grzegorczyk J, Pawliczak R, Kornatowski T, Wagrowska-Danilewicz M, Danilewicz M. Decreased apoptosis and distinct profile of infiltrating cells in the nasal polyps of patients with aspirin hypersensitivity. Allergy 2002; 57:493–500.
50. Sladek K, Szczeklik A. Cysteinyl leukotrienes overproduction and mast cell activation in aspirin-provoked bronchospasm in asthma. Eur Respir J 1993; 6:391–9.

7

Mucociliary Transport in Chronic Rhinosinusitis

Fuad M. Baroody
Section of Otolaryngology–Head and Neck Surgery,
Departments of Surgery and Pediatrics, Pritzker School of Medicine,
University of Chicago, Chicago, Illinois, U.S.A.

INTRODUCTION

Mucociliary transport is critical in clearing the nasal cavity and paranasal sinuses of secretions and foreign particles. Mucociliary transport can be affected in many disease states and conditions that are associated with chronic rhinosinusitis (CRS). Normal nasal and paranasal sinus mucociliary clearance will be discussed in this chapter as well as disease states that might interfere with normal transport in the context of CRS.

PARANASAL SINUS ANATOMY

The paranasal sinuses are four pairs of cavities that are named after the skull bones in which they are located: frontal, ethmoid (anterior and posterior), maxillary, and sphenoid (Fig. 1). All sinuses contain air and are lined by a thin layer of respiratory mucosa composed of ciliated, pseudostratified, columnar epithelial cells with goblet mucous cells interspersed among the columnar cells.

Frontal Sinuses

At birth, the frontal sinuses are indistinguishable from the anterior ethmoid cells and they grow slowly after birth so that they are barely seen anatomically at one year of age. After the fourth year, the frontal sinuses begin to enlarge and can usually be demonstrated radiographically in children over six years of age. Their size continues to increase into the late teens. The frontal sinuses are usually pyramidal structures in the vertical part of the frontal bone. They open via the frontal recess into the anterior part of the middle meatus, or directly into the anterior part of the infundibulum. The natural ostium is located directly posterior to the anterior attachment of the middle turbinate to the lateral nasal wall. They are supplied by the supraorbital and supratrochlear arteries, and branches of the ophthalmic artery, which in turn is a branch of the internal carotid artery. Venous drainage is via the superior ophthalmic vein into the cavernous sinus. The sensory innervation of the mucosa is supplied via the supraorbital and supratrochlear branches of the frontal nerve, derived from the ophthalmic division of the trigeminal nerve.

Ethmoid Sinuses

At birth, the ethmoid and maxillary sinuses are the only sinuses that are large enough to be clinically significant as a cause of rhinosinusitis. By the age of 12, the ethmoid air cells have almost reached their adult size and form a pyramid with the base located posteriorly. The lateral wall of the sinus is the lamina papyracea, which also serves as the paper thin medial wall of the orbit.

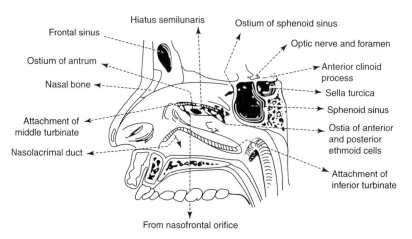

Frontal sinus

Hiatus semilunaris

Ostium of sphenoid sinus

Optic nerve and foramen

Ostium of antrum

Anterior clinoid process

Nasal bone

Sella turcica

Sphenoid sinus

Attachment of middle turbinate

Ostia of anterior and posterior ethmoid cells

Nasolacrimal duct

Attachment of inferior turbinate

From nasofrontal orifice

FIGURE 1 A detailed view of the lateral wall of the nose. Parts of the inferior and middle turbinates have been removed. Visualized are the various openings into the inferior, middle, and superior meati as well as drainage sites of the various paranasal sinuses *Source*: From Ref. 57.

The medial wall of the sinus functions as the lateral nasal wall. The superior boundary of the ethmoid sinus is formed by the horizontal plate of the ethmoid bone which separates the sinus from the anterior cranial fossa. This horizontal plate is composed of a thin, medial portion named the cribriform plate, and a thicker, more lateral portion named the fovea ethmoidalis, which forms the ethmoid roof. The posterior boundary of the ethmoid sinus is the anterior wall of the sphenoid sinus. The ethmoidal air cells are divided into an anterior group that drains into the ethmoidal infundibulum of the middle meatus and a posterior group that drains into the superior meatus which is located inferior to the superior turbinate. The ethmoidal infundibulum is a three-dimensional cleft running anterosuperiorly to posteroinferiorly, and the two-dimensional opening to this cleft is the hiatus semilunaris. The bulla ethmoidalis (an anterior group of ethmoidal air cells) borders the ethmoid infundibulum posteriorly and superiorly, the lateral wall of the nose resides laterally, and the uncinate process borders anteromedially. The uncinate process is a thin semilunar piece of bone, the superior edge of which is usually free but can insert into the lamina papyracea or the fovea ethmoidalis and the posteroinferior edge of which usually lies just lateral to the maxillary sinus ostium. The ethmoid sinuses receive their blood supply from both the internal and external carotid circulations. The branches of the external carotid circulation that supply the ethmoids are the nasal branches of the sphenopalatine artery, and the branches of the internal carotid circulation are the anterior and posterior ethmoidal arteries, derived from the ophthalmic artery. Venous drainage can also be directed via the nasal veins, branches of the maxillary vein or via the ophthalmic veins, tributaries of the cavernous sinus. The latter pathway is responsible for cavernous sinus thrombosis after ethmoid sinusitis. The sensory innervation of these sinuses is supplied by the ophthalmic and maxillary divisions of the trigeminal nerve.

Maxillary Sinuses

The size of the maxillary sinus is estimated to be 6–8 cm^3 at birth. The sinus then grows rapidly until three years of age and then more slowly until the seventh year. Another growth acceleration occurs until about age 12. By then, pneumatization has extended laterally as far as the lateral wall of the orbit and inferiorly so that the floor of the sinus is even with the floor of the nasal cavity. Much of the growth that occurs after the twelfth year is in the inferior direction, with pneumatization of the alveolar process after eruption of the secondary dentition. By adulthood, the floor of the maxillary sinus is usually 4–5 mm inferior to that of the nasal cavity. The maxillary sinus occupies the body of the maxilla and has a capacity of around 15 mL. Its anterior wall is the facial surface of the maxilla and the posterior wall corresponds to the infratemporal surface of the maxilla. Its roof is the inferior orbital floor and is about twice as wide as its floor, formed by the alveolar process of the maxilla. The medial wall of the sinus forms part of the lateral nasal wall and has the ostium of the sinus which is located within the infundibulum of the middle meatus, with accessory ostia occurring in 25–30% of individuals. Mucociliary clearance within the maxillary sinus moves secretions in the direction of the natural ostium. The major blood supply of the maxillary sinuses is via branches of the maxillary artery with a small contribution from the facial artery. Venous drainage occurs anteriorly via the anterior facial vein into the jugular vein or posteriorly via the tributaries of the maxillary vein which also eventually drains into the jugular system. Innervation of the mucosa of the maxillary sinuses is via several branches of the maxillary nerve, which primarily carry sensory fibers. Another contribution to the innervation via the maxillary nerve are postganglionic, parasympathetic secretomotor fibers originating in the facial nerve and carried to the sphenopalatine ganglion in the pterygopalatine fossa via the greater petrosal nerve and the nerve of the pterygoid canal.

Sphenoid Sinuses

At birth, the size of the sphenoid sinus is small and is little more than an evagination of the sphenoethmoid recess. By the age of seven, the sphenoid sinuses have extended posteriorly to the level of the sella turcica. By the late teens most of the sinuses have aerated to the dorsum sellae and some further enlargement may occur in adults. The sphenoid sinuses are frequently asymmetric because the intersinus septum is bowed or twisted. Depending on the extent of pneumatization, the optic nerve, internal carotid artery, nerve of the pterygoid canal, maxillary nerve, and sphenopalatine ganglion may all appear as impressions indenting the walls of the sphenoid sinuses. The sphenoid sinus drains into the sphenoethmoid recess above the superior turbinate and the ostium typically lies 10 mm above the floor of the sinus. The blood supply is via branches of the internal and external carotid arteries and the venous drainage follows that of the nasopharynx and the nasal cavity into the maxillary vein and pterygoid venous plexus. The first and second divisions of the trigeminal nerve supply the mucosa of the sphenoid sinus.

Function of the Paranasal Sinuses

Many theories exist related to the function of the paranasal sinuses. Some of these theories include imparting additional voice resonance, humidifying and warming inspired air, secreting mucus to keep the nose moist, and providing thermal insulation for the brain. While none of these theories have been supported by objective evidence, it is commonly believed that the paranasal sinuses form a collapsible framework to help protect the brain from frontal blunt trauma. While the function of the paranasal sinuses might not be completely understood, they are the frequent target of infections, both acute and chronic.

NASAL/SINUS EPITHELIUM

Nasal and sinus epithelium consists of three types of cells: basal, goblet, and columnar, which are either ciliated or nonciliated.

Basal Cells

Basal cells lie on the basement membrane and do not reach the airway lumen. They have an electron-dense cytoplasm and bundles of tonofilaments. Among their morphologic specializations are desmosomes, which mediate adhesion between adjacent cells, and hemidesmosomes, which help anchor the cells to the basement membrane (1). These cells have long been thought to be progenitors of the columnar and goblet cells of the airway epithelium but experiments in rat bronchial epithelium suggest that the primary progenitor cell of airway epithelium might be the nonciliated columnar cell population (2). Currently, basal cells are believed to help in the adhesion of columnar cells to the basement membrane. This is supported by the fact that columnar cells do not have hemidesmosomes and attach to the basement membrane only by cell-adhesion molecules, i.e., laminin.

Goblet Cells

The goblet cells arrange themselves perpendicular to the epithelial surface (3). The mucous granules give the mature cell its characteristic goblet shape, in which only a narrow part of the tapering basal cytoplasm touches the basement membrane. The nucleus is situated basally, with the organelles and secretory granules that contain mucin toward the lumen. The luminal surface, covered by microvilli, has a small opening, or stoma, through which the granules secrete their content. The genesis of goblet cells is controversial, some experimental studies supporting a cell of origin unrelated to epithelial cells, and others supporting either the cylindrical nonciliated columnar cell population or undifferentiated basal cells as the cells of origin (3). There are no goblet cells in the squamous, transitional, or olfactory epithelia of adults and they are irregularly distributed but present in all areas of pseudostratified columnar epithelium (3).

Columnar Cells

These cells are related to neighboring cells by tight junctions apically and, in the uppermost part, by interdigitations of the cell membrane. The cytoplasm contains numerous mitochondria in the apical part. All columnar cells, ciliated and nonciliated, are covered by 300 to 400 microvilli, uniformly distributed over the entire apical surface. These are not precursors of cilia but are short and slender fingerlike cytoplasmic expansions that increase the surface area of the epithelial cells, thus promoting exchange processes across the epithelium. The microvilli also prevent drying of the surface by retaining moisture essential for ciliary function (4). In humans, ciliated epithelium lines the majority of the airways from the nose to the

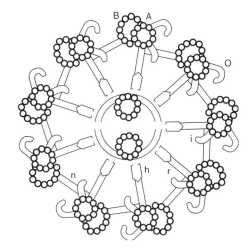

FIGURE 2 Normal ciliary ultrastructure. Cross section of a cilium is depicted with the nine peripheral and one central pair of microtubules. The outer pairs are composed of A and B subunits. The outer dynein arms (o), inner dynein arms (i), radial spokes (r), spoke heads (h), and nexin links (n) are labeled. *Source*: From Ref. 52.

respiratory bronchioles, as well as the paranasal sinuses, the eustachian tube, and parts of the middle ear.

In addition to microvilli, ciliated columnar epithelial cells have between 50 and 200 cilia. Cilia are cellular projections that show intrinsic motility resulting in propulsion of surface fluid. In humans, they are 5 μm long, have an average diameter of 0.2 μm, and consist of a shaft covered by cell membrane. The shaft, also called axoneme, consists primarily of microtubules made of the globular protein tubulin. They are arranged as nine peripheral doublets and two central singlets (nine plus two arrangement). The peripheral doublets are connected to each other by nexin links and by spokes to the central sheet that surrounds the two central singlets (Fig. 2). Half of the peripheral microtubules have two dynein arms (an outer and an inner). These proteins contain adenosine triphosphatase activity that provides the energy to the dynein arms bridging the space between two peripheral doublets and creating ciliary motion (4). The part of the cilium beneath the cell surface consists of a basal body, a basal foot, and a rootlet that is an extension of a microtubule from the basal body in the apical cytoplasm. The peripheral microtubules continue from the axoneme into the basal body; however, their arrangement changes, and the central microtubules and dynein arms are lost at the cell surface. The basal foot projects from the side of the basal body as a short cone, parallel to the cell surface, and points in the direction of the effective stroke of the cilium and of mucus transport.

NASAL MUCUS AND MUCOCILIARY TRANSPORT

A 10- to 15-μm deep layer of mucus covers the entire nasal cavity (5). It is slightly acidic, with a pH between 5.5 and 6.5. The mucous blanket consists of two layers: a thin, low viscosity, periciliary layer (sol phase) that envelops the shafts of the cilia, and a thick, more viscous, layer (gel phase) riding on the periciliary layer. The gel phase can also be envisioned as discontinuous plaques of mucus. The distal tips of the ciliary shafts contact these plaques when they are fully extended. Insoluble particles caught on the mucous plaques move with them as a consequence of ciliary beating. Soluble materials such as droplets, formaldehyde, and CO_2 dissolve in the periciliary layer. Thus nasal mucus effectively filters and removes nearly 100% of particles greater than 4 μm in diameter (6–8). An estimated 1–2 L of nasal mucus, composed of 2.5–3% glycoproteins, 1–2% salts, and 95% water, are produced per day. Mucin, one of the glycoproteins, gives mucus its unique attributes of protection and lubrication of mucosal surfaces.

The sources of nasal secretions are multiple and include anterior nasal glands, seromucous submucosal glands, epithelial secretory cells (of both mucous and serous types), tears, and transudation from blood vessels. Transudation increases in pathologic conditions as a result of the effects of inflammatory mediators that increase vascular permeability. A good example is the increased vascular permeability seen in response to allergen challenge of subjects with allergic rhinitis as measured by increasing levels of albumin in nasal lavages after provocation (9). In contrast to serum, immunoglobulins make up the bulk of the protein in mucus; other substances in nasal secretions include lactoferrin, lysozyme, antitrypsin, transferrin, lipids, histamine and other mediators, cytokines, antioxidants, ions (Cl, Na, Ca, K), cells, and bacteria. Mucus functions in mucociliary transport, and substances will not be cleared from the nose without it, despite adequate ciliary function. Furthermore, mucus provides immune and mechanical mucosal protection and its high water content plays a significant role in humidifying inspired air.

Mucociliary transport is unidirectional based on the unique characteristics of cilia. Cilia in mammals beat in a biphasic, or to-and-fro, manner. The beat consists of a rapid effective stroke during which the cilium straightens, bringing it in contact with the gel phase of the mucus, and a slow recovery phase during which the bent cilium returns in the periciliary or sol layer of the mucus, thus propelling it in one direction (Fig. 3).

Metachrony is the coordination of the beat of individual cilia which prevents collision between cilia in different phases of motion and results in the unidirectional flow of mucus. Ciliary beating produces a current in the superficial layer of the periciliary fluid in the direction of the effective stroke. The mucous plaques move as a result of motion of the periciliary fluid layer and the movement of the

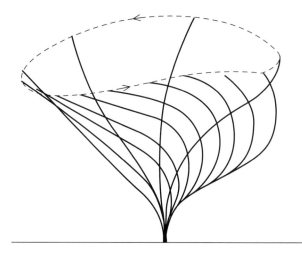

FIGURE 3 A schematic diagram of motion of a single cilium during the rapid forward beat and the slower recovery phase. *Source*: From Ref. 15.

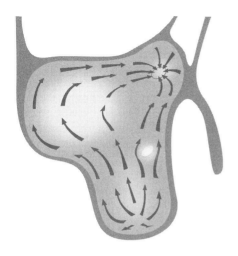

FIGURE 4 Normal clearance pathway of the maxillary sinus toward the natural ostium *Source*: From Ref. 58.

extended tips of the cilia into the plaques. Thus, the depth of the periciliary fluid is the key factor in mucociliary transport. If excessive, the extended ciliary tips fail to contact mucous plaques, and the current of the periciliary fluid provides the only means of movement.

In the nose, mucociliary transport moves mucus and its contents toward the nasopharynx, with the exception of the anterior portion of the inferior turbinates, where transport is anterior. This anterior current prevents many of the particles deposited in this area from progressing further into the nasal cavity. The particles transported posteriorly toward the nasopharynx are periodically swallowed. Mucociliary transport, however, is not the only mechanism by which particles and secretions are cleared from the nose. Sniffing and nose blowing help in moving airway secretions backward and forward, respectively. Sneezing results in a burst of air, accompanied by an increase in watery nasal secretions that are then cleared by nose blowing and sniffing.

In the paranasal sinuses, mucus production is less than that of the nasal mucosa. Mucociliary transport within the maxillary sinus of human cadavers, studied immediately after death by introducing India ink into the sinus and observing its movement, is star-shaped, radiating from the bottom of the sinus in various directions toward the normal ostium (Fig. 4) (10). This pattern persists even after creating an inferior antrostomy. In the frontal sinus, mucociliary transport sweeps in a large curve rising from the medial portion toward the roof and curving laterally and downward to the nasofrontal duct (11). No precise description is available as to the patterns of mucociliary transport within the ethmoid and sphenoid sinuses.

ASSESSMENT OF MUCOCILIARY ACTIVITY

Most assessments of ciliary activity are performed using one of two techniques: measurement of ciliary beat frequency (CBF) *in vivo* or in tissue explants, and measuring clearance by applying a tracer directly to the tissue and following clearance of the tracer and then reporting on the velocity of its movement as a direct reflection of mucociliary transport.

Ciliary Beat Frequency

Most modern measurements of CBF are made using a microscope with a small aperture that allows a light beam to be interrupted by ciliary beat. The interruptions are measured and the frequency of the ciliary beat is calculated (12). Most studies are performed in explants which have limitations including the fact that the specimen is separated from the host, and the specimens are immersed in a suitable buffer that has a different composition and viscosity than normal mucus. Most studies in humans have indicated a CBF of approximately 1000 beats/min (13) with no differences between healthy males and females (14).

Mucociliary Clearance/Transport (MCT)

Respiratory cilia beat about 1000 times per minute, which translates to surface materials being moved at a rate of 3–25 mm per minute. Both the beat rate and propelling speed vary. Several substances have been used to measure nasal mucociliary clearance, and the most utilized are sodium saccharin, dyes, or tagged particles. The dye and saccharin methods are similar, consisting of placing a strong dye or saccharin sodium on the nasal mucosa just behind the internal ostium and recording the time it takes to reach the pharyngeal cavity; this interval is termed nasal mucociliary transport time. With saccharin, the time is recorded when the subject reports a sweet taste, whereas, with a dye, when it appears in the pharyngeal cavity. Combining the two methods reduces the disadvantages of both—namely, variable taste thresholds in different subjects when using saccharin and repeated pharyngeal inspection when using the dye—and makes them more reliable. The use of tagged particles involves placement of an anion exchange resin particle about 0.5 mm in diameter tagged with a 99Tc ion on the anterior nasal mucosa behind the area of anterior mucociliary movement, and following its subsequent clearance with a gamma camera or multicollimated detector. This last method permits continuous monitoring of movement.

Studies of several hundred healthy adult subjects by the tagged particle or saccharin methods have consistently shown that 80% exhibit clearance rates of 3–25 mm/min (average = 6 mm/min), with slower rates in the remaining 20% (15). The latter subjects have been termed "slow clearers." The findings of a greater proportion of slow clearers in one group of subjects living in an extremely cold climate raise the possibility that the differences in clearance may be related to an effect of inspired air (15). In diseased subjects, slow clearance may be due to a variety of factors, including the immotility of cilia, transient or permanent injury to the mucociliary system by physical trauma, viral infection, dehydration, or excessively viscid secretions secondary to decreased ions and water in the mucus paired with increased amounts of DNA from dying cells, as in cystic fibrosis.

Effects of the Environment on MCT

Exposure to a variety of environmental stimuli might have an effect on mucociliary transport. Tobacco smoke exposure in animal models results in a negative impact on CBF (16). In a human study, Agius et al. obtained nasal brushings from inferior turbinates of tobacco-exposed subjects and controls and determined CBF using a computerized photometric technique (17). Nasal CBF in tobacco smoke-exposed patients (active or passive smokers) was significantly less than in non smoke-exposed controls. When mucociliary transit time was measured using the saccharin test in human subjects, smokers who had been smoking for more than

5 years at more than one pack per day had a significantly prolonged time (16.5 min) compared with normal controls (12 min) (18).

The effects of allergic rhinitis on mucociliary clearance have been evaluated, but a consensus has not been reached. Holmstrom et al. measured nasal beat frequency ex vivo before and 20 minutes after antigen provocation and found that the CBF was decreased (19). In in vitro studies, Schuil et al. showed no effect of histamine and leukotriene C4 on ciliary beat frequency (20). Guerico et al. showed no effect if antigen was sprayed or inhaled but found that direct instillation slowed mucociliary clearance (21). Ogino et al. (22) and Mahakit and Pumhirun (18), using the saccharin dye test in independently performed studies, showed no difference in clearance between patients with allergic rhinitis and healthy controls. In contrast, Mori et al., using the same saccharin test, showed that allergen challenge accelerated the clearance time (23). Most studies of viral infections show an adverse effect on mucociliary transport. In artificially induced colds, normal subjects were exposed to rhinovirus and mucociliary transport rate assessed using radioactively-labeled resin beads (24). Mucus transport was decreased at two days, and was maximally impaired at 72 hours with significantly slower mucociliary transport times noted from 9 to 11 days after infection. Another study evaluated the effects of natural acute viral upper respiratory infections on mucociliary transport time using dyed saccharin tests (25). Nasal airflow was decreased and mucociliary transport time prolonged during the cold compared to the post cold convalescent period.

MUCOCILIARY CLEARANCE IN CHRONIC SINUSITIS
Nasal Mucociliary Transport
There are several studies that describe nasal mucociliary transport in patients with chronic sinusitis and fewer studies that describe mucociliary activity within the sinuses themselves. Majima et al. measured nasal mucociliary clearance in both healthy subjects and patients with chronic sinusitis using the saccharin technique and reported a significantly slower transit time in patients with chronic sinusitis (26). Saline nebulization seemed to restore nasal mucociliary clearance in the patients with chronic sinusitis but had no effect on transport in the healthy controls. In a related study, the same group attempted to elucidate the contribution of ciliary abnormalities versus mucus properties in the observed slowed clearance. They collected nasal mucus from 38 patients with chronic sinusitis, placed it on a frog's palate in vitro preparation, and mucociliary transport was measured (27). They also measured nasal mucociliary clearance by means of the saccharin method and found two subgroups of patients, one with clearance within the normal range and one with slower than normal mucociliary clearance. Mucociliary transport rate on the frog's palate was not different between the two groups suggesting that factors other than rheologic properties of mucus control nasal mucociliary clearance in patients with chronic sinusitis.

Wilson et al. measured nasal mucociliary clearance by the saccharin method and CBF by a photometric technique in four groups of subjects: normal controls, patients with bronchiectasis without nasal symptoms, patients with chronic mucopurulent sinusitis, and patients with chronic mucopurulent sinusitis and bronchiectasis (13). Nasal mucociliary clearance was prolonged in both groups of patients with mucopurulent sinusitis, and cilia from these groups were found to beat more slowly in vitro. Passali et al. measured nasal mucociliary transport time using a combined charcoal powder, saccharin technique in patients with three different nasal pathologies: hypertrophy of the nasal turbinates, septal deviations, and chronic sinusitis (28). Patients with chronic sinusitis had symptoms lasting more than 3 months and the diagnosis was confirmed by computed tomography (CT) examinations after prolonged antibiotic therapy. They compared their values to previously reported reference values obtained from normal individuals and noted a significantly slower transport time for patients with chronic sinusitis but not the other two groups. They speculated that the inflammation associated with chronic sinusitis leads to increased viscoelasticity of the mucus and a slower clearance rate. Although this is a plausible explanation, the authors had no evidence that the structure of the cilia was preserved in the chronic sinusitis patients, and, thus, such an abnormality cannot be completely ruled out in patients with chronic sinusitis.

Cilia Within the Sinuses

In an attempt to evaluate the cilia within the sinus cavities in patients with chronic sinusitis, Nuutinen et al. evaluated CBF ex vivo in surgical specimens from 150 patients with chronic sinusitis (29). They also obtained similar measurements of ciliary activity in normal mucosa in 26 controls obtained from various surgical sites (sphenoid and maxillary sinuses, mastoids, and middle turbinates). In 23% of the patients, no ciliary activity was seen, whereas the CBF in the rest of the patients was not different from controls. Although the authors had no good explanation for the lack of ciliary activity in a proportion of the sinusitis patients, the remainder of their data suggests that primary ciliary immotility is not a significant contributor to the slowed clearance seen in subjects with chronic sinusitis. King examined the clearance of contrast medium infused into the maxillary sinus and noted a decline of mucociliary transport in chronic sinusitis (30).

Several investigators have assessed the morphology of ciliated epithelium in patients with chronic sinusitis. Fontolliet and Terrier obtained 34 sinus biopsies in 28 subjects investigated for chronic sinusitis (31). The specimens were further classified as being normoplastic versus hyperplastic and were evaluated by electron microscopy for ultrastructural abnormalities. The incidence of ultrastructural ciliary abnormalities was low at 2% of the specimens. By contrast, compound cilia were found in approximately two-thirds of the cases, and microtubular abnormalities occurred in almost 50%. These same abnormalities were also observed in control biopsies, were independent of the sinusitis type (normoplastic vs. hyperplastic), and did not correlate with mucociliary transport within the maxillary sinus which was comparable between the patients with sinusitis and controls. In contrast, Ohashi and Nakai studied maxillary sinus mucosa obtained at the time of surgery in 16 patients with chronic sinusitis using electron microscopy and found swelling of the ciliary membrane, formation of compound cilia, dropping of epithelial cells, and squamous metaplasia (32). Unlike the previous study, the abnormalities seemed to correlate with measures of ciliary function by CBF.

Al-Rawi et al. studied 32 patients (18 adults and 14 children) with chronic sinusitis who had failed maximal medical treatment and confirmed the diagnosis by CT scan (33). They performed biopsies of the middle turbinates and submitted the tissues to light and electron microscopic study. Ciliated cells were found in 72% of patients with 28% of patients having no cilia. Foci of normal ciliated epithelium were found in only 19% of patients, often in epithelial invaginations, which the authors speculate protected the cilia from exposure to inflammatory and bacteriologic influences associated with chronic sinusitis. In 87% of cases with ciliated cells, variable numbers of cilia (usually a small proportion) exhibited ultrastructural defects including compound cilia and microtubule and dynein arm defects. All patients showed variable loss of differentiated epithelial cells ranging from denuded epithelium to squamous metaplasia. The authors speculate that as normal ciliogenesis was found in 72% of the patients, the ciliary abnormalities detected were secondary to the chronic disease process seen in chronic sinusitis as opposed to being its cause.

In another approach to assess the importance of cilia in chronic sinusitis, Guo et al. obtained tissue biopsies from 28 patients with chronic sinusitis and quantified the ciliary area (percentage of mucosal surface occupied by cilia) by scanning electron microscopy (34). They also obtained CT scans and quantified the degree of opacity of the maxillary sinus. They found that the greater the opacity of the maxillary sinus, the more the ciliated area of the sinus decreases, suggesting a potential role for cilia in chronic sinusitis pathophysiology.

Thus, most of the studies reviewed suggest slower MCT in the nose and paranasal sinuses in patients with CRS as well as some ciliary morphologic abnormalities in these chronically ill patients. Most studies also suggest that ciliary abnormalities, when present, are likely to be secondarily rather than primarily, responsible for the disease.

Effects of Mediators on MCT

As many authors speculate that substances released from inflammatory cells in CRS might be responsible for the alteration of ciliary function, it is interesting to review the effect of some of these mediators on ciliary function. Georgitis et al. performed maxillary sinus lavages in subjects with chronic sinusitis as well as nasal lavages from allergic subjects out of season and from another group of allergic subjects after allergen challenge (35). They detected higher levels of histamine, leukotriene C_4, and prostaglandin D_2 in the lavages of the patients with sinusitis and the allergics after challenge compared to the asymptomatic allergics out of season. Ganbo et al. studied the effect of leukotriene C_4 and D_4 on ciliary activity of human paranasal sinus mucosa in vitro by obtaining ethmoid sinus mucosa from subjects who suffered from facial trauma. They incubated the mucosa with 10^{-8} M of LTC_4 or LTD_4 for a time period of 6 hours and measured ciliary activity using an inverted microscope (36). Both mediators resulted in progressive inhibition of ciliary activity from baseline and compared to control, with LTD_4 resulting in a significant effect by one hour of incubation and LTC_4 by four hours of incubation. The magnitude of the effect of LTD_4, the metabolite, was larger than that of its precursor, LTC_4. They were also able to show in the incubation medium a progressive increase in the concentration of LTD_4, and a decrease in that of LTC_4, supporting the metabolism of one to the other. In another study, the effect of histamine and PGE_1 on CBF was studied in explants from the guinea pig trachea, human adenoid tissue, and rabbit maxillary sinus mucosa (37). The different tissues had slightly different responses to the mediators and, of interest to this chapter, PGE_1 produced a strong dose-dependent increase in CBF while histamine had no significant effect in rabbit maxillary sinus explants. The same group studied the effect of histamine on mucociliary activity in the rabbit maxillary sinus in vivo by injecting histamine and various other antagonists and agonists in the maxillary artery and measuring mucociliary activity in the maxillary sinus using a photoelectric technique (38). They showed a dose-dependent stimulatory effect of histamine on mucociliary activity, which was inhibited by the H_1 receptor antagonist pyrilamine but was not affected by either atropine or pretreatment with the H_2 receptor antagonist cimetidine. The contribution of the H_2 receptor to this histamine effect was further ruled out by showing no effect of the specific agonist, dimaprit, on mucociliary activity. These in vivo studies support a stimulatory effect of histamine on mucociliary activity that is mediated by H_1 receptors, but not H_2 or cholinergic receptors.

Harlin et al. illustrated the deposition of eosinophil-derived major basic protein (MBP) in the sinus epithelium and basement membrane area in patients with CRS and proposed this as an important mechanism leading to epithelial damage and loss of mucociliary function (39). This study was corroborated by a more recent study showing the dramatic degranulation of eosinophils in mucus of patients with CRS (40). The highest levels of eosinophil-derived MBP were actually found in mucus rather than in the tissues, and this places the MBP in a critical location for causing epithelial and potentially ciliary damage.

EFFECT OF SINUS SURGERY ON MUCOCILIARY TRANSPORT
Animal Studies
Multiple experimental manipulations have been performed in animal models to address regeneration of ciliated epithelium and status of mucociliary transport after surgical interventions which include stripping of the mucosa and widening the natural sinus ostia. Most of these experiments were performed in rabbit maxillary sinuses. In rabbits, Min et al. stripped the maxillary sinus mucosa in one maxillary sinus and, in the same animals, either widened the maxillary antrostomy surgically or left it untouched (41). The contralateral sinus was not manipulated and used as control. They then examined the histologic characteristics of the regenerated mucosa as well as mucociliary transport of India ink particles 6, 8, 10, and 12 weeks after the original manipulation. Mucociliary transport times were significantly reduced in the manipulated groups compared to control. The reduction persisted at 12 weeks after the initial injury and did not differ in the groups where the sinus ostium was widened or left untouched. Histopathologic changes showed the mucosa to be regenerated with ciliated epithelia in 88% of both surgical groups with no differences across the time intervals. Submucosal fibrosis was found in 75% of the specimens from both surgical groups. In the regenerated mucosa, however, there was a decrease in ciliary density and abnormal ciliary characteristics such as edema, abnormal microtubules, and compound cilia as observed by electron microscopy. These are speculated to have resulted in reduced mucociliary transport time despite the absence of significant alterations of the histology by light microscopy.

Human Studies
Hafner et al. studied nasal mucociliary transport using the saccharin test and CBF of nasal specimens obtained from normal controls and patients with severe chronic sinusitis with/without polyposis before and around 6 months after endoscopic sinus surgery (42). The mucociliary transport time was significantly longer in the subjects with sinusitis preoperatively compared to normals and improved to within the normal range on postoperative evaluation. CBF was also less in the patients with sinusitis compared to normal controls, but did not change on postoperative assessment. The authors hypothesize that the decrease in CBF and

the lack of improvement after surgery are a reflection of a possible mucosal disorder with a ciliotoxic effect. In a study of the effects of endoscopic sinus surgery on actual maxillary sinus mucociliary transport, Asai et al. evaluated 74 patients who underwent endoscopic sinus surgery for chronic sinusitis at least 3 months after the surgical procedure (43). They placed a saccharin granule on the lateral wall of the bottom of the maxillary sinus mucosa and recorded taste perception by the patients in the sitting position. They also classified the maxillary sinuses into four groups (normal, mild, moderate, and severe disease) on the basis of mucosal edema and swelling. Mucociliary transport time was progressively prolonged with observed disease severity in the maxillary sinuses. In some patients, a second evaluation was performed and showed improved (shortened) mucociliary transport time in 64% of the cases. In general, there was a correlation between mucosal disease severity and mucociliary transport but that was not observed in all specimens. Inanli et al. compared the electron microscopic appearance of maxillary sinus specimens of subjects with chronic sinusitis at the time of surgery and 12 weeks later and compared them to that of controls (44). They also measured nasal mucociliary transport using the saccharin test in the same patients. Their results show slower nasal clearance in the subjects at the time of surgery which improved significantly at 12 weeks postoperatively but was still slower than normal controls. Furthermore, significant loss of cilia and ciliary abnormalities were seen in the patients' specimens obtained at the time of surgery compared to control specimens. There was some improvement in ciliary number and structure 3 months after surgery but the mucosal appearance was clearly not yet back to normal. This study suggests abnormalities in maxillary sinus ciliary structure and nasal ciliary function in patients with CRS. These abnormalities were already showing signs of improvement and reversal three months post endoscopic sinus surgery but were still not comparable to normal values.

In another attempt at evaluating mucociliary transport after sinus surgery, Ikeda et al. introduced technetium 99m-labeled Tc-human serum albumin into the maxillary sinus and measured rate of clearance from the sinus using a gamma camera (45). This was performed in some patients with chronic sinusitis prior to surgery, in some four days after surgery and in yet another group of operated patients with healed mucosal at 6–14 months postoperatively. There was significantly more rapid clearance of the radiolabel from the maxillary sinuses of the subjects with heared mucosal compared to before, or four days after the procedure suggesting improved sinus mucociliary transport after resolution of mucosal disease by successful surgical intervention. In biopsies obtained from the sinus mucosa, significant ciliary abnormalities (total loss, partial loss, and short height) were noted in the mucosa of the actively inflamed patients and these changes were reversed to a large degree in the biopsies obtained after the procedure. An improvement in the mucociliary clearance of maxillary sinuses has also been shown to improve as soon as three weeks postoperatively, and will improve to a larger extent in patients with less severe disease (46). Thus, the majority of these studies suggest a negative impact of CRS on nasal and sinus mucociliary transport which is reversed at various time intervals after surgical drainage.

PRIMARY CILIARY DYSKINESIA (PCD)

Primary ciliary dyskinesia refers to a condition caused by congenitally dyskinetic cilia. Affected patients suffer from derangements of mucociliary transport and experience chronic otitis media, rhinosinusitis, and bronchiectasis with male patients additionally being afflicted with infertility. Information and understanding of this condition was acquired over the past century by clinical and pathologic observation of affected individuals. In 1901, Oeri first described a clinical association between bronchiectasis and situs inversus (47), followed in 1904 by Siewert who expanded the description by reporting a patient with sinusitis, bronchiectasis, and situs inversus (48). In 1933, Kartagener described four patients with sinusitis, bronchiectasis, situs inversus, and male infertility and the syndrome bearing his name was thereafter characterized (49). In 1975, Camner et al. demonstrated that sperm immobility in patients with Kartagener syndrome was caused by abnormal/ deficient dynein arms in the flagellar microtubules and that these patients had impaired transport in the tracheobronchial tree (50,51). Pedersen and Mygind further demonstrated an absence of nasal and bronchial mucociliary clearance associated with an absence of dynein arms in both nasal and bronchial cilia in patients with the syndrome (52).

In normal individuals, functional cilia are responsible for dextrorotation of embryonic viscera. In patients with dynein deficiency, dysfunctional cilia leave visceral rotation to chance and consequently, approximately half of these patients will have situs inversus. PCD is a term used to encompass all congenital forms of ciliary motility disorders. Patients usually have chronic otitis, sinusitis, and bronchiectasis but only half exhibit situs inversus (Kartagener's syndrome). PCD is inherited as an autosomally recessive disease and occurs in approximately 1 : 20,000 live births. The diagnosis is usually suspected in children with chronic otitis, sinusitis and bronchiectasis, and is confirmed by electron microscopic examination of cilia that can be obtained from nasal, adenoid, or bronchial biopsies. In addition to the original description of absent or deficient dynein arms of the cilia of these patients, other defects have been characterized which include: complete or partial loss of radial spokes and abnormal numbers and configurations of microtubules. Electron microscopy in the diagnosis of PCD is challenging for the following reasons: the specimens need to be preserved in special media, tissue processing and pathologic examination might delay the result for several days, tissue specimens may lack sufficient cilia, and accurate diagnosis is based on a relatively subjective evaluation of the specimen and largely depends on the expertise of the examining pathologist. In a report by leading ultrastructural pathologists, it was acknowledged that the current knowledge and technical capabilities are inadequate for the diagnosis of ciliary dysfunction (53). A quantitative and objective method of diagnosis based on the average count of dynein arms present in biopsy specimens has been devised that appears to increase the likelihood of making the diagnosis of PCD (54). To bypass some of the limitations of electron microscopy in the diagnosis of PCD, Bent and Smith obtained tracheal biopsies in patients suspected to have the disorder and immediately examined them under light microscopy at 400× magnification in the operating room (55). When ciliary motility was clearly present and synchronized, PCD was excluded without using electron microscopy. Lack of identifiable ciliated epithelium warranted a second biopsy that was submitted for electron microscopic examination. In three of twenty cases reviewed that showed abnormal cilia on light microscopy, the diagnosis of PCD was confirmed by electron microscopy. In the other 17 of 20 patients, the cilia appeared normal on light microscopy and the diagnosis of PCD was excluded without electron microscopic examination. This approach might miss some cases where motion is observed erroneously under light microscopy and where electron microscopy might have picked up abnormalities diagnostic of PCD. A study where both electron and light microscopy were performed on all specimens would help address this concern.

Once the diagnosis is established, patients are treated with multiple modalities which include hydration, physical therapy, postural drainage, bronchodilators, antibiotics, interval influenza and pneumococcal vaccines. Surgical interventions for chronic ear infections and CRS include placement of ventilation tubes and endoscopic sinus surgery, respectively. Although these procedures do not address the underlying problem, some reports suggest an improvement in the symptoms after surgical intervention (56).

SUMMARY

In conclusion, this chapter provides a review of paranasal sinus anatomy and discusses the physiology of mucociliary transport and abnormalities observed in patients with CRS. Normal mucociliary transport is essential for the maintenance of healthy sinuses. This is well illustrated by PCD in which a congenital abnormality in ciliary function leads to, among other manifestations, CRS and bronchiectasis. A decrease in mucociliary clearance has been demonstrated in most studies of CRS, with the bulk of evidence suggesting that the decrease is secondary rather than a primary event. Mucostasis, hypoxia, microbial products, and mediators and toxic proteins generated during chronic inflammation probably all contribute to diminished mucociliary function. These factors decrease mucociliary function by direct toxic effects on cilia, ciliary loss, other ultrastructural alterations in the epithelium and changes in the viscoelastic properties of mucus. Studies of patients before and after surgical restoration of sinus ventilation have shown that mucociliary function improves gradually over 1–6 months postoperatively. The slower than normal rate of recovery of mucociliary clearance after surgery highlights the importance of careful postoperative medical and surgical management which is discussed in Chapters 19 and 20.

REFERENCES

1. Evans MJ, Plopper GG. The role of basal cells in adhesion of columnar epithelium to airway basement membrane. Am Rev Respir Dis 1988; 138:481.
2. Evans MJ, Shami S, Cabral-Anderson LJ, et al. Role of nonciliated cells in renewal of the bronchial epithelium of rats exposed to NO_2. Am J Pathol 1986; 123:126.
3. Tos M. Goblet cells and glands in the nose and paranasal sinuses. Proctor DF, Andersen IB eds. The Nose. Amsterdam: Elsevier Biomedical Press BV; 1982.
4. Mygind N, Pedersen M, Nielsen M. Morphology of the upper airway epithelium. In: Proctor DF, Andersen IB, eds. The Nose. Amsterdam: Elsevier Biomedical Press BV, 1982: 71–96.
5. Wilson WR, Allansmith MR. Rapid, atraumatic method for obtaining nasal mucus samples. Ann Otol Rhinol Laryngol 1976; 85:391.
6. Andersen I, Lundqvist G, Proctor DF. Human nasal mucosal function under four controlled humidities. Am Rev Respir Dis 1979; 119:619.
7. Fry FA, Black A. Regional deposition and clearance of particles in the human nose. Aerosol Sci 1973; 4:113.
8. Lippmann M. Deposition and clearance of inhaled particles in the human nose. Ann Otol Rhinol Laryngol 1970; 79:519.
9. Baumgarten C, Togias AG, Naclerio RM, et al. Influx of kininogens into nasal secretions after antigen challenge of allergic individuals. J Clin Invest 1985; 76:191.

10. Messerklinger W. Uber die drainage der menschlichen nasennebenhollen unter normallen und pathologichen bedingungen. Monatscher Ohrenhelik 1966; 100:56–68.
11. Drettner B. The paranasal sinuses. In: Proctor DF Andersen I, eds. The Nose: Upper Airway Physiology and the Atmospheric Environment, Chapter 6. Amsterdam: Elsevier Biomedical Press, 1982: 145–62.
12. Dalhamn T, Rylander R. Frequency of ciliary beat measured with a photosensitive cell. Nature 1962; 196:592–3.
13. Wilson R, Sykes DA, Currie D, et al. Beat frequency of cilia from sites of purulent infection. Thorax 1986; 41:453–8.
14. Phillips PP, McCaffrey TV, Kern EB. Measurement of human nasal ciliary motility using computerized microphotometry. Otolaryngol Head Neck Surg 1990; 103:420–6.
15. Proctor DF. The mucociliary system. In: Proctor DF, Andersen IB, eds. The Nose: Upper Airway Physiology and the Atmospheric Environment. Amsterdam: Elsevier Biomedical Press BV, 1982; pp. 245–278.
16. Kaminski EJ, Fancher OE, Calandra JC. In vivo studies of the ciliostatic effects of tobacco smoke. Arch Environ Health 1968; 16:188–93.
17. Agius AM, Smallman LA, Pahor AL. Age, smoking and nasal ciliary beat frequency. Clin Otolaryngol Allied Sci 1998; 23:227–30.
18. Mahakit P, Pumhirun P. A preliminary study of nasal mucociliary clearance in smokers, sinusitis and allergic rhinitis patients. Asian Pac J Allergy Immunol 1995; 13:119–21.
19. Holmstrom M, Lund VJ, Scadding G. Nasal ciliary beat frequency after nasal allergen challenge. Am J Rhinol 1992; 6:101–5.
20. Schuil PJ, van Gelder JME, ten Berge M, et al. Histamine and leukotriene C_4 effects on in vitro ciliary beat frequency of human upper respiratory cilia. Eur Arch Otorhinolaryngol 1994; 251:325–8.
21. Guercio JP, Birch S, Fernandez RJ, et al. Deposition of ragweed pollen and extract on nasal mucosa of patients with allergic rhinitis: effect on nasal airflow resistance and nasal mucus velocity. J Allergy Clin Immunol 1980; 66:61–9.
22. Ogino S, Nose M, Irifune M, et al. Nasal mucociliary clearance in patients with upper and lower respiratory diseases. Otorhinolaryngology 1993; 55:352–5.
23. Mori S, Fujieda S, Kimura Y, et al. Nasal challenge activates the mucociliary transport system on not only the ipsilateral but also the contralateral side of the nose in patients with perennial allergic rhinitis. Otorhinolaryngology 2000; 62:303–6.
24. Sakakura Y, Sasaki Y, Hornick RB, et al. Mucociliary function during experimentally induced rhinovirus infections in man. Ann Otol Rhinol Laryngol 1973; 82:203–11.
25. Alho OP. Nasal airflow, mucociliary clearance, and sinus functioning during viral colds: effects of allergic rhinitis and susceptibility to recurrent sinusitis. Am J Rhinol 2004; 18:349–55.
26. Majima Y, Sakakura Y, Matsubara T, Murai S, Miyoshi Y. Mucociliary clearance in chronic sinusitis: related human nasal clearance and in vitro bullfrog palate clearance. Biorheology 1983; 20:251–62.
27. Majima Y, Sakakura Y, Matsubara T, Miyoshi Y. Possible mechanisms of reduction of nasal mucociliary clearance in chronic sinusitis. Clin Otolaryngol Allied Sci 1986; 11:55–60.
28. Passali D, Ferri R, Becchini G, Passali GC, Bellussi L. Alterations of nasal mucociliary transport in patients with hypertrophy of the inferior turbinates, deviations of the nasal septum and chronic sinusitis. Eur Arch Otorhinolaryngol 1999; 256:335–37.
29. Nuutinen J, Rauch-Toskala E, Saano V, Joki S. Ciliary beating frequency in chronic sinusitis. Arch Otolaryngol Head Neck Surg 1993; 119:645–7.
30. King E. A clinical study of the functioning of the maxillary sinus mucosa. Ann Otol 1935; 44:480–2.
31. Fontolliet C, Terrier G. Abnormalities of cilia and chronic sinusitis. Rhinology 1987; 25:57–62.
32. Ohashi Y, Nakai Y. Functional and morphological pathology of chronic sinusitis mucous membrane. Acta Otolaryngol Suppl (Stockh) 1983; 397:11–48.
33. Al-Rawi MM, Edelstein DR, Erlandson RA. Changes in nasal epithelium in patients with severe chronic sinusitis: a clinicopathologic and electron microscopic study. Laryngoscope 1998; 108:1816–23.

34. Guo Y, Majima Y, Hattori M, Seki S, Sakakura Y. A comparative study of the ciliary area of the maxillary sinus mucosa and computed tomographic images. Eur Arch Otorhinolaryngol 1998; 255:202–4.
35. Georgitis JW, Matthews BL, Stone B. Chronic sinusitis: characterization of cellular influx and inflammatory mediators in sinus lavage fluid. Int Arch Allergy Immunol 1995; 106:416–21.
36. Ganbo T, Hisamatsu K, Inoue H, Mizukoshi A, Goto R, Murakami Y. The effects of leukotrienes C_4 and D_4 on ciliary activity of human paranasal sinus mucosa in vitro. Rhinology 1995; 33:199–202.
37. Khan R, Dolata J, Lindberg S. Effects of inflammatory mediators on ciliary function in vitro. Rhinology 1995; 33:22–25.
38. Dolata J, Lindberg S, Mercke U. Histamine stimulation of mucociliary activity in the rabbit maxillary sinus. Ann Otol Rhinol Laryngol 1990; 99:666–71.
39. Harlin SL, Ansel DG, Lane SR, Myers J, Kephart GM, Gleich GJ. A clinical and pathologic study of chronic sinusitis: the role of the eosinophil. J Allergy Clin Immunol 1988; 81:867–75.
40. Ponikau JU, Sherris DA, Kephart GM, et al. Striking deposition of toxic eosinophil major basic protein in mucus: implications for chronic rhinosinusitis. J Allergy Clin Immunol 2005; 116:362–9.
41. Min YG, Kim IT, Park SH. Mucociliary activity and ultrastructural abnormalities of regenerated sinus mucosa in rabbits. Laryngoscope 1994; 104:1482–6.
42. Hafner B, Davris S, Riechelmann H, Mann WJ, Amedee RG. Endonasal sinus surgery improves mucociliary transport in severe chronic sinusitis. Am J Rhinol 1997; 11:271–4.
43. Asai K, Haruna S, Otori N, Yanagi K, Fukami M, Moriyama H. Saccharin test of maxillary sinus mucociliary function after endoscopic sinus surgery. Laryngoscope 2000; 110:117–22.
44. Inanli S, Tutkun A, Batman C, Okar I, Uneri C, Sehitoglu MA. The effect of endoscopic sinus surgery on mucociliary activity and healing of maxillary sinus mucosa. Rhinology 2000; 38:120–3.
45. Ikeda K, Oshima T, Furukawa M, et al. Restoration of the mucociliary clearance of the maxillary sinus after endoscopic sinus surgery. J Allergy Clin Immunol 1997; 99:48–52.
46. Dal T, Onerci M, Caglar M. Mucociliary function of the maxillary sinuses after restoring ventilation: a radioisotopic study of the maxillary sinus. Eur Arch Otorhinolaryngol 1997; 254:205–2.
47. Oeri R. Bronchiectasis in situs inversus. Frankfurter Zeitschrift fur Pathologie 1901; 3:393–8.
48. Siewert A. Uber einen fall von bronchiectasie bei einem patienten mit situs inversus viscrum. Berliner Klinische Wochenschrift 1904; 41:139–41.
49. Kartagener M. Zur pathogenese der bronchiectasien. I mitteilung: bronchiectasien bei situs viscerum inversus. Betr Klin Tuberk 1933; 83:498–501.
50. Camner P, Mossberg B, Afzelius, BA. Evidence for congenitally non-functioning cilia in the tracheobronchial tree in two subjects. Am Rev Respir Dis 1975; 112:807–9.
51. Afzelius BA. A human syndrome caused by immotile cilia. Science 1976; 193:317–9.
52. Pedersen H, Mygind N. Absence of axonemal arms in nasal mucosa cilia in Kartagener's syndrome. Nature 1976; 262:494–5.
53. Mierau GW, Agostini R, Beals TF, et al. The role of electron microscopy in evaluating ciliary dysfunction: report of a workshop. Ultrastruct Pathol 1992; 16:245–54.
54. Teknos TN, Metson R, Chasse T, Balercia G, Dickersin GR. New developments in the diagnosis of Kartagener's syndrome. Otolaryngol Head Neck Surg 1997; 116:68–74.
55. Bent JP III, Smith RJH. Intraoperative diagnosis of primary ciliary dyskinesia. Otolaryngol Head Neck Surg 1997; 116:64–7.
56. Parsons DS, Greene BA. A treatment for primary ciliary dyskinesia: efficacy of functional endoscopic sinus surgery. Laryngoscope 1993; 103:1269–72.
57. Montgomery WW. Surgery of the ethmoid and sphenoid sinuses. In: Montgomery WW, ed. Surgery of the Upper Respiratory System. Philadelphia: Lea and Febiger, 1971; 1:41–93.
58. Stammberger H. Secretion transportation. In: Stammberger H. Functional Endoscopic Sinus Surgery. Philadelphia: B.C. Decker, 1991:17–47.

8

Chronic Rhinosinusitis with Glandular Hypertrophy

James N. Baraniuk
Georgetown University Proteomics Laboratory, Washington, D.C., U.S.A.

Sonya Malekzadeh
Department of Otolaryngology–Head and Neck Surgery, Georgetown University, Washington, D.C., U.S.A.

Begona Casado
Georgetown University Proteomics Laboratory, Washington, D.C., U.S.A.

INTRODUCTION

Chronic rhinosinusitis (CRS) can be divided into two mutually exclusive histological subtypes based on the presence of polyps or glandular hypertrophy (1). In CRS with nasal polyps the full thickness and organs of normal nasal mucosa are replaced with an edematous, generally eosinophilic, epithelium-coated "bag" of interstitial matrix "ground substance." In contrast, the histological findings in CRS without nasal polyps include glandular hypertrophy and a mononuclear and potentially neutrophilic inflammatory pattern that accounts for the thickening of the mucosa in this CRS subset. The pathophysiological processes involved in glandular hypertrophy and nasal polyposis are contrasted in order to highlight the distinct mechanisms that lead to these contrasting phenotypes (1–7).

In CRS with nasal polyps Chronic rhinosinussitis with nasal polyps (CRS with NP) the full thickness and organs of normal nasal mucosa are replaced with an edematous, generally eosinophilic, epithelium-coated "bag" of interstitial matrix "ground substance". This material has not been fully characterized. In contrast, the histological findings in CRS without nasal polyps Chronic rhinosinussitis without nasal polyps (CRS without NP) include glandular hypertrophy and a mononuclear and potentially neutrophilic inflammatory pattern that thickening the mucosa (1–4). The typical mucosal structures of sub-basement membrane superficial vasculature, submucosal glands, nerves, and deep venous sinusoids are maintained. However, there is a transition away from the usual mixed leukocytic infiltrate found in normal inferior turbinates and an extensive expansion of the mucosal volume containing submucosal serous and mucous cells. Differences in patterns of mRNA (8,9) and protein (10,11) expression have begun to accelerate our understanding of potential mechanisms that may explain these two distinct pathological processes. This histopathological distinction is clinically important since CRS is a heterogenous chronic disorder that persists for over 20 years of follow-up despite current surgical and topical glucocorticoids treatment (12). Different treatments may be required for each phenotype.

NASAL POLYPS VERSUS NONPOLYPOID CRS WITH GLANDULAR HYPERTROPHY

Evidence for this dualistic pathology was provided by histological studies. Middle turbinate biopsies were stained for mucous cells with Alcian Blue (1), and the results stratified by computed tomography (CT) scan severity using the May CT scan classification system (13). The ratio of Alcian Blue staining glands to total mucosal area was $6.88 \pm 0.48\%$ (mean $\pm$ SEM, N = 22) in normal (May CT scan class 0), symptomatic May class I osteomeatal complex disease (OMC) and May class II (mild ethmoid disease) subjects (1–4) (Figs. 1 and 2). The upper 95th percentile (>11.5%) was set as a threshold for glandular hypertrophy. The threshold was exceeded in four of seven class III (moderate bilateral disease) subjects ($17.7\% \pm 1.4\%$, $P < 0.0001$). The other three of seven class III subjects had visual and histological evidence of eosinophilic, edematous polyps that replaced the normal nasal mucosa. The ratio was reduced in pansinusitis (May class IV, n = 6/ 6) to $3.0\% \pm 0.8\%$ ($P < 0.001$) with polypoid degeneration of the full thickness of the mucosa. There were clear associations between (i) pansinusitis and polyposis (May class IV), (ii) multi-sinus mucosal thickening (May class III) with either, *but never both*, gland hypertrophy or polyposis, (iii) early polyp changes in some class II subjects, and (iv) minimal CT scan changes (May classes 0–II; no polyps) with minimal histological changes. Our work has been confirmed (14), and is consistent with Eichel's radiologic classification of hyperplastic rhinosinusitis $\pm$ nasal polyps (15). Furthermore, distinct mRNA patterns for "edematous" and "glandular" polyps have recently been described by genomic microarray studies (9).

PATHOGENESIS OF NASAL POLYPOSIS

Pathogenic mechanisms in nasal polyposis (16–18) are discussed extensively in this text. However, it is critical to reinforce the distinction between CRS with NP and CRS without NP. In a retrospective analysis, we found that polyp and nonpolyp

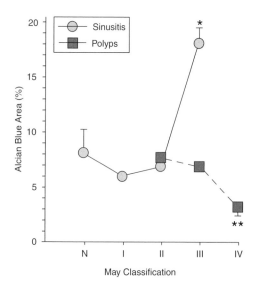

FIGURE 1 Percent Alcian Blue-stained area vs. May CT scan class. Histopathology worsened with sinusitis severity. Histology was normal in normal (class 0), mild sinusitis (classes I and II) except for one class II subject with polypoid changes. Significant glandular hypertrophy (% Alcian Blue stained mucus cell area >11.5%) occurred in class III. Nasal polyps were identified visually and by microscopy in class II, class III, and all class IV subjects. By definition, there was no histological overlap between polyps and glandular hypertrophy. Therefore, distinct pathogenic mechanisms were responsible for the two subtypes.

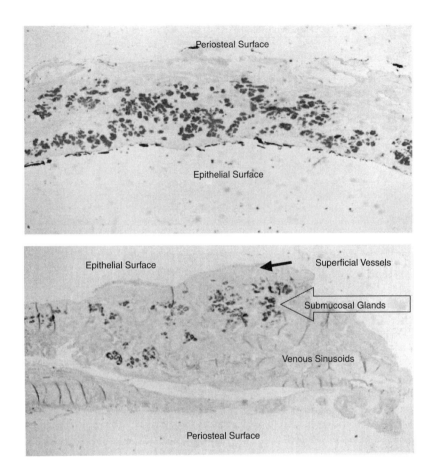

FIGURE 2 Alcian Blue-stained middle turbinate. *Top:* Glandular hypertrophy in May CT class III. Alcian Blue-stained mucous cells (dark) were increased in area indicating submucosal gland hypertrophy. Normal superficial vessels and deep venous sinusoids were present in the lamina propria (lower) and periostial (upper) regions. *Bottom:* May grade II sinusitis. Normal mucous and serous cells were seen in the glands. The superficial and deep venous sinusoids were normal. Polyps (see Preliminary Data) have few glands or vessels, but many eosinophils in an edematous tissue matrix.

groups were best discriminated by forced expiratory volume in 1 second/forced vital capacity (FEV_1/FVC) (66.7 ± 4.7% vs. 80.7 ± 4.0%, respectively; mean ± 95% CI; P = 0.0002 by two-tailed unpaired *t*-tests with Bonferroni corrections for multiple comparisons), total lung capacity (TLC) (111.1 ± 5.9% vs. 96.1 ± 8.1%; P = 0.006), and forced expiratory flow between 25% and 75% ($FEF_{25-75\%}$) (52.2 ± 11.0% vs. 70.4 ± 12.2%; P < 0.05) (19). Clinical asthma was equally prevalent, but the polyp group had more severe disease. Aspirin sensitivity was the next discriminator, and was present in 11 of 33 polyp and 1 of 41 (aspirin-induced urticaria only) nonpolyp subjects. These findings reinforce the hypothesis that distinct mechanisms are responsible for polypoid and nonpolypoid CRS. The importance of the mechanism (s) of aspirin sensitivity is clear given the increased severity of the "systemic" upper

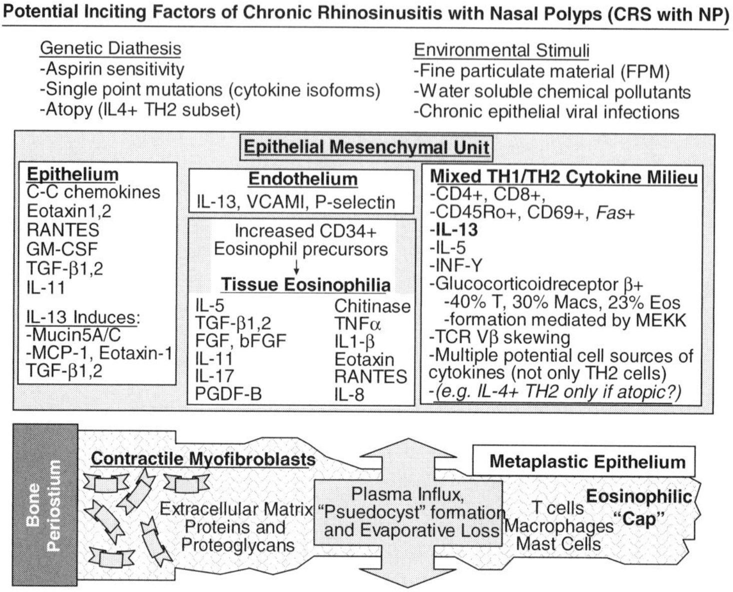
Potential Inciting Factors of Chronic Rhinosinusitis with Nasal Polyps (CRS with NP)
Genetic Diathesis
-Aspirin sensitivity
-Single point mutations (cytokine isoforms)
-Atopy (IL4+ TH2 subset)
Environmental Stimuli
-Fine particulate material (FPM)
-Water soluble chemical pollutants
-Chronic epithelial viral infections
Epithelial Mesenchymal Unit
Epithelium
C-C chemokines
Eotaxin1,2
RANTES
GM-CSF
TGF-β1,2
IL-11
IL-13 Induces:
-Mucin5A/C
-MCP-1, Eotaxin-1
TGF-β1,2
Endothelium
IL-13, VCAMI, P-selectin
Increased CD34+
Eosinophil precursors
Tissue Eosinophilia
IL-5
TGF-β1,2
FGF, bFGF
IL-11
IL-17
PGDF-B
Chitinase
TNFα
IL1-β
Eotaxin
RANTES
IL-8
Mixed TH1/TH2 Cytokine Milieu
-CD4+, CD8+,
-CD45Ro+, CD69+, Fas+
-IL-13
-IL-5
-INF-Y
-Glucocorticoidreceptor β+
-40% T, 30% Macs, 23% Eos
-formation mediated by MEKK
-TCR Vβ skewing
-Multiple potential cell sources of cytokines (not only TH2 cells)
-(e.g. IL-4+ TH2 only if atopic?)
Bone Periostium
Contractile Myofibroblasts
Extracellular Matrix
Proteins and
Proteoglycans
Plasma Influx,
"Psuedocyst" formation
and Evaporative Loss
Metaplastic Epithelium
Eosinophilic
"Cap"
T cells
Macrophages
Mast Cells

FIGURE 3 Chronic rhinosinusitis with nasal polyps (CRS with NP). We propose that specific environmental and microbial stimuli acting in a host with the appropriate genetic diathesis will lead to CRS with NP (upper panel). Regional epithelial activation leads to local dysregulation of the epithelial-mechenchymal unit (middle panel). The cellular influx of eosinophils, mast cells, and different types of T cells generates a mixed "TH1/TH2" cytokine mileu. Atopic subjects also express IL-4. The distinct polyp histology will result from the constrained pattern of cytokine secretion, eosinophil chemoattraction and juxtacrine inflammation, plasma flux into the polypoid pseudocyst, differentiation and contraction of myofibroblasts (lower panel). This process has many parallels with bronchial and bronchiolar remodeling in asthma.

and lower airway disease in "Triad Asthma (Triad Sinusitis?)." Mechanisms of polyposis stand in sharp contrast to those responsible for nonpolypoid CRS.

Bachert et al. demonstrated very early polypoid changes in the middle turbinate (medial wall of the OMC). A "cap" of eosinophils was found under the epithelial basement membrane (Fig. 3) (6,7). The cause of the primary influx of eosinophils and other polyp-related cells is the fundamental issue underlying polyp pathogenesis. Chronic epithelial cell activation in chronic bronchitis by adenovirus or other pathogens has been proposed by Ogawa et al. (20). Similar mechanisms may lead to the predominantly ethmoid–OMC region of origin for polyps. This region is also the area of highest deposition of toxic inhalants, particularly water-soluble chemical toxins (e.g., aldehydes) and particulate (e.g., diesel particles, pollen grains, and fungal spores) (21,22). However, it would be anticipated that the general population is exposed to a similar pattern of toxicants, but clinical experience demonstrates that only a small proportion develop CRS. This suggests that underlying co-morbid factors including genetic predispositions are also operating. These topics are discussed elsewhere in this book.

Once activated, epithelial or other sentinel cells can generate chemoattractant factors such as regulated upon activation, normal T-cell expressed and secreted (RANTES) (23–27), eotaxin ($2 > 1,3$) (28,29), and monocyte chemotactic proteins MCP-3 and MCP-4 (27,30). These will promote the influx of eosinophils. Newly arrived, differentiating, and activated mucosal eosinophils may promote their own survival and further cellular influx by autocrine and paracrine release of granulocyte macrophase-colony stimulating factor (GM-CSF) (23,31,32), Interleukin-5 (IL-5) (23,29,33), eotaxin ($2 > 1,3$) (27,28), RANTES (23–27), transforming growth factor β (TGF-β) (25,34–36), and platelet-derived growth factor (PDGF)-B (37). Continued epithelial and potentially mast cell and lymphocyte-derived mediators may add to this eosinopoeitic milieu.

Tissue destruction by the eosinophil cationic proteins (38) and halide free radicals may destroy normal tissue elements such as vessels and glands. Leukotriene C_4 (LTC_4) (39) may promote vascular leak that generates an albumin and fibronectin pseudocyst under the eosinophil cap (16). We propose that evaporation of water from the surface of the polyp generates an osmotic and capillary pressure gradient that will "wick" ever greater amounts of plasma ultrafiltrate from adjacent normal mucosa through the polyp. Water influx and evaporation will increase the concentration of salts and other nonvolatile plasma components within the polyp matrix. These will contribute to the osmotic gradient and provide a continuous "sink" for additional plasma transudation (40).

Myofibroblasts (41) differentiate from tissue fibroblasts beneath the pseudocyst. Eosinophilic and other cell cytokines such as TGF-β2 ($>$-β1, -β3) (24–26,33,42), PDGF-A $>$ PDGF-B (37), basic fibroblast growth factor (FGF) (43), insulin-like growth factor-1 (44), endothelin-1 (45), IL-11 (46), vascular endothelial growth factor (VEGF) (47,48) and keratinocyte growth factor (KGF) (49–53) are likely of importance. Contraction of myofibroblast α-1-smooth muscle actin (54) may extrude the pseudocyst gel into the airway lumen (34,37,54,55). Polyp pathology extends deep to the periostium with the loss of glands, vessels, and nerves (56). Denervation may enhance fibrosis (57,58).

Total IgE concentrations were significantly higher in polyps than nonpolyp tissues, and correlated significantly with IL-5, eosinophil cationic protein (ECP), LTC4/D4/E4, sCD23 soluble Fcε receptor II (sFcεRII) and eosinophil density. Eotaxin and collagen types I and III were also increased (7,28,35). Mast cells activated by IgE or anaphylactoid histamine releasing factor mechanisms (e.g., cytokines, complement 3a (C3a)) or other non-IgE-dependent mechanisms are likely to play an important role as multilogistic modeling demonstrated that nasal lavage fluid tryptase, histamine, and ECP levels were most predictive of polyposis (59,60). Macrophage, type 1 T helper lympocytes (TH1), and natural killer (NK) cell function may be dysregulated since interferon-γ (INF-γ) and IL-12 can be elevated in both allergic and nonallergic CRS (61–63).

Several polyp classification systems have been proposed based on the predominance of eosinophils or neutrophils (64), or more complex mechanisms and co-morbid asthma (1,7,46). Neutrophils predominate in children, and in particular those with cystic fibrosis where *Pseudomonas* and *Staphylococcus* sp. are important pathogens. The factors that lead to predominantly neutrophilic polypoid infiltrates (64) may include the neutrophil chemoattractants IL-8, C3b (immune complex activation), and leukotriene B (LTB4). However, the relevance and preeminence of these potential mechanisms are poorly understood.

An alternative system is based on the concomitant IgE response in CRS (7). (i) Nonatopic polypoid asthmatics have aspirin sensitivity [Widel's syndrome (65); Samter's syndrome (66)], and high cysteinyl leukotriene 1 receptor expression (67), but no specific IgE. (ii) Subjects with polyps, allergic rhinitis and asthma have IgE to dust mites, molds, and other perennial aeroallergens, and may be more susceptible to allergic fungal sinusitis (68). (iii) Asthmatics with high IgE levels have multiclonal, antigen-specific IgE to *Staphylococcus aureus* enterotoxins A and B superantigens (6). As yet unknown precipitating insults or innate immunity deficiencies may permit *S. aureus* colonization and successful evasion of the adaptive immune system. *Staphylococcus aureus* colonizes the nares of 33–50% of chronic sinusitis subjects compared to 22–33% of nonsinusitis controls (69,70).

PATHOGENESIS OF GLANDULAR HYPERTROPHY

Based on our recent studies, we believe the glandular hypertrophy phenotype best describes nonpolypoid CRS. However, because some of the early literature on NP described a "glandular" histologic variant, we shall also discuss this literature as a background to our studies.

Factors responsible for glandular hypertrophy and dysfunction in CRS (71) have just begun to be investigated. In part, this is because the histological similarities to normal inferior turbinates have led to its designation as "hyperplastic" or "hypertrophic" sinusitis (72). In these earlier studies, glandular hypertrophy may have been mistaken for microglandular adenosis, analogous to tubular carcinoma of the breast (73), seromucous maxillary sinusitis (SMMS) (74), or the elongated epithelial invaginations within polyps (13,14). "Glandular polyps" with an increased area of submucosal glands (9,75–77) were differentiated from "edematous polyps" (78). However, there are no data to define these putative phenotypes of "polyps", nor long-term follow-up studies to determine if "early" glandular polyps (9) eventually generated macroscopic "edematous" polyps. In fact, microscopic edema and eosinophilia may appear in the middle turbinate in the earliest stages of polyposis (7,16). This lack of informed opinion occurred despite the millions of sinus operations that have had "routine" histological examinations. Detailed analysis of glandular hypertrophy began with the systematic analyses provided by Biedlingmaier et al. (5), Malekzadeh et al. (1–3), and Majima et al. (79). Majima et al. demonstrated that submucosal gland density in inferior turbinates of chronic sinusitis subjects was increased compared to nonrhinitic controls (79). Goblet cell density was not different. Malekzadeh et al. (1) concluded that the so-called "glandular polyps" were more likely to represent submucosal gland hypertrophy than polyp formation, as had been previously sugggested (72).

Quantitative histochemical assessments have now been coupled with demographic and clinical analysis in larger populations to identify multiple CRS subtypes. Multifactorial analysis has allowed for identification of distinct phenotypes with aspirin sensitivity and asthma, frontal sinus disease, and glandular hypertrophy (80). Principal components analysis of CT scan extent of disease and symptoms permitted classification of 474 patients with chronic perennial and persistent rhinosinusitis (81). A chronic rhinitis group shared nasal obstruction, anterior and posterior nasal discharge, sneezing, and facial congestion with the other groups, but did not have sinus involvement on CT scan. This group may have a component of neural hyperalgesia and allodynia that heightens their symptomatic perceptions from this visceral mucosa (82–85). A second group experienced localized anterior ethmoid sinusitis and complained of cacosmia (the sensation of pain on inhalation). Those with sinusitis localized to other regions tended to have more severe, chronic facial pain. Subjects with diffuse rhinosinusitis due to nasal polyposis had anosmia and loss of taste but generally lacked facial pain and cacosmia. These studies reinforce the hypothesis that separate pathophysiological mechanisms lead to distinct phenotypes of CRS.

Mucous Cells

Malekzadeh et al. (1) demonstrated a relationship between the percent area of Alcian Blue staining mucous material in submucosal glands and the extent of maxillary and other large sinus disease detected by CT scan. Their tissue was obtained from the lateral middle turbinate that forms the medial wall of the osteomeatal complex. The data indicated hypertrophy of the mucin-secreting mucous cells in comparison with both normal middle turbinate mucosa and nasal polyps (Fig. 1). The degree of glandular hypertrophy increased in proportion to the extent of the sinusitis (CT scan).

Alcian Blue at pH 2.5 stains the carboxylate side chains of sialic acid (neuraminic acid) (Fig. 2) (86,87). Sialic acid groups terminate the highly branched O-linked glycoconjugate side chains of "acidic" mucins. These carboxylate groups are oriented away from the glycoconjugate and greatly increase the size of the mucin hydration shell and electrostatic interactions between these tenaciously adherent glycoproteins and particulate, microbial, or cellular materials. Very highly acidic, sulfated mucins stain with pH 1.0 Alcian Blue.

Mucins are long chain proteins that may be anchored in the membrane (transmembrane mucins 1, 3A, 3B, 4, 12, 17), or secreted into the gel or sol phases. Several mucins have been cloned but remain poorly characterized in airways (mucins 8, 9, 13, 15, 16, I, tracheobronchial mucin (TBM)). The transmembrane mucins are important for intercellular and matrix interactions. *Muc4* mRNA may be a marker of ciliated cells (88) or an indicator of epithelial regeneration after acute injury (89). The acidic, gel-forming mucin genes map to 11p5.5, and are differentially expressed in goblet (*muc5A/C, muc2*) and glandular mucous (*muc5B*) cells (90). *Muc6* mRNA has not been detected in airways. *Muc7* is probably a "neutral mucin" secreted from serous cells into the sol phase (91). These mucins are of great functional importance for airway epithelial lining fluid rheology, humidification, lubrication, particle adhesion, and host defense. They form "gel rafts" that are pulled along by ciliary motion. The secreted mucins have multiple cysteine residues in their N- and C-terminal regions. These form disulfide links to create the gel phase of mucus. The middle region of the polypeptide contains multiple, repeated sequences rich in serine and threonine repeats. These amino acids are the sites for O-glycosylation. The cysteine-rich, cross-linking areas may become cleaved from the adhesive carbohydrate-rich domain and so release the "sticky sponge" into the freely mobile phase of epithelial lining fluid mucus (88). The mucin fragment and any adherent foreign material may be removed from mucoclots and expelled or carried posteriorly and digested in the stomach. The material may also become phagocytosed by macrophages or other dedicated mucosal antigen-presenting cells and localized, tissue-specific immune responses generated against the ensnared foreign antigens.

Mucins in CRS express more sialic acid, SO_4, and galactose, and less mannose in their polysaccharide side chains (92). Sialylation may be regulated by TNF-α (93). Proteomic methods demonstrated the induction of glycosyl sulfotransferase in acute sinusitis subjects after 1 week of treatment (10). This finding suggested that further acidification of mucous cell acidic mucins was a host response to viral, bacterial, and potentially other mucosal injury. It may also be an indication of mucous and goblet cell hyperplasia and/or hypertrophy in both acute and CRS.

We propose that acidic mucin hypersecretion in CRS with glandular hypertrophy plays an unintended role in pathogenesis. The tightly crosslinked mucins may congeal with fibrinogen, albumin, lysozyme, DNA and other materials to form indigestible barriers, or mucoclots, that are intended to prevent microbial spread and repair mucosal epithelial and basement membrane lesions. They may become irreversibly attached to the sinus mucosa, and eventually become buried under newly generated basement membranes and epithelium during remission and convalescence. We propose that these form the cores of post-infectious mucocoeles. The mucocoagulant may also become the substrate for microbial growth and formation of biofilms. If so, these "protective barriers" would be subverted to protect the colonizing microbes rather than the host.

Muc5A/C and *muc5B* mRNAs are most significantly upregulated in CRS without nasal polyps (94). *Muc4*, *muc7*, and *muc8* are upregulated in chronic ethmoid sinusitis in a process that may require retinoic acid (95). However, IL-4 and IL-13 may downregulate *muc5A/C* and upregulate *muc8* mRNA expression in nasal polyps (96). Mucin expression has been assessed in idiopathic nonallergic rhinitis ("vasomotor rhinitis"). The only difference from normal turbinate mucosa was a slightly lower in situ hybridization signal for *muc1* mRNA in nonallergic rhinitis (97).

Nuclear factor for κ chain production by B lymphocytes (NFκB) is a key mucin transcriptional regulator (98). Protein kinase (PKC), cyclic GMP guanosyl mano phosphate (cGMP)-dependent phosphokinase, and myristoylated alanine-rich C kinase substrate (MARCKS) mediate mucin granule exocytosis (98). Rodent mucous cell proliferation and mucin gene expression are upregulated by epithelial growth factor (EGF) (99–103), TNF-α (104), IL-9 (105,106), IL-4 (107,108), and IL-13 (109–111). IL-9 expression is strongly linked to expression of the calcium-activated chloride channel (HCLCA1) and mucus production in bronchial epithelium from asthmatics (112). EGF may also regulate goblet cell proliferation (100).

Serous Cells

About one-third of the total nasal lavage protein is synthesized by submucosal gland serous cells in normal nasal mucosa. These glands secrete antimicrobial proteins (86,113–116) including lysozyme (∼14% of total nasal protein) (117), lactoferrin, secretory leukocyte protease inhibitor (SLPI) (118), and proteases. The latter include neutral endopeptidase, which degrades neuropeptides and bradykinin (119), membrane-bound puromycin-resistant aminopeptidase M (120), and secreted glandular kallikrein which cleaves plasma kininogen to release bradykinin (121).

A major task of glandular serous cells is the secretion of antigen-specific IgA (15% of nasal mucus total protein). IgA-producing plasma cells express CCR10 (122). In the lactating breast, these cells migrate towards the CCL28 chemokine that is up-regulated on secretory mammary gland epithelium. The IgA is secreted as a dimer ([IgA]$_2$-joining chain) that diffuses to the interstitial side of the epithelium, and binds to the polymeric immunoglobulin receptor (poly Ig R) expressed on this surface. TNF-α up-regulates expression of poly Ig R (123). The complex is translocated to the luminal side of the acinar cell, and then exocytosed as secretory IgA (sIgA: J-[IgA]$_2$-poly Ig R) (124,125). We propose that CCL28 and CCR10 may be responsible for the close proximity of IgA-producing plasma cells to submucosal gland serous cells in human nasal mucosa and in CRS with glandular hypertrophy.

The lipocalin superfamily of lipid-binding proteins contains important components of the innate immune system (126). Lipocalin 1 (LCN1) is secreted from glands. Lipocalin 2, or neutrophil granule-associated lipocalin, is packaged with elastase in neutrophil secretory granules. The PLUNC (Palate, Lung, Upper airways, Nasal Clone) protein family is well represented in glandular cells (11,126,127). There are two general forms with a lipid-binding domain with or without a cell binding domain. The "short PLUNCs" such as SPLUNC1 (the "classic" PLUNC) (11,127) have only the lipid binding, eight-fold β-barrel domain. Lung specific X protein (LUNX) is a purported lung cancer marker that differs from SPLUNC1 by one amino acid. It is likely a polymorphism of this gene. SPLUNC proteins may sequester lipopolysaccharide or other microbial lipids to protect against cellular overactivation by LPLUNCs or CD14 (128) that activate toll-like receptor-4 (TLR-4) (129). TLR-2 and TLR-4 mRNA expression were not significantly different between normal and sinusitis tissues (130). SPLUNC2 and SPLUNC3 mRNA were detected in human nasal mucosa (126), but their proteins were not (10,11,127). Related families of odorant binding proteins are released into the mucus of the olfactory region and may bind excessive amounts of inhaled odorants so that a lower concentration of odorant can interact with olfactory nerve receptors without causing neural desensitization and tachyphylaxis (131).

The "Long PLUNCs" such as LPLUNC1 (von Ebner's gland protein), bacteriocidal/permeability inhibitory protein (BPLI 1, LPLUNC2), and lipopolysaccharide (LPS) binding protein (LBP) (132,133) have two domains. When lipids slide into the lipocalin pocket of one domain, the second domain unfolds. This domain may bind to uncharacterized cellular proinflammatory receptors. The polypeptide tether between the domains may be cleaved by elastase or other proteases to release the ligand domain so it can diffuse and activate its receptors, while the first domain and its captured lipid are expelled, or swallowed and destroyed in the gastrointestinal tract.

The cationic antimicrobial factor human β-defensin (HBD) 1 may be constitutively expressed by normal nasal epithelium and glands (134). HBD2 is inducible, and nasal polyp epithelium has been shown to express HBD2 mRNA and immunoreactive protein, indicating upregulation during inflammation (135). HBD3 had negligible expression in nasal and sinusitis tissue (130).

GENOMICS AND PROTEOMICS: TRANSCRIPTOMES AND PROTEOMES IN CRS

Genomic methods of Northern blotting and in situ hybridization assess mRNA expression one mRNA at a time. They have now been augmented by more extensive screening by mRNA microarray analysis and other advanced methods that assess expression patterns from the entire genome (136).

Fritz et al. studied nasal mucosal biopsies from a small group of allergic rhinitis subjects with (N = 3) and without (N = 4) nasal polyps (8). Apparently polyp tissue was not examined. mRNAs that showed greater than two fold difference in expression (fluorescence intensity) and P < 0.05 between the two groups were considered significant. Their intent was to examine the transcriptome (list of significantly altered mRNAs) in nasal turbinate tissue that might contribute to polyp formation without being influenced by changes occurring inside NP. Mammoglobin was the most highly increased mRNA in the polyp group. It was localized to the cytoplasm of distal serous demilunes in submucosal glands. This raises the possibility that glandular hypertrophy was surveyed in this study. *Fos* was elevated as has been shown previously (137). Lipophilin B, tryptase beta 1, kallikrein 8, glutathione *S*-transferase theta 2, purinergic receptor P2Y, pyrimidinergic receptor P2Y, retinoblastoma-binding protein 8, allograft inflammatory factor 1, prostaglandin D2 synthase, and cystatin S were among the significantly increased mRNAs. mRNAs that were decreased by more than three fold were butyrophilin 3, prostate stem cell antigen, pro-platelet basic protein, T cell receptor gamma constant 2, myosin light polypeptide 4, and soluble acid phosphatase 1.

Nasal polyp tissue expressed different mRNAs. Liu et al. compared NP to normal nasal turbinate tissue to define the differentially expressed polypoid transcriptome (9). They found 192 mRNAs that were upregulated and 156 that were downregulated in polyps. Thirty-nine were greater than five fold higher, but only 10 were greater than five fold lower, in polyps than normal tissue. The highest fold-changes were confirmed by quantitative reverse transcriptase polymerase chain reaction (RT-PCR). Histological analysis of the lamina propria divided the polyps into edematous, eosinophilic, and glandular subtypes. The "glandular polyps" had more glands than normal turbinates. Again this calls into question whether these so-called "glandular polyps" were more likely to represent submucosal gland hypertrophy than polyp formation, as was found in the study by Malekzadeh et al. (1).[a] The mRNAs showing the largest differences were from the glandular polyp set and included increased levels of deleted in malignant brain tumor 1 (DMBT1), lactoferrin, prolactin-induced protein (PIP), and statherin. Immunohistochemistry localized lactoferrin, PIP, and statherin to the serous cells of submucosal glands. Statherin may maintain oral mineral homeostasis. PIP may have many functions, including fibronectin-specific aspartyl protease activity. Lactoferrin is an avid iron-sequestering molecule. DMBT1 may have been present in either serous or mucous cells of glands. DMBT1 is a member of the multiple scavenger receptor cysteine-rich (SRCR) superfamily. DMBT1 or its splice variant gp340 may bind serous and epithelial cell trefoil proteins 1 and 3 (138), *Streptococcus mutans*, and influenza virions. Clara cell protein 10 (CC10), and CC16, (uteroglobulin) were the most downregulated mRNA in NP.

Proteomics is the general title for broad-spectrum identification of the list of proteins that are unique to a given tissue or that may be differentially altered under distinct experimental conditions (139,140). Simple examples include differences in protein concentrations or distributions of immunohistochemical protein expression. More advanced methods employ a two stage process. First, a sample is fractionated. Methods include two-dimensional gel electophoresis and liquid chromatography. Second, mass spectrometry is used to identify the mass/charge ratio for all proteins or trypsin-digested peptides from a gel peak or chromatography

---

[a]In the Editor's experience (DLH), some non-cystic fibrosis nasal polyps with otherwise typical histologic appearance have an abundance of glands. Whether these truly represent a "glandular variant" of nasal polyps is debatable and has not been exhaustively investigated.

fraction. Matrix-assisted laser desorption ionization–time-of-flight (MALDI–ToF) is an example of one-dimensional mass spectrometry. More elaborate two-dimensional mass spectrometry methods permit peptide sequencing. These sequences are used for precise identification of the protein and any polymorphisms, splice variants, or post-translational modifications that may be present. Most results are qualitative, and should be considered an indication of the detectability of a given protein. Detectability is determined by the relative abundance of a protein in a mixture compared to the high-abundance proteins such as albumin and immunoglobulins, the protein's susceptibility to trypsin (or other endoprotease) digestion (no digestion = no peptides for sequencing), and the chemical properties of the peptides that enable chromatographic and mass spectrometric separation and sequencing.

Proteomics and genomics assess different aspects of tissues, and have a poor concordance. For example, the proteome and transcriptome specific for LPS-stimulated neutrophils had a concordance of only 28% (141). Further analysis was more disconcerting. The neutrophils expressed 923 genes, with 100 increasing three fold and 56 decreasing three-fold after 4 hours of LPS. Two-dimensional gel electrophoresis revealed about 1200 "protein spots", but comparison of 12 replicate runs identified only 125 reproducible spots. Spot intensity increased by 1.5-fold for an average of 24 spots (19%), and decreased 1.5-fold in 22 spots (17%) per replicate. These "significantly altered" protein spots were sequenced by MALDI–ToF and then compared to the Affymetrix 7070 chip results. Only 18 proteins and mRNAs matched. Of these, two showed concordant increases and three concordant decreases for both protein and mRNA (5/18 = 28% concordance). When placed in the perspective of the 156 significantly altered mRNAs and 46 protein spots, these five concordant results may have occurred as a result of chance (probability of 5/46 potential mRNA-protein matches = 0.11 = P > 0.05, not significant). In contrast, two new proteins were identified by proteomics that were not present on the Affymetrix 7070 chip. This is a limitation of presumptively assuming that these chips can detect all gene transcripts. In a simpler case, platelets have 2928 mRNAs (microarray result) that can be translated into 82 proteins (proteomic result) (142). However, only 57 of the proteins matched the mRNA results.

The proteins expressed in acute sinusitis and acute exacerbations of CRS (10) have been compared to those expressed in nasal secretions from healthy subjects (11). As expected (143), plasma contributed albumin, immunoglobulins, transferrin, plasminogen, haptoglobin, C3 complement factor, apolipoprotein A1, α-1-antitrypsin, and other antiproteases (detected in >30% of samples) (11). Submucosal gland serous cell products (117) were abundant including polymeric immunoglobulin receptor, IgA, lysozyme, lactoferrin, LPLUNC1, LPLUNC2 (bacterial/permeability-increasing protein-like 1), SPLUNC1, lipocalin 1, proline-rich protein 4, prolactin-induced protein, and mammoglobin. Mucous cell MUC5A/C and MUC5B were also detected.

Sinusitis nasal lavage fluid proteins were similar to those in normal lavage fluid, but many were present in more samples (e.g., serous cell proteins). This suggested that higher concentrations of some proteins may have been present in sinusitis (10). Conversely, immunoglobulins and mucins were detected less frequently in sinusitis.

Many proteins such as plasma-derived fibrinogen-β and -γ were detected only on the day of initial presentation. IL-17E was detected only in sinusitis (10).

IL-17E can activate NFκB and stimulate secretion of IL-8 in vitro (144). Over-expression of IL-17E in a murine model led to high serum levels of IL-2, IL-4, IL-5, GM-CSF, eotaxin, and interferon-γ (145). Eosinophilia and B lymphocyte hyperpla-sia resulted. B-cell lymphocytosis was associated with significant elevations of serum IgM, IgG, and IgE. However, antigen challenge caused antigen-specific IgA and IgE, but not IgG, production. Matrix metalloprotease-27 (MMP-27) (146), which has also been associated with B lymphocytes (147), was detected acutely (10). S100 calcium-binding proteins A12 (S100A12; EN-RAGE: extracellular newly identified receptor for advanced glycation end products binding protein; calgranu-lin C) and S100A9 (calgranulin B) were other markers of inflammation in sinusitis as has been described in type 2 diabetes (148). 5-Lipoxygenase (5-LO), lipocalin 2 (neutrophil gelatinase-associated lipocalin, NGAL), and myeloperoxidase were consistent with an influx of neutrophils. The autocrine neutrophil chemokine IL-8 was increased in concentration in acute sinusitis, but would have too low a concentration for detection by mass spectrometry (51). Curiously, α-1B adrenergic receptors were detected in acute sinusitis. This suggested that inflammation- or stressor-activated mechanisms may release catecholamines from adrenal or sympa-thetic sources. The site of receptor expression has not been identified as yet. Glycosylsulphotransferase was detected only on day six indicating a long-duration conversion to the secretion of highly acidified mucins.

Serine protease inhibitor (SERPINB) (squamous cell carcinoma antigen 2; SCCA2) protein was also detected more readily in the sinusitis group. SERPINB inhibits dust mite proteases and may protect against other microbial serine proteases (149). SERPINB mRNA is highly upregulated by IL-4 and IL-13 (150). The recurring association of IL-4, IL9, and IL-13 implies roles for TH2 lymphocytes (151), mast cells and eosinophils in sinusitis as has been shown for allergic rhinitis and asthma. IL-4 also causes the dose-limiting sensation of nasal congestion when administered parenterally to humans (152). The mechanism does not appear to involve changes in vascular permeability or parasympathetic cholinergic glandular secretory reflexes. Activation of a specific set of "congestion" neurons is one possible explanation.

The sources of the proteins contained within the combined nasal and sinusitis proteome are depicted in Figure 4. Plasma plus the immunoglobulins accounted for 31% of the different types of proteins in the lavage fluids. Cytoske-letal, transmembrane, and cell surface proteins contributed an equal proportion. The final third were secreted from submucosal glands and epithelium (10% from serous and 4% from mucous cells), were present in the nucleus and other cellular sites (11%), or were inflammatory proteins detected only in acute sinusitis (11%).

CELL CYTOKINES ASSOCIATED WITH CRS WITH GLANDULAR HYPERTROPHY

The presence of IL-4, IL-5, IL-9, IL-13, and other cytokines suggest that TH2–IgE–mast cell–eosinophil mechanisms of atopy have a strong influence on the development of CRS. However, many of the studies describing the presence of these cytokines were performed without stratification of patients by the clinical expression of atopic disease or histological diagnosis. Neither the detection of "Th2 cytokines" nor eosinophils is proof positive that atopy initiates or accent-uates the development of any of the phenotypes of sinusitis that have been discussed. Allergic rhinitis has been diagnosed based on positive allergy skin tests

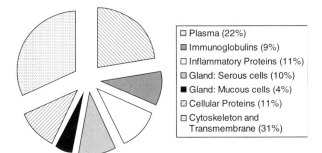

FIGURE 4 Diversity of origins for the combined nasal and sinusitis lavage fluid proteome. Plasma and immunoglobulins, and cytoskeletal and transmembrane proteins each contributed about one third of the total proteins detected in this proteome. Inflammatory proteins were only found on the day of presentation with acute sinusitis. The number of serous and mucous cell proteins was relatively small, but they were present in high concentrations and detected in most samples.

or radioallergosorbent test (RAST) results in 84% of endoscopic sinus surgery patients (153), 54% of CRS outpatients (154), and 37% of children with sinusitis (155). Perennial allergic rhinitis may be more closely linked to sinusitis (156). In retrospect, these studies were flawed by their simplicity. There is now a necessity to stratify patients according to the presence of nasal polyps and atopy that specifically affects the target organ (i.e., allergic rhinitis) as opposed to other sites (skin as in eczema or the gastrointestinal tract as in food allergy), or even the presence of potentially suppressed, asymptomatic allergy (157,158).

Atopy may modify glandular cytokine production. Methacholine nasal provocation in house dust mite allergic rhinitis subjects caused a significant increase in IL-6 concentration in mucus, indicating its release from glands (159). Both IL-6 and IL-8 were immunolocalized to glands, the apical portions of epithelial cells, and cells in the lamina propria (160). GM-CSF-immunoreactive material was more strongly localized to the basal part of epithelial cells, basement membrane, glandular ducts, and leukocytes. If atopy can augment cytokine production in allergic rhinitis, then it would be anticipated to have similar effects in CRS with glandular hypertrophy. An increased prevalence of atopy is predicted in the glandular hypertrophy phenotype.

Serous cells of glands synthesize IL-17, macrophage migration inhibitory factor (161), EGF, the EGF-receptor, and other EGF-R ligands (Fig. 5) (99–103,162). EGF and nerve growth factor (NGF) were increased in salivary gland secretions during oral inflammation suggesting that EGF and NGF secretion in mucus may be up-regulated in CRS with glandular hypertrophy (163). Glands and epithelium synthesize and store IL-16 that is secreted after stimulation by IL-9 (164). These mechanisms may be greatly magnified in the presence of glandular hypertrophy in CRS. ECP, IL-1β, TNF-α, and GM-CSF stimulated glandular exocytosis from human turbinate explants, suggesting that they may play similar roles in vivo (165). Corticosteroids significantly reduced the cytokine-induced glandular output.

A role for TGF- β1 was inferred by the detection of actin-γ1 and -γ2 that are regulated by this cytokine, and TGF-β II receptor (10) in acute sinusitis (166). These proteins and α2-smooth muscle actin may be markers of myofibroblast differentiation. TGF-β1 protein ($P = 0.0008$) and mRNA ($P = 0.025$) levels were

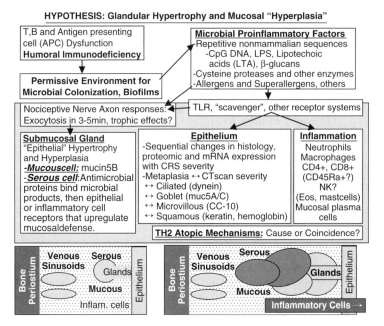

FIGURE 5 Hypothetical mechanism of CRS with glandular hypertrophy. Humoral immunodeficiency plays a permissive role in the colonization and infection of the sinuses (upper left). Microbial factors may stimulate glandular hypertrophy by several pathways (middle panel). We propose that microbial virulence factors activate epithelial cells either directly via toll-like or other receptor systems. Secreted innate immune proteins such as lipocalins that bind lipopolysaccharide (LPS), lipotechoic acid (LTA), β-glucans, and related materials may serve as sentinels to detect colonization, and activate epithelial and inflammatory pathways. Neutrophils become activated as indicated by our proteomic data. Acquired immune cell mechanisms may be activated, but not eliminate the microbial colonization. The inflammatory milieu of acidosis and hypoxia will depolarize specific subsets of nociceptive nerves. We have shown that their activation leads to rapid glandular exocytosis (3–5 min) by the axon response mechanism. Exocytosis of mucin, antimicrobial innate immune proteins and secretory IgA will attempt to eliminate the microbes, but may only provide a substrate for biofilm formation. This chronic process will lead to epithelial metaplasia (e.g., loss of cilia proteins, increased inflammatory keratins), neutrophil and mononuclear inflammation, and serous and mucous cell hypertrophy with mucosal thickening (bottom).

significantly higher in nonpolypoid CRS than nasal polyp samples (76). Extensive TGF-β1-immunoreactive material was found in the fibrotic extracellular matrix of nonpolypoid CRS tissues. In contrast, no TGF-β1 staining was found in the pseudocyst region of nasal polyps. Watelet et al. proposed that TGF-β1 expression with fibrosis may differentiate nonpolypoid CRS from nasal polyposis (76).

The cellular infiltrates in CRS with NP and CRS without NP are distinct. When nasal polyps were absent, CD38[+] lymphocytes and elastase-staining neutrophils were the predominant leukocytes in the tissue (167). Polyps also contained neutrophils, but had higher tissue concentrations of albumin and IL-5, and high densities of ECP staining eosinophils.

A role for macrophages in CRS with NP and CRS without NP has been based on the detection of IL-12 mRNA (168). This has suggested analogies to smokers with chronic bronchitis, as CD68$^+$ macrophages and CD8$^+$ lymphocytes that lacked IL-4 and IL-5 ("T$_{C1}$" lymphocytes) were the predominant epithelial inflammatory cells in that disorder (169–171). These cells and their cytokines were not associated with glands. This finding suggests that gland hypertrophy may be stimulated by alternative pathways that do not involve "Th2" cytokines. For example, salivary glands in Sjogren's syndrome are surrounded by mononuclear cells. They appear to secrete INF-γ that induces interferon-inducible T cell α chemoattractant (I-TAC or CXCL11) from the ductal epithelium (172). CXCL11 is absent from normal salivary glands. This Th1 mechanism may be active in other autoimmune disorders as well (173). We predict that upregulation of CXCL11 in CRS with glandular hypertrophy will provide indirect support for mechanisms involving INF-γ and its potential sources in CD4$^+$ Th1, CD8$^+$ Tc1-like, or NK cells in this subset of CRS. CXCL11 is not anticipated in nasal polyposis because of their reduced glandular volume, and the supposition that most of the "glandular" material represents invagination of surface epithelium during polyp formation (16).

Interferon-γ—induced activation of ductal epithelium may also increase arachidonic acid metabolism in CRS with glandular hypertrophy. Cycloxygenase-1 (Cox-1) and Cox-2 immunoreactive materials were detected in the ductal epithe-lium of submucosal glands. More intense Cox-1 staining was present in the epithelial lining in sinusitis compared to normal turbinate tissue (174). The exact prostaglandin, thromboxane, and other products have yet to be established. The pattern of Cox expression may be different from aspirin sensitivity in polyposis.

CRS with NP and CRS without NP also differ in the expression of MMP (175). NP demonstrate MMP-9-positive inflammatory cells in pseudocysts, more intense MMP-9 and MMP-7 immunoreactive material in blood vessels, and higher tissue concentrations of MMP-7 compared to control turbinates and nonpolypoid CRS. In contrast, the concentrations of tissue MMP-9 and tissue inhibitor of metalloproteinase-1 protein (TIMP-1) were equally elevated in both types of CRS compared to control tissue. The authors suggest that differences in the regulation of enzyme expression and activities may help account for the distinct patterns of tissue remodeling observed in polypoid and nonpolypoid CRS.

HYPOTHESIS
Humoral Immune Defects Lead to Glandular Hypertrophy in CRS

We hypothesize that humoral immunodeficiencies are one of the fundamental factors underlying CRS with glandular hypertrophy (Fig. 5). In a retrospective analysis, we assessed the frequencies of low immunoglobulin isotype levels in CRS with NP and CRS without NP subjects (Table 1) (176). Absent IgE has been associated with CRS (177). Since there is no consensus for a lower limit of normal, we assumed that IgE < 10 IU/mL was indicative of a dysfunctional capacity to synthesize antigen-specific IgE. The lower limits of normal established by clinical laboratories were used to qualitatively define immune deficits for the other immunoglobulin isotypes. The CRS without nasal polyp group had significantly more subjects with IgE < 10 IU/mL and low IgG1, IgG3, and IgM. These frequen-cies were much higher than previously reported. However, previous reports did not stratify CRS subjects according to presumed histological subtype as done here.

TABLE 1 Frequencies of Qualitatively Low Antibody Levels for CRS with Nasal Polyps (CRS with NP) and CRS Without Nasal Polyps (CRS Without NP; Presumed Glandular Hypertrophy) Groups

Serum concentration below normal	CRS with NP	CRS without NP	ANOVA
Number per group	39	36	
IgE <10 IU/mL	3	21	0.000003
IgG1	8	21	0.0020
IgG2	2	5	0.2
IgG3	4	11	0.028
IgG4	2	7	0.058
IgA	3	6	0.2
IgM	3	9	0.042

Immunodeficiencies are more prevalent in CRS than control populations (178–180). Reduced total IgG was found in 18% , and IgA in 17% (180). Anergy to delayed-type hypersensitivity skin tests was detected in 40%. Common variable hypogammaglobulinemia was diagnosed in 10%. These findings suggest dysfunction of antigen presentation, T cell help, and/or B cell heavy chain switching and immunoglobulin secretion. We hypothesize that the humoral deficits play a "permissive" role by allowing novel and increasingly aggressive, virulent pathogens to occupy "unprotected" mucosal ecological niches in the sinuses (Fig. 5) Specific types of microbes may take advantage of the loss of secretory IgA, or IgG1- and IgG3-mediated immune complex, complement activation and Fcγ-receptor-mediated opsonization (181). Dysfunctional host defense mechanisms in IgE deficiency are unclear (182) but could involve low occupancy of FCεR-II on eosinophils and macrophages (183).

We further hypothesize that the colonizing microbes shed LPS, lipotechoic acids, β-glucans, CpG-rich DNA, and other products that are bound by the PLUNC and other families of innate immune proteins (125–129,131,132). These proteins then activate leukocytes and epithelial cells via toll-like receptor and other mechanisms. This may lead to paracrine release of cytokines and other innate immune biological response modifiers that initiate and promulgate glandular hypertrophy.

Epithelial Metaplasia in CRS

Evidence to support the changing ecological niches has been provided by the correlation between CT scan severity and epithelial metaplasia documented by scanning electron microscopy (5). Normal epithelium is dominated by ciliated cells. Narrowing of the OMC (May class 1) was associated with the replacement of ciliated goblet cells. The result was epithelial mucin hypersecretion with decreased mucociliary activity. Progression to May class 3 was associated with differentiation to microvillous cells. In pansinusitis (May class 4), there was squamous metaplasia with denuded basement membranes and local hemorrhage. We propose that gram-negative and anaerobic microbes that become blood-borne during brushing of the teeth and bowel movements may gain access to the sinuses through the injured mucosa.

Subsequent Progression to Glandular Hypertrophy

We hypothesize that activation of innate immune proteins by microbial factors is the first active step leading to epithelial metaplasia and glandular hypertrophy. These microbial factors may stimulate TLR and other mechanisms leading to epithelial chemokine release and the influx of leukoctyes. Any of a series of dysfunctional Th1, Th2, CD8, NK, B, or antigen-presenting cell activities could play permissive roles for microbial colonization. Recruitment of cells possessing dysfunctional mechanisms of action, or of secondary, but less effective immune mechanisms may accentuate the local immune deficit. The consequences may be an exhuberant immune response, but one that is inappropriate or unable to eliminate the colonizing microbes. This situation may be analogous to that of leprosy (184). Tuberculoid leprosy is the more well contained form of *Mycobacterium leprae* infection. It is characterized by appropriate Th1 and granulomatous macrophage responses that stop the spread of the organism. In contrast, the absence of effective Th1 defenses with recruitment of Th2-like responses occurs in lepromatous leprosy. Hypergammaglobulinemia and eosinophilia lead to ineffective killing of this intraphagolysozomal parasite. The ensuing attempts to eliminate the mycobacterium lead to tissue necrosis without limiting the spread of the microbe. *Mycobacterium avium—intracellulare* may be another model (185). Defects in INF-γ and IL-12 signaling pathways lead to ineffective Th1 responses. The absence of protective immunity may lead to the default recruitment of other, less effective antimicrobial mechanisms that lead to disease progression. In each of these situations and in CRS is it probable that the recruitment and activation of macrophages, neutrophils, eosinophils, endothelium, glands, and fibroblasts would lead to novel combinations of cytokines and other regulatory molecules that further stimulate the innate immune system. Glandular hypertrophy that maximizes exocytosis of mucins and serous cell antimicrobial proteins and cytokines may be the end result of such a defective mucosal immune response.

CONCLUSION

This review has summarized a number of observations that may contribute to the phenotype of CRS with glandular hypertrophy. As discussed, we believe that glandular hypertrophy is a key histologic abnormality in CRS and one that distinguishes CRS without NP from CRS with NP. Increased tissue area of Alcian Blue staining mucous (>11.5% of area) and serous cells (threshold not established) represent the cornerstone for glandular hypertrophy. Products of glandular exocytosis would be anticipated to be higher in this subtype compared to nasal polyposis. Polyps are associated with a 10-fold increase in albumin transudation compared to normal (40). If the glands are capable of responding to secretagogues such as methacholine (71) or hypertonic saline (83), then provocations with these agents may lead to glandular exocytosis in CRS without NP and negligible responses from polyps that lack glands, nerves, and vessels. Other features of this phenotype, such as indices of macrophage, neutrophil, eosinophil, and myofibroblast proliferation, are not yet elucidated, but may offer additional histochemical tools to distinguish glandular hypertrophy from polyposis. Immunohistochemical detection of TGF-β1 and associated submucosal fibrosis appears to be another marker of glandular hypertrophy (76). Immunodeficiency and atopy certainly impact on the histologic phenotype and must be used to stratify subjects for histopathologic studies. Multivariate and principal component analysis will be extremely valuable tools for dissecting and organizing the data derived from genomic, proteomic, histologic, cytokine, atopy, immunodeficiency, asthmatic, and other clinical data (80,81). The advanced methods discussed above require that investigators consider the multifactorial causes of CRS in much more sophisticated and nuanced fashion. The result will be a set of better defined disorders that can be classified by pathophysiological mechanisms, and one that can be approached in a more individualized and targeted manner than is currently the case.

ACKNOWLEDGMENTS

Supported by Public Health Service Award RO1 AI42403, and 1 M01-RR13297-01A1 from the General Clinical Research Center Program of the National Center for Research Resources, National Institutes of Health.

REFERENCES

1. Malekzadeh S, Hamburger MD, Whelan PJ, Biedlingmaier JF, Baraniuk JN. Density of middle turbinate subepithelial mucous glands in patients with chronic rhinosinusitis. Otolaryngol Head Neck Surg 2002; 127:190–5.
2. Malekzadeh S, Hamburger M, Biedlingmaier JF, Baraniuk JN. Density of middle turbinate subepithelial mucous glands in patients with chronic sinusitis and polyposis. Otolaryngology Society, Southern Meeting, 1997.
3. Malekzadeh S, Hamburger M, Biedlingmaier JF, Trifillis A, Baraniuk JN. Epithelial and glandular metaplasia in the middle turbinates of chronic sinusitis patients correlate with CT scan severity (May classification). J Allergy Clin Immunol 1998; 101:S250.
4. Malekzadeh S, McGuire JF. The new histologic classification of chronic rhinosinusitis. Curr Allergy Asthma Rep 2003; 3:221–6.
5. Biedlingmaier JF, Trifillis A. Comparison of CT scan and electron microscopic findings on endoscopically harvested middle turbinates. Otolaryngol Head Neck Surg 1998; 118:165–73.
6. Bachert C, Gevaert P, van Cauwenberge P. Nasal polyposis—a new concept on the formation of polyps. ACI Int 1999; 11:130–5.
7. Bachert C, Gevaert P, Holtappels G, Cuvelier C, van Cauwenberge P. Nasal polyposis: from cytokines to growth. Am J Rhinol 2000; 14:279–90.
8. Fritz SB, Terrell JE, Conner ER, Kukowska-Latallo JF, Baker JR. Nasal mucosal gene expression in patients with allergic rhinitis with and without nasal polyps. J Allergy Clin Immunol 2003; 112:1057–63.
9. Liu Z, Kim J, Sypek JP, et al. Gene expression profiles in human nasal polyp tissues studied by means of DNA microarray. J Allergy Clin Immunol 2004; 114:783–90.
10. Casado B, Pannell LK, Viglio S, Iadarola P, Baraniuk JN. Analysis of the sinusitis nasal lavage fluid proteome using capillary liquid chromatography interfaced to electro-spray ionization quadrupole-time of flight tandem mass spectrometry. Electrophoresis 2004; 25:1386–93.
11. Casado B, Pannell KL, Iadarola P, Baraniuk J. Identification of human nasal mucous proteins using proteomics. Proteomics 2005; 5:2949–2959.
12. Vento SI, Ertama LO, Hytonen ML, Wolff CH, Malmberg CH. Nasal polyposis: clinical course during 20 years. Ann Allergy Asthma Immunol 2000; 85:209–14.
13. May M, Levine HL. Endoscopic Sinus Surgery. York: Thiem Medical Publishing, 1993:105–25.
14. Cousin JN, Har-El G, Li J. Is there a correlation between radiographic and histologic findings in chronic sinusitis? J Otolaryngol 2000; 29:170–3.
15. Eichel BS. A proposal for a staging system for hyperplastic rhinosinusitis based on the presence or absence of intranasal polyposis. ENT J 1999; 78:262–8.

16. Mygind N, Lildholdt T. Nasal Polyposis. An Inflammatory Disease and Its Treatment. Copenhagen: Munksgaard, 1997;1–183.
17. Settipane GA, Lund VJ, Bernstein JM, Tos M. Nasal Polyps: Epidemiology, Pathogenesis and Treatment. Providence, RI: OceanSide Publications, 1997:1–189.
18. Lennard CM, Mann EA, Sun LL, Chang AS, Bolger WE. Interleukin-1 beta, interleukin-5, interleukin-6, interleukin-8, and tumor necrosis factor-alpha in chronic sinusitis: response to systemic corticosteroids. Am J Rhinol 2000; 14:367–73.
19. White K, Baraniuk JN. Chronic sinusitis subtypes and airway function. J Allergy Clin Immunol 2004; 113:S203.
20. Ogawa E, Elliott WM, Hughes F, Eichholtz TJ, Hogg JC, Hayashi S. Latent adenoviral infection induces production of growth factors relevant to airway remodeling in COPD. Am J Physiol Lung Cell Mol Physiol 2004; 286:L189–L197.
21. Shusterman D. Toxicology of nasal irritants. Curr Allergy Asthma Rep 2003; 3:258–65.
22. Saijo R, Majima Y, Hyo N, Takano H. Particle deposition of therapeutic aerosols in the nose and paranasal sinuses after transnasal sinus surgery: a cast model study. Am J Rhinol 2004; 18:1–7.
23. Hamilos DL, Leung DY, Huston DP, Kamil A, Wood R, Hamid Q. GM-CSF, IL-5 and RANTES immunoreactivity and mRNA expression in chronic hyperplastic sinusitis with nasal polyposis (NP). Clin Exp Allergy 1998; 28:1145–52.
24. Fakhri S, Frenkiel S, Hamid QA. Current views on the molecular biology of chronic sinusitis. J Otolaryngol 2002; 31:S2–9.
25. Lee CH, Lee KS, Rhee CS, Lee SO, Min YG. Distribution of RANTES and interleukin-5 in allergic nasal mucosa and nasal polyps. Ann Otol Rhinol Laryngol 1999; 108:594–8.
26. Allen JS, Eisma R, LaFreniere D, Leonard G, Kreutzer D. Characterization of the eosinophil chemokine RANTES in nasal polyps. Ann Otol Rhinol Laryngol 1998; 107:416–20.
27. Bartels J, Maune S, Meyer JE, et al. Increased eotaxin-mRNA expression in non-atopic and atopic nasal polyps: comparison to RANTES and MCP-3 expression. Rhinology 1997; 35:171–4.
28. Minshall EM, Cameron L, Lavigne F, et al. Eotaxin mRNA and protein expression in chronic sinusitis and allergen-induced nasal responses in seasonal allergic rhinitis. Am J Respir Cell Mol Biol 1997; 17:683–90.
29. Kamil A, Ghaffar O, Lavigne F, Taha R, Renzi PM, Hamid Q. Comparison of inflammatory cell profille and Th2 cytokine expression in the ethmoid sinuses, maxillary sinuses, and turbinates of atopic subjects with chronic sinusitis. Otolaryngol Head Neck Surg 1998; 118:804–9.
30. Wright ED, Frenkiel S, Ghaffar O, et al. Monocyte chemotactic protein expression in allergy and non-allergy-associated chronic sinusitis. J Otolaryngol 1998; 27:281–7.
31. Hamilos DL, Leung DL, Wood R, et al. Chronic hyperplastic sinusitis: association of tissue eosinophilia with mRNA expression of granulocyte-macrophage colony-stimulating factor and interleukin-3. J Allergy Clin Immunol 1993; 92:39–48.
32. Ohno I, Lea R, Finotto S, et al. Granulocyte/macrophage colony-stimulating factor (GM-CSF) gene expression by eosonophils in nasal polyposis. Am J Respir Cell Mol Biol 1991; 5:505–10.
33. Hamilos DL, Leung DY, Wood R, et al. Evidence for distinct cytokine expression in allergic versus nonallergic chronic sinusitis. J Allergy Clin Immunol 1995; 96:537–44.
34. Montesano R, Orci L. Transforming growth factor-β stimulates collagen-matrix contraction by fibroblasts: implications for wound healing. Proc Natl Acad Sci U S A 1988; 85:4894–7.
35. Coste A, Lefaucher JP, Wang QP, et al. Expression of the transforming growth factor beta isoforms in inflammatory cells of nasal polyps. Arch Otol Head Neck Surgery 1998; 124:1361–6.
36. Eisma RJ, Allen JS, LaFreniere D, Leonard G, Kreutzer DL. Eosinophil expression of transforming growth factor-beta and its receptors in nasal polyposis: role of the cytokines in this disease process. Am J Otolaryngol 1997; 18:405–11.
37. Clark RAF, Folkvord JM, Hart CE, Murray MJ, McPherson JM. Platelet isoforms of platelet-derived growth factor stimulate fibroblasts to contract collagen matrices. J Clin Invest 1989; 84:1036–40.

38. Rasp G, Thomas PA, Bujia J. Eosinophil inflammation of the nasal mucosa in allergic and non-allergic rhinitis measured by eosinophil cationic protein levels in native nasal fluid and serum. Clin Exp Allergy 1994; 24:1151–6.
39. Georgitis JW, Matthews BL, Stone B. Chronic sinusitis: characterization of cellular influx and inflammatory mediators in sinus lavage fluid. Int Arch Allergy Immunol 1995; 106:416–21.
40. Biewenga J, Stoop AE, van der Heijden HA, van der Baan S, van Kamp GJ. Albumin and immunoglobulin levels in nasal secretions of patients with nasal polyps treated with endoscopic sinus surgery and topical corticosteroids. J Allergy Clin Immunol 1995; 96:334–40.
41. Gabbiani G. Evolution and clinical implications of the myofibroblast concept. Cardiovas Res 1998; 38:545–8.
42. Montesano R, Orci L. Transforming growth factor-β stimulates collagen-matrix contraction by fibroblasts: implications for wound healing. Proc Natl Acad Sci U S A 1988; 85:4894–7.
43. Powers MR, Qu Z, LaGesse PC, Liebler JM, Wall MA, Rosenbaum JT. Expression of basic fibroblast growth factor in nasal polyps. Ann Otol Rhinol Laryngol 1998; 107:891–7.
44. Petruson B, Hansson HA, Petrusson K. Insulin-like growth factor I immunoreactivity in nasal polyps. Arch Otolaryngol Head Neck Surg 1988; 114:1272–5.
45. Zhang S, Smartt H, Holgate ST, Roche WR. Growth factors secreted by bronchial epithelial cells control myofibroblast proliferation: an in vitro co-culture model of airway remodeling in asthma. Lab Invest 1999; 79:395–405.
46. Tang W, Geba GP, Zheng T, et al. Targeted expression of IL-11 in the murine airway causes lymphocytic inflammation, bronchial remodeling, and airways obstruction. J Clin Invest 1996; 98:2845–53.
47. Coste A, Brugel L, Maitre B, et al. Inflammatory cells as well as epithelial cells in nasal polyps express vascular endothelial growth factor. Eur Respir J 2000; 15: 367–72.
48. Wittekindt C, Hess A, Bloch W, Sultanie S, Michel O. Immunohistochemical expression of VEGF and VEGF receptors in nasal polyps as compared to normal turbinate mucosa. Eur Arch Otorhinolaryngol 2002; 259:294–8.
49. Ishibashi T, Tanaka T, Nibu K, Ishimoto S, Kaga K. Keratinocyte growth factor and its receptor messenger RNA expression in nasal mucosa and nasal polyps. Ann Otol Rhinol Laryngol 1998; 107:85–89.
50. Ghaffar O, Lavigne F, Kamil A, Renzi P, Hamid Q. Interleukin-6 expression in chronic sinusitis: colocalization of gene transcripts to eosinophils, macrophages, T Lymphocytes, and mast cells. Otolaryngol Head Neck Surg 1998; 118: 504–11.
51. Rudack C, Stoll W, Bachert C. Cytokines in nasal polyposis, acute and chronic sinusitis. Am J Rhino 1998; 12:383–8.
52. Zhang S, Howarth PH, Roche WR. Cytokine production by cell cultures from bronchial subepithelial myofibroblasts. J Pathol 1996; 180:95–101.
53. Mullol J, Xaubet A, Gaya A, et al. Cytokine gene expression and release from epithelial cells. A comparison study between healthy nasal mucosa and nasal polyps. Clin Exp Allergy 1995; 25:607–15.
54. Singer AJ, Clark RAF. Cutaneous wound healing. New Engl J Med 1999; 341:738–46.
55. Schiro JA, Chan BM, Roswit WT, et al. Integrinα2β1 (VLA-2) mediates reorganization and contraction of collagen matrices by human cells. Cell 1999; 67:403–10.
56. Gungor A, Baroody FM, Naclerio RM, White SR, Corey JP. Decreased neuropeptide release may play a role in the pathogenesis of nasal polyps. Otolaryngol Head Neck Surg 1999; 121:585–90.
57. Norlander T, Bolger WE, Stierna P, Uddman R, Carlsoo B. A comparison of morphological effects on the rabbit nasal and sinus mucosa after surgical denervation and topical capsaicin application. Eur Arch Otorhinolaryngol 1996; 253:205–13.
58. Carver TW Jr, Srinathan SK, Velloff CR, Perez Fontan JJ. Increased type I procollagen mRNA in airways and pulmonary vessels after vagal denervation in rats. Am J Respir Cell Mol Biol 1997; 17:691–701.

59. Di Lorenzo G, Drago A, Esposito Pellitteri M, et al. Measurement of inflammatory mediators of mast cells and eosinophils in native nasal lavage fluid in nasal polyposis. Int Arch Allergy Immunol 2001; 125:164–75.

60. Bhattacharyya N, Vyas DK, Fechner FP, Gliklich RE, Metson R. Tissue eosinophilia in chronic sinusitis: quantification techniques. Arch Otolaryngol Head Neck Surg 2001; 127:1102–5.

61. Kassim SK, Elbeigermy M, Nasr GF, Khalil R, Nassar M. The role of interleukin-12, and tissue antioxidants in chronic sinusitis. Clin Biochem 2002; 35:369–75.

62. Wright ED, Christodoulopoulos P, Frenkiel S, Hamid Q. Expression of interleukin (IL)-12 (p40) and IL-12 (beta 2) receptors in allergic rhinitis and chronic sinusitis. Clin Exp Allergy 1999; 29:1320–5.

63. Jyonouchi H, Sun S, Le H, Rimell FL. Evidence of dysregulated cytokine production by sinus lavage and peripheral blood mononuclear cells in patients with treatment-resistant chronic rhinosinusitis. Arch Otolaryngol Head Neck Surg 2001; 127:1488–94.

64. Kountakis SE, Arango P, Bradley D, Wade ZK, Borish L. Molecular and cellular staging for the severity of chronic rhinosinusitis. Laryngoscope 2004; 114:1895–905.

65. Widel F, Abrami P, Lermoyez J. Anaphylaxie et idiosyncrasie. Presse Med 1922; 30:189–93.

66. Samter M, Beers RF. Intolerance to aspirin: Clinical studies and consideration of its pathogenesis. Ann Int Med 1968; 68:975–83.

67. Sousa AR, Parikh A, Scadding G, Corrigan CJ, Lee TK. Leukotriene receptor expression on nasal mucosal inflammatory cells in aspirin-sensitive rhinosinusitis. N Engl J Med 2002; 347:1493–9.

68. Marple BF. Allergic fungal rhinosinusitis: current theories and management strategies. Laryngoscope 2001; 111:1006–19.

69. Kremer B, Jacobs JA, Soudijn ER, van der Ven AJ. Clinical value of bacteriological examinations of nasal and paranasal mucosa in patients with chronic sinusitis. Eur Arch Otorhinolaryngol 2001; 258:220–5.

70. Perl TM, Cullen JJ, Wenzel RP, et al. and the Mupirocin And The Risk of Staphylococcus aureus Study Team. Intranasal mupirocin to prevent postoperative *Staphylococcus aureus* infections. N Engl J Med 2002; 346:1871–7.

71. Jeney EV, Raphael GD, Meredith SD, Kaliner MA. Abnormal cholinergic parasympathetic responsiveness in the nasal mucosa of patients with recurrent sinusitis. J Allergy Clin Immunol 1990; 86:10–18.

72. Larsen PL, Tos M, Mogensen C. Nasal glands and goblet cells in chronic hypertrophic rhinitis. Am J Otolaryngol 1986; 7:28–33.

73. Eusebi VV. Microglandular adenosis arising in a chronic paranasal sinusitis. Histopathology 2000; 37:474.

74. Assimakopoulos D, Danielides V, Kontogiannis N, Skevas A, Evangelou A, Van Cauwenberge P. Seromucous maxillary sinusitis (SMMS): a clinicophysiological approach. Acta Otorhinolaryngol Belg 2001; 55:65–9.

75. Kakoi H, Hiraide F. A histological study of formation and growth of nasal polyps. Acta Otolaryngol 1987; 103:137–44.

76. Watelet JB, Claeys C, Perez-Novo C, Gevaert P, Van Cauwenberge P, Bachert C. Transforming growth factor beta1 in nasal remodeling: differences between chronic rhinosinusitis and nasal polyposis. Am J Rhinol 2004; 18:267–72.

77. Caye-Thomasen P, Hermansson A, Tos M, Prellner K. Polyps pathogenesis—a histopathological study in experimental otitis media. Acta Otolaryngol 1995; 115:76–82.

78. Leprini S, Garaventa G, Pallestrini R, Leprini E, Pallestrini EA. Analysis of the cellular infiltrate and epithelial class I and II molecular expression in edematous type nasal polyps. Allergy 2004; 59:54–60.

79. Majima Y, Masuda S, Sakakura Y. Quantitative study of nasal secretory cells in normal subjects and patients with chronic sinusitis. Laryngoscope 1997 107:1515–8.

80. Facon F, Paris J, Guisiano B, Dessi P. Multifactorial analysis of preoperative functional symptoms in nasal polyposis (report of 403 patients). Rev Laryngol Otol Rhinol (Bord) 2003; 124:151–9.

81. Bonfils P, Halimi P, Le Bihan C, Nores JM, Avan P, Landais P. Correlation between nasosinusal symptoms and topographic diagnosis in chronic rhinosinusitis. Ann Otol Rhinol Laryngol 2005; 114:74–83.
82. Adam G. Visceral Perception: Understanding Internal Organs. New York: Plenum Press, 1998.
83. Baraniuk JN, Petrie KN, Le U, et al. Neuropathology in rhinosinusitis. Am J Respir Crit Care Med 2005; 171:5–11.
84. Naranch K, Park Y-J, Repka-Ramirez SM, Velarde A, Clauw D, Baraniuk JN. A tender sinus does not always mean sinusitis. Otolaryngol Head Neck Surg 2002; 127:387–97.
85. Acquardo MA, Montgomery WW. Treatment of chronic paranasal sinus pain with minimal sinus CT changes. Ann Otol Rhinol Laryngol 1996; 105:607–14.
86. Ali M, Maniscalco J, Baraniuk JN. Spontaneous release of submucosal gland serous and mucous cell macromolecules from human nasal explants in vitro. Am J Physiol Lung Cell Mol Physiol 1996; 14:L595–600.
87. Pon DJ, van Staden CJ, Rodger IW. Hypertrophic and hyperplastic changes of mucus-secreting epithelial cells in rat airways: assessment using a novel, rapid, and simple technique. Am J Respir Cell Mol Biol 1994; 10:625–34.
88. Davies JR, Herrmann A, Russell W, Svitacheva N, Wickstrom C, Carlstedt I. Respiratory tract mucins: structure and expression patterns. Novartis Found Symp 2002; 248:76–88.
89. Bhattacharyya SN, Dubick MA, Yantis LD, et al. In vivo effect of wood smoke on the expression of two mucin genes in rat airways. Inflammation 2004; 28:67–76.
90. Copin MC, Buisine MP, Devisme L, et al. Normal respiratory mucosa, precursor lesions and lung carcinomas: differential expression of human mucin genes. Front Biosci 2001; 6:D1264–75.
91. Sharma P, Dudus L, Nielsen PA, et al. MUC5B and MUC7 are differentially expressed in mucous and serous cells of submucosal glands in human bronchial airways. Am J Respir Cell Mol Biol 1998; 19:30–7.
92. Kaneko T, Komiyama K, Horie N, Tsuchiya M, Moro I, Shimoyama T. A histochemical study of inflammatory lesions of the maxillary sinus mucosa using biotinylated lectins. J Oral Sci 2000; 42:87–91.
93. Delmotte P, Degroote S, Merten MD, et al. Influence of TNF-alpha on the sialylation of mucins produced by a transformed cell line MM-39 derived from human tracheal gland cells. Glycoconj J 2001; 18:487–97.
94. Kim DH, Chu HS, Lee JY, Hwang SJ, Lee SH, Lee HM. Up-regulation of MUC5AC and MUC5B mucin genes in chronic rhinosinusitis. Arch Otolaryngol Head Neck Surg 2004; 130:747–52.
95. Jung HH, Lee JH, Kim YT, Lee SD, Park JH. Expression of mucin genes in chronic ethmoiditis. Am J Rhinol 2000; 14:163–70.
96. Seong JK, Koo JS, Lee WJ, et al. Upregulation of MUC8 and downregulation of MUC5AC by inflammatory mediators in human nasal polyps and cultured nasal epithelium. Acta Otolaryngol 2002; 122:401–7.
97. Aust MR, Madsen CS, Jennings A, Kasperbauer JL, Gendler SJ. Mucin mRNA expression in normal and vasomotor inferior turbinates. Am J Rhinol 1997; 11:293–302.
98. Rogers DF. The airway goblet cell. Int J Biochem Cell Biol 2003; 35:1–6.
99. Takeyama K, Fahy JV, Nadel JA. Relationship of epidermal growth factor receptors to goblet cell production in human bronchi. Am J Respir Crit Care Med 2001; 163: 511–6.
100. Burgel PR, Escudier E, Coste A, et al. Relation of epidermal growth factor receptor expression to goblet cell hyperplasia in nasal polyps. J Allergy Clin Immunol 2000; 106:705–712.
101. Reindel JF, Gough AW, Pilcher GD, Bobrowski WF, Sobocinski GP, de la Iglesia FA. Systemic proliferative changes and clinical signs in cynomolgus monkeys administered a recombinant derivative of human epidermal growth factor. Toxicol Pathol 2001; 29:159–73.
102. Takeyama K, Dabbagh K, Lee HM, et al. Epidermal growth factor system regulates mucin production in airways, Proc Natl Acad Sci USA 1999; 16:3081–6.

103. Amishima M, Munakata M, Nasuhara Y, et al. Expression of epidermal growth factor and epidermal growth factor receptor immunoreactivity in the asthmatic human airway. Am J Respir Crit Care Med 1998; 157:1907–12.
104. Levine SJ, Larivee P, Logun C, Angus CW, Ognibene FP, Shelhammer JH. Tumor necrosis factor-alpha induces mucin hypersecretion and MUC-2 gene expression by human airway epithelial cells. Am J Respir Cell Mol Biol 1995; 12:196–204.
105. Louahed J, Toda M, Jen J, et al. Interleukin-9 upregulates mucus expression in the airways. Am J Respir Cell Mol Biol 2000; 22:649–56.
106. Longphre M, Li D, Gallup M, et al. Allergen-induced IL-9 directly stimulates mucin transcription in respiratory epithelial cells. J Clin Invest 1999; 104:1375–82.
107. Dabbagh K, Takeyama K, Lee HM, Ueki IF, Lausier JA, Nadel JA. IL-4 induces mucin gene expression and goblet cell metaplasia in vitro and in vivo. J Immunol 1999; 162:6233–7.
108. Temann UA, Prasad B, Gallup MW, et al. A novel role for murine IL-4 expression and mucin hypersecretion. Am J Respir Cell Mol Biol 1997; 16:471–8.
109. Wills-Karp M, Luyimbazi J, Xu X, et al. Interleukin-13: central mediator of allergic asthma. Science 1999; 282:2258–61.
110. Whittaker L, Niu N, Temann UA, et al. Interleukin-13 mediates a fundamental pathway for airway epithelial mucus induced by CD4 T cells and interleukin-9. Am J Respir Cell Mol Biol 2002; 27:593–602.
111. Cohn L, Whittaker L, Niu N, Homer RJ. Cytokine regulation of mucus production in a model of allergic asthma. Novartis Found Symp 2002; 248:201–13; discussion 213–20, 277–82.
112. Toda M, Tulic MK, Levitt RC, Hamid Q. A calcium-activated chloride channel (HCLCA1) is strongly related to IL-9 expression and mucus production in bronchial epithelium of patients with asthma. J Allergy Clin Immunol 2002; 109:246–50.
113. Sharma P, Dudus L, Nielsen PA, et al. MUC5B and MUC7 are differentially expressed in mucous and serous cells of submucosal glands in human bronchial airways. Am J Respir Cell Mol Biol 1998; 19:30–7.
114. Wickstrom C, Davies JR, Eriksen GV, Veerman EC, Carlstedt I. MUC5B is a major gel-forming, oligomeric mucin from human salivary gland, respiratory tract and endocervix: identification of glycoforms and C-terminal cleavage. Biochem J 1998; 334:685–93.
115. Copin MC, Buisine MP, Devisme L, et al. Normal respiratory mucosa, precursor lesions and lung carcinomas: differential expression of human mucin genes. Front Biosci 2001; 6:D1264–75.
116. Kim CH, Song KS, Kim SS, Kim HU, Seong JK, Yoon JH. Expression of MUC5AC mRNA in the goblet cells of human nasal mucosa. Laryngoscope 2000; 110:2110–3.
117. Raphael GD, Jeney EV, Baraniuk JN, Kim I, Meredith SD, Kaliner MA. The pathophysiology of rhinitis: lactoferrin and lysozyme in nasal secretions. J Clin Invest 1989; 84:1528–35.
118. Lee CH, Igarashi Y, Hohman RJ, Kaulbach H, White MV, Kaliner MA. Distribution of secretory leukoprotease inhibitor in the human nasal airway. Am Rev Respir Dis 1993; 147:710–6.
119. Baraniuk JN, Ohkubo K, Kwon OJ, et al. Localization of neutral endopeptidase mRNA in human nasal mucosa. J Appl Physiol 1993; 74:272–9.
120. Ohkubo K, Baraniuk JN, Hohman R, Merida M, Hersh LB, Kaliner MA. Aminopeptidase activity in human nasal mucosa. J Allergy Clin Immunol 1998; 102:741–50.
121. Hamaguchi Y, Ohi M, Sakakura Y, Miyoshi Y. Purification of glandular kallikrein in maxillary mucosa from humans suffering from chronic inflammation. Enzyme 1985; 33:41–8.
122. Wilson E, Butcher CE. CCL28 controls immunoglobulin (Ig)A plasma cell accumulation in the lactating mammary gland and IgA antibody transfer to the neonate. J Exp Med 2004; 200:805–9.
123. Kvale D, Lovhaug D, Sollid LM, Brandtzaeg P. Tumor necrosis factor-alpha upregulates expression of secretory component, the epithelial receptor for polymeric Ig. J Immunol 1988; 140:3086–9.
124. Brandtzaeg P. Immunocompetent cells of the upper airway: functions in normal and diseased mucosa. Eur Arch Otorhinolaryngol 1995; 252(Suppl. 1):S8–21.

125. Meredith SD, Raphael GD, Baraniuk JN, Banks SM, Kaliner MA. The pathophysiology of rhinitis. III. The control of IgG secretion. J Allergy Clin Immunol 1989; 84:920–30.

126. Bingle CD, Craven L. Characterisation of the human plunc gene, a gene product with an upper airways and nasopharyngeal restricted expression pattern. Biochim Biophys Acta 2000; 1493:363–7.

127. Casado B, Pannell L, Iadarola P, Baraniuk J. Identification of lipocalin family proteins in nasal secretions. Exp Lung Res 2003; 29(Suppl.):93–121.

128. Koppelman GH, Postma DS. The genetics of CD14 in allergic disease. Curr Opin Allergy Clin Immunol 2003; 3:347–52.

129. Dabbagh K, Lewis DB. Toll-like receptors and T-helper-1/T-helper-2 responses. Curr Opin Infect Dis 2003; 16:199–204.

130. Claeys S, de Belder T, Holtappels G, et al. Human beta-defensins and toll-like receptors in the upper airway. Allergy 2003; 58:748–53.

131. Pelosi P. Odorant-binding proteins. Crit Rev Biochem Mol Biol 1994; 29:199–228.

132. Weber JR, Freyer D, Alexander C, et al. Recognition of pneumococcal peptidoglycan: an expanded, pivotal role for LPS binding protein. Immunity 2003; 19:269–79.

133. Weiss J. Bactericidal/permeability-increasing protein (BPI) and lipopolysaccharide-binding protein (LBP): structure, function and regulation in host defence against Gram-negative bacteria. Biochem Soc Trans 2003; 31:785–90.

134. Lee SH, Lim HH, Lee HM, Choi JO. Expression of human beta-defensin 1 mRNA in human nasal mucosa. Acta Otolaryngol 2000; 120:58–61.

135. Chen PH, Fang SY. Expression of human beta-defensin 2 in human nasal mucosa. Eur Arch Otorhinolaryngol 2004; 261:238–41.

136. Saito H, Abe J, Matsumoto K. Allergy-related genes in microarray: an update review. J Allergy Clin Immunol 2005; 116:56–9.

137. Baraniuk JN, Wong G, Ali M, Sabol M, Troost T. Glucocorticoids decrease c-fos expression in human nasal polyps in vivo. Thorax 1998; 53:577–82.

138. Lee SH, Lee SH, Oh BH, Lee HM, Choi JO, Jung KY. Expression of mRNA of trefoil factor peptides in human nasal mucosa. Acta Otolaryngol 2001; 121:849–53.

139. Yates JR III. Mass spectrometry from genomics to proteomics TIG 2000; 16:5–8.

140. Patterson SD, Aebersold RH. Proteomics: the first decade and beyond. Nat Genet 2003; 33(Suppl.):311–23.

141. Fessler MB, Malcolm KC, Duncan MW, Worthen GS. A genomic and proteomic analysis of activation of the human neutrophil by lipopolysaccharide and its mediation by p38 mitogen-activated protein kinase. J Biol Chem 2002; 277:31291–302.

142. McRedmond JP, Park SD, Reilly DF, et al. Integration of proteomics and genomics in platelets: a profile of platelet proteins and platelet-specific genes. Mol Cell Proteomics 2004; 3:133–44.

143. Rapheal GD, Meredith SD, Baraniuk JN, Druce HM, Banks SM, Kaliner MA. The pathophysiology of rhinitis. II. Assessment of the sources of protein in histamine-induced nasal secretions. Am Rev Respir Dis 1989; 139:791–800.

144. Kempuraj D, Frydas S, Conti P, et al. Interleukin-25 (or IL-17E): a new IL-17 family member with growth factor/inflammatory actions. Int J Immunopathol Pharmacol 2003; 16:185–8.

145. Kim MR, Manoukian R, Yeh R, et al. Transgenic overexpression of human IL-17E results in eosinophilia, B-lymphocyte hyperplasia, and altered antibody production. Blood 2002; 100:2330–40.

146. Clark HF, Gurney AL, Abaya E, et al. The secreted protein discovery initiative (SPDI), a large-scale effort to identify novel human secreted and transmembrane proteins: a bioinformatics assessment. Genome Res 2003; 13:2265–70.

147. Bar-Or A, Nuttall RK, Duddy M, et al. Analyses of all matrix metalloproteinase members in leukocytes emphasize monocytes as major inflammatory mediators in multiple sclerosis. Brain 2003; 126:2738–49.

148. Kosaki A, Hasegawa T, Kimura T, et al. Increased plasma S100A12 (EN-RAGE) levels in patients with type 2 diabetes. J Clin Endocrinol Metab 2004; 89:5423–8.

149. Sakata Y, Arima K, Takai T, et al. The squamous cell carcinoma antigen 2 inhibits the cysteine proteinase activity of a major mite allergen, Der p 1. J Biol Chem 2004; 279:5081–7.

150. Yuyama N, Davies DE, Akaiwa M, et al. Analysis of novel disease-related genes in bronchial asthma. Cytokine 2002; 19:287–96.
151. Whittaker L, Niu N, Temann UA, et al. Interleukin-13 mediates a fundamental pathway for airway epithelial mucus induced by CD4 T cells and interleukin-9. Am J Respir Cell Mol Biol 2002; 27:593–602.
152. Emery BE, White MV, Igarashi Y, et al. The effect of IL-4 on human nasal mucosal responses. J Allergy Clin Immunol 1992; 90:772–81.
153. Emanuel IA, Shah SB: Chronic rhinosinusitis: Allergy and sinus computed tomography relationships. Otolaryngol Head Neck Surg 2000; 123:687–91.
154. Benninger MS. Rhinitis, sinusitis, and their relationships to allergies. Am J Rhinol 1992; 6:37–43.
155. Rachelefsky GS: Chronic sinusitis. The disease of all ages. Am J Dis Child 1989; 143:886–8.
156. Kalfa VC, Spector SL, Ganz T, Cole AM. Lysozyme levels in the nasal secretions of patients with perennial allergic rhinitis and recurrent sinusitis. Ann Allergy Asthma Immunol 2004; 93:288–92.
157. von Bubnoff D, Fimmers R, Bogdanow M, Matz H, Koch S, Bieber T. Asymptomatic atopy is associated with increased indoleamine 2,3-dioxygenase activity and interleukin-10 production during seasonal allergen exposure. Clin Exp Allergy 2004; 34:1056–63.
158. von Bubnoff D, Hanau D, Wenzel J, et al. Indoleamine 2,3-dioxygenase-expressing antigen-presenting cells and peripheral T-cell tolerance: another piece to the atopic puzzle? J Allergy Clin Immunol 2003; 112:854–60.
159. Ohkubo K, Ikeda M, Pawankar R, Gotoh M, Yagi T, Okuda M. Mechanisms of IL-6, IL-8, and GM-CSF release in nasal secretions of allergic patients after nasal challenge. Rhinology 1998; 36:156–61.
160. Tabary O, Zahm JM, Hinnrasky J, et al. Selective up-regulation of chemokine IL-8 expression in cystic fibrosis bronchial gland cells in vivo and in vitro. Am J Pathol 1998; 153:921–30.
161. Delbrouck C, Gabius HJ, Vandenhoven G, Kiss R, Hassid S. Budesonide-dependent modulation of expression of macrophage migration inhibitory factor in a polyposis model: evidence for differential regulation in surface and glandular epithelia. Ann Otol Rhinol Laryngol 2004; 113:544–51.
162. Lee HM, Choi JH, Chae SW, Hwang SJ, Lee SH. Expression of epidermal growth factor receptor and its ligands in chronic sinusitis. Ann Otol Rhinol Laryngol 2003; 112:132–8.
163. Ruhl S, Hamberger S, Betz R, et al. Salivary proteins and cytokines in drug-induced gingival overgrowth. J Dent Res 2004; 83:322–6.
164. Little FF, Cruikshank WW, Center DM. IL-9 stimulates release of chemotactic factors from human bronchial epithelial cells. Am J Respir Cell Mol Biol 2001; 25:347–52.
165. Roca-Ferrer J, Mullol J, Xaubet A, et al. Proinflammatory cytokines and eosinophil cationic protein on glandular secretion from human nasal mucosa: regulation by corticosteroids. J Allergy Clin Immunol 2001; 108:87–93.
166. Untergasser G, Gander R, Lilg C, Lepperdinger G, Plas E, Berger P. Profiling molecular targets of TGF-beta1 in prostate fibroblast-to-myofibroblast transdifferentiation. Mech Ageing Dev 2005; 126:59–69.
167. Rudack C, Sachse F, Alberty J. Chronic rhinosinusitis–need for further classification? Inflamm Res 2004; 53:111–7.
168. Davidsson A, Danielsen A, Viale G, et al. Positive identification in situ of mRNA expression of IL-6, and IL-12, and the chemotactic cytokine RANTES in patients with chronic sinusitis and polypoid disease. Clinical relevance and relation to allergy. Acta Otolaryngol 1996; 116:604–10.
169. Jeffery PK. Comparison of the structural and inflammatory features of COPD and asthma. Giles F. Filley Lecture. Chest 2000; 117(5 Suppl. 1):251S–60S.
170. Jeffery PK. Differences and similarities between chronic obstructive pulmonary disease and asthma. Clin Exp Allergy 1999; 29(Suppl. 2):14–26.
171. Zhu J, Majumdar S, Oui Y, et al. Interleukin-4 and interleukin-5 gene expression and inflammation in the mucus-secreting glands and subepithelial tissue of smokers with

chronic bronchitis. Lack of relationship with CD8(+) cells. Am J Respir Crit Care Med 2001; 164:2220–8.

172. Ogawa N, Kawanami T, Shimoyama K, Ping L, Sugai S. Expression of interferon-inducible T cell alpha chemoattractant (CXCL11) in the salivary glands of patients with Sjogren's syndrome. Clin Immunol 2004; 112:235–8.

173. Rotondi M, Lazzeri E, Romagnani P, Serio M. Role for interferon-gamma inducible chemokines in endocrine autoimmunity: an expanding field. J Endocrinol Invest 2003; 26:177–80.

174. Gosepath J, Brieger J, Gletsou E, Mann WJ. Expression and localization of cyclooxygenases (Cox-1 and Cox-2) in nasal respiratory mucosa. Does Cox-2 play a key role in the immunology of nasal polyps? J Investig Allergol Clin Immunol 2004; 14:114–8.

175. Watelet JB, Bachert C, Claeys C, Van Cauwenberge P. Matrix metalloproteinases MMP-7, MMP-9 and their tissue inhibitor TIMP-1: expression in chronic sinusitis vs. nasal polyposis. Allergy 2004; 59:54–60.

176. Baraniuk, JN, White K. Immunodeficiency in subtypes of chronic sinusitis. J Allergy Clin Imunol 2004; 113:S203.

177. Smith JK, Krishnaswamy GH, Dykes R, Reynolds S, Berk SL. Clinical manifestations of IgE hypogammaglobulinemia. Ann Allergy Asthma Immunol 1997; 78:313–8.

178. Finocchi A, Angelini F, Chini L, et al. Evaluation of the relevance of humoral immunodeficiencies in a pediatric population affected by recurrent infections. Pediatr Allergy Immunol 2002; 13:443–7.

179. Litzman J, Sevcikova I, Stikarovska D, Pikulova Z, Pazdirkova A, Lokaj J. IgA deficiency in Czech healthy individuals and selected patient groups. Int Arch Allergy Immunol 2000; 123:177–80.

180. Chee L, Graham SM, Carothers DG, Ballas ZK. Immune dysfunction in refractory sinusitis in a tertiary care setting. Laryngoscope 2001; 111:233–5.

181. Lund VJ, Scadding GK. Immunologic aspects of chronic sinusitis. J Otolaryngol 1991; 20:379–81.

182. Smith JK, Krishnaswamy GH, Dykes R, Reynolds S, Berk SL. Clinical manifestations of IgE hypogammaglobulinemia. Ann Allergy Asthma Immunol 1997; 78:313–8.

183. Abdelilah SG, Bouchaib L, Morita M, et al. Molecular characterization of the low-affinity IgE receptor Fc epsilonRII/CD23 expressed by human eosinophils. Int Immunol 1998; 10:395–404.

184. Modlin RL. Learning from leprosy: insights into contemporary immunology from an ancient disease. Skin Pharmacol Appl Skin Physiol 2002; 15:1–6.

185. Cosma CL, Sherman DR, Ramakrishnan L. The secret lives of the pathogenic mycobacteria. Annu Rev Microbiol 2003; 57:641–76.

9

Bacterial Infection and Antibiotic Treatment in Chronic Rhinosinusitis

Itzhak Brook

Georgetown University School of Medicine, Washington, D.C., U.S.A.

INTRODUCTION

Rhinosinusitis generally occurs following an acute viral upper respiratory tract infection. It is estimated that almost nine out of ten patients with a cold develop viral rhinosinusitis. Acute bacterial infection of the sinuses occurs in 0.5–2% of these individuals, which brings about the development of acute bacterial rhinosinusitis in about 20 million Americans yearly (1,2).

The oropharynx is colonized by aerobic and anaerobic bacteria which can also include potential pathogenic bacteria capable of causing respiratory tract infections including rhinosinusitis (3). Establishing the correct microbiology of all the forms of rhinosinusitis is of great clinical importance as it can assist in the selection of adequate antimicrobial therapy. This chapter outlines the microbiology and management of chronic rhinosinusitis (CRS).

THE ORAL CAVITY NORMAL FLORA

The human body mucosal and epithelial surfaces, including the oropharynx, are colonized by aerobic and anaerobic bacteria (3). The predominant members of the oropharyngeal flora are anaerobic bacteria, which outnumber their aerobic counterparts in ratios of 10–100 to one. The number of anaerobes at a site is generally inversely related to the oxygen tension (3). Familiarity with the composition of the oropharyngeal flora is helpful in predicting which organisms may become involved in an infection adjacent to that site and can assist in the selection of proper empirical antimicrobial therapy.

The normal flora does not serve as a potential source of pathogenic bacteria, but can serve as a beneficial protector from colonization or subsequent invasion by potentially pathogenic bacteria. The formation of the normal oropharyngeal flora is initiated at birth and reaches adult composition by 1–2 years (3). However, colonization with potential respiratory pathogens is more commonly observed in young children, especially during a viral infection.

The most predominant group of facultative microorganisms native to the oropharynx are the alpha-hemolytic streptococci which include the species *Streptococcus mitis, Streptococcus milleri, Streptococcus sanguis, Streptococcus intermedius, Streptococcus salivarius,* and several others (4). Other groups of organisms native to the oropharynx are *Moraxella catarrhalis* and *Haemophillus influenzae,* organisms that are capable of producing beta-lactamase. The oropharynx also contains *Staphylococcus aureus* and *Staphylococcus epidermidis* both of which can also produce beta-lactamase.

The normal oropharynx is seldom colonized by gram-negative *Enterobacteriaceae*. In contrast, hospitalized patients are generally heavily colonized by these organisms (5). The shift from predominantly gram-positive to gram-negative bacteria is thought to contribute to the high incidence of sinus infection caused by gram-negative bacteria in patients with chronic illnesses.

Anaerobic bacteria are present in large numbers in the oropharynx, particularly in patients with poor dental hygiene, caries, or periodontal disease. Anaerobic bacteria outnumber their aerobic counterparts in ratios of 10:1 to 100:1. Anaerobes can adhere to tooth surfaces and contribute through the elaboration of metabolic byproducts to the development of both caries and periodontal disease (4). The predominant anaerobes are *Peptostreptococcus, Veillonella, Bacteroides*, and pigmented *Prevotella, Porphyromonas*, and *Fusobacterium* spp (4). These bacteria can serve as a potential cause of various chronic respiratory tract infections including otitis and rhinosinusitis, aspiration pneumonia, lung abscesses, and oropharyngeal and dental abscesses.

Over half of pigmented *Prevotella, Porphyromonas*, and *Fusobacterium* spp. produce beta-lactamase especially in patients who had recently received a beta-lactam antibiotic (6). The rate of recovery of beta-lactamase-producing bacteria (BLPB) in the oropharynx has increased in the past two decades, as they were isolated in over half of the patients with head and neck infections including rhinosinusitis (6). BLPB have the potential of causing infections by themselves as well as protecting not only themselves from the activity of penicillins but also penicillin-susceptible co-pathogens. This "protection" phenomenon occurs when the enzyme beta-lactamase is released into the infected tissues or abscess cavity in sufficient amount to degrade the beta-lactam ring of penicillin before it can eradicate the susceptible bacteria (7). The high incidence of recovery of BLPB in upper respiratory tract infections may be due to their selection during antimicrobial therapy with beta-lactam agents and is of special significance in CRS (see below). Penicillin-resistant bacterial flora can emerge even after a short course of penicillin therapy (8,9).

INTERFERING FLORA

The nasopharynx of healthy individuals is colonized by relatively nonpathogenic aerobic and anaerobic organisms (10), some capable of interfering with the growth of potential bacterial pathogens (11). This phenomenon is called "bacterial interference." These interfering organisms include the aerobic alpha-hemolytic streptococci (mostly *S. mitis* and *S. sanguis*) (12) and several species of anaerobic bacteria (including *Prevotella melaninogenica* and *Peptostreptococcus anaerobius*) (13). Many of these interfering organisms can produce bactericidal proteins known as "bacteriocins." The presence of organisms with interfering potential may play a role in the prevention of colonization by pathogens and the occurrence of upper respiratory infections. Nasopharyngeal colonization with respiratory tract pathogens can occur in healthy individuals and in young children during viral respiratory illnesses (14,15). The number of interfering organisms is also lower in children that are prone to rhinosinusitis (16). The absence of such organisms can explain the higher colonization with pathogens in these children.

Exposure to antimicrobial agents can influence the nasopharyngeal flora (17). Members of the oral flora with interfering capability (e.g., aerobic and anaerobic streptococci, as well as penicillin-susceptible *P. melaninogenica* strains) can become resistant to amoxicillin, but stay susceptible to amoxicillin-clavulanate. Beta-lactamase-producing *P. melaninogenica* strains are susceptible to amoxicillin–clavulanate and can be eradicated by this agent. All these interfering organisms are more resistant to higher generation cephalosporin therapy. Therapy with narrow spectrum antibiotics, such as the oral second generation or extended spectrum cephalosporins, does not eliminate organisms with interfering capabilities, nor does amoxicillin (17) or amoxicillin–clavulanate (18,19).

MICROBIOLOGY OF RHINOSINUSITIS

The pattern of rhinosinusitis as well as otitis media evolves in several clinical and microbiological phases (Fig. 1). Viral infection that generally resolves within 7–10 days initiates the proccess (20). In a small number of patients a secondary acute infection due to aerobic bacteria (i.e., *Streptoccus pneumoniae, H. influenzae,* and *M. catarrhalis*) emerges, and if resolution does not take place, oral flora anaerobic bacteria become predominant over time.

The changes in types of bacteria as the infection becomes chronic were demonstrated by serial endoscopic culture in five patients with nonresolving maxillary rhinosinusitis (21) (Fig. 2). Most isolates from the first cultures were aerobic or facultative bacteria—*S. pneumoniae, H. influenzae* and *M. catarrhalis*. Failure to respond to antimicrobial therapy was associated with the appearance of resistant aerobic and anaerobic bacteria. These included *Fusobacterium nucleatum,* pigmented *Prevotella, Porphyromonas* and *Peptostreptococcus* spp. Eradication of the infection was finally accomplished by administration of effective antimicrobial agents and in three individuals also by surgical evacuation.

These data show that as the infection becomes chronic, the aerobic and facultative organisms are replaced by anaerobic bacteria (21). This transition may be the result of the selective pressure of the antimicrobial therapy that enhances the survival of resistant organisms, and from the slow development of conditions that are appropriate for the growth of anaerobic bacteria, which include the reduction in oxygen tension, and an increase in acidity within the sinus cavity. These changes are caused by the long-standing edema and swelling, which reduce blood supply, and by the removal of oxygen and production of bicarbonate by the aerobic bacteria (22). Another explanation for the slower emergence of anaerobes

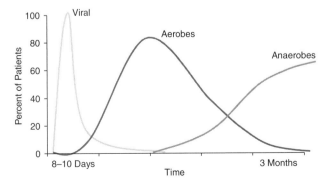

FIGURE 1 The changes over time of the viral and bacterial causes of sinusitis.

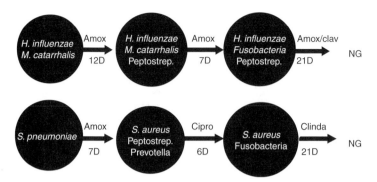

FIGURE 2 Dynamics of rhinosinusitis: changes in bacteria recovered from the sinuses of two patients over time (20). *Abbreviations:* Amox, amoxicillin; Amox/clav, amoxicillin/clavulanic-acid; Clinda, clindamycin; cipro, ciprofloxacin; NG, no growth on culture.

is that expression of some of their virulence factors such as a capsule is a gradual process (23).

Bacteriology of Acute Rhinosinusitis

Bacteria can be recovered from two-thirds of patients with acute maxillary, ethmoid, frontal, and sphenoid rhinosinusitis, and the infection is polymicrobial in about a third of the patients (24). The organisms isolated from children and adults with community-acquired acute purulent rhinosinusitis are the common respiratory pathogens (*S. pneumoniae, M. catarrhalis, H. influenzae,* and beta-hemolytic streptococci) and those considered as part of the normal nasal flora (*S. aureus*) (Table 1) (25–27). *S. aureus* is a common pathogen in sphenoid rhinosinusitis (27), anaerobic bacteria were rarely recovered, and when they were found it was mostly

TABLE 1 Microbiology of Rhinosinusitis (% Patients)

	Maxillary		Ethmoid		Frontal		Splenoid	
Bacteria	Acute	Chronic (N = 66)	Acute (N = 26)	Chronic (N = 17)	Acute (N = 15)	Chronic (N = 13)	Acute (N = 16)	Chronic (N = 7)
Aerobic								
S. aureus	4	14	15	24	–	15	56	14
S. pyogenes	2	8	8	6	3	–	6	–
S. pneumoniae	31	6	35	6	33	–	6	–
H. infuenzae	21	5	27	6	40	15	12	14
M. catarrhalis	8	6	8	–	20	–	–	
Enterobacteriaceae	7	6	–	47	–	8	–	28
P. aeruginosa	2	3	–	6	–	8	6	14
Anaerobic								
Peptostreptococcus sp.	2	56	15	59	3	38	19	57
P. acnes		29	12	18	3	8	12	29
Fusobacterium sp.	2	17	4	47	3	31	6	54
Prevotella and Porphyromonas sp.	2	47	8	82	3	62	6	86
B. fragilis		6	–	–	–	15	–	–

Source: From Refs. 1, 41, 42, 78–80.

in acute rhinosinusitis associated with dental infection, mainly of the roots of the premolar or molar teeth (28,29).

Pseudomonas aeruginosa and other gram-negative rods are rarely isolated from community-acquired rhinosinusitis, but are common in rhinosinusitis of nosocomial origin (especially in association with nasal tubes or catheters), immunocompromised patients, those with human immunodeficiency virus infection, and patients with cystic fibrosis (30).

Bacteriology of CRS

Even though the cause of the inflammation in CRS is uncertain, the presence of bacteria within the sinuses in this patient population has been well documented (31,32). Most clinicians believe that bacteria plays a major role in the etiology and pathogenesis of CRS and prescribe antimicrobial therapy for the treatment of this infection.

Numerous studies reported the recovery of bacterial pathogens from patients with CRS. Unfortunately, most of these did not utilize adequate methods for the recovery of anaerobes. Significant differences exist in the microbial pathogens recovered in chronic when compared with acute rhinosinusitis. *Staphylococcus aureus*, *S. epidermidis*, and anaerobic and gram-negative bacteria predominate in chronic infection. However, the role of some of the low-virulence bacteria, such as *S. epidermidis*, a common colonizer of the nasal cavity, is questionable (33,34).

Gram-negative enteric bacilli were also reported in several studies (35–38). These organisms included *Pseudomonas aeruginosa*, *Klebsiella pneumoniae*, *Proteus mirabilis*, *Enterobacter* spp., and *Escherichia coli*. These may have been selected out following the administration of antimicrobials in patients with CRS.

When adequate methods are utilized, anaerobic bacteria can be isolated in more than half of all the patients with CRS (Table 2); while the pathogens that are common in acute rhinosinusitis (e.g., *S. pneumoniae*, *H. influenzae*, and *M. catarrhalis*) are rarely isolated (39–43). Polymicrobial infection is present in over two-third of patients with CRS, where the infection is synergistic (23) and more difficult to cure using narrow-spectrum antimicrobials. Chronic rhinosinusitis

TABLE 2 Anaerobes in CRS

Reference	Country	# Patients (N)	Anaerobes % pts.	Anaerobes % organisms
Frederick and Braude (64)	USA	83	75	52
Van Cauwenberge et al. (65)	Belgium	66	39	39
Karma et al. (66)	Finland	40 (adult)	–	19
Brook (41)	USA	40	100	80
Berg et al. (67)	Sweden	54 (adult)	≥33	42
Tabaqchali (71)	UK	35	70	39
Brook (43)	USA	72	88	71
Fiscella and Chow (68)	USA	15 (adult)	38	48
Erkan et al. (74)	Turkey	126 (adult)	88	71
		93 (ped.)	93	74
Ito et al. (73)	Japan	10	60	82
Klossek et al. (76)	France	394	26	25
Finegold et al. (42)	USA	150 (adult)	56	48

Source: From Refs. 41–43, 64–76.

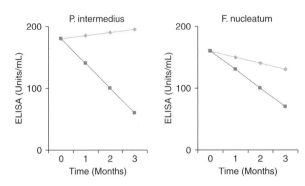

FIGURE 3   Serum antibodies to *P. intermedius* and *F. nucleatum* in 23 patients with CRS. *Source:* From Ref. 48.

caused by anaerobes possesses a greater risk of serious local (e.g., mucocele, osteomyelitis, and abscess) and intracranial complications which can also be attributed to these organisms (44).

Scientific support for the importance of anaerobes in CRS is provided by several observations: the ability to induce CRS in a rabbit by inoculation of *Bacteroides fragilis* into the sinus (45) the rapid emergence of serum immunoglobulin-G (IgG) antibodies against this organism (46), and the detection of antibodies (IgG) in individuals with CRS to two anaerobic organisms that were also found in their sinuses (*F. nucleatum* and *P. intermedius*) (47). The antibody concentrations declined in those who were cured, but did not decline in those who failed therapy (Fig. 3).

In addition to their role as pathogens, many gram-negative anaerobes that produce the enzyme beta-lactamase (e.g., *Prevotella, Porphyromonas,* and *Fusobacterium* spp.) can shield other co-pathogens, including aerobic pathogens, from beta-lactam antibiotics (7,48). The beta-lactamase enzyme activity within the sinus cavity and the potential for the presence of the 'shielding' phenomenon were demonstrated in acutely and chronically inflamed sinus fluids (48). Beta-lactamase producing bacteria (BLPB) were recovered in four of ten acute rhinosinusitis aspirates and in 10 of 13 CRS aspirates (Table 3). The predominant BLPB present in acute infection were *H. influenzae* and *M. catarrhalis*, and those isolated in CRS were *S. aureus, B. fragilis, Prevotella* and *Fusobacterium* spp (48). "Free" beta-lactamase was found in 86% of aspirates that contained these BLPB, and was associated with persistence of even penicillin-susceptible pathogens despite penicillin therapy.

Studies in Children

Ten studies of the microbiology of CRS in children were performed in the past 25 years 1981 and 2000 (41,49–57). Four were prospective (49,50,54,56) and six were retrospective. Sampling was performed by transnasal aspiration in all except two studies. The nose was sterilized prior to obtaining a culture in only five of the studies and bacterial quantitation was rarely performed. Antibiotics were administered prior to culture in six studies. *Staphyloccus epidermidis* and alpha-hemolytic streptococci which are members of the normal nasal flora were the main isolates in two of the studies. It is therefore difficult to ascertain the pathologic significance of these organisms. *Haemophillus influenzae, S. pneumoniae,* and *M. catarrhalis* were recovered in about 60% of cases in the remaining studies, especially in those where the criteria for entry included purulent secretions. Anaerobic bacteria were

TABLE 3   Beta-Lactamase (BL) Detected in Aspirates from Four Patients with CRS

Organism	Patient no.			
	1	2	3	4
Staphylococcus aureus (BL+)		+		+
Streptococcus pneumoniae	+			
Peptostreptococcus spp	+			+
Propionibacterium acnes	+			
Fusobacterium spp (BL+)		+		+
Fusobacterium spp (BL−)		+		+
Prevotella spp (BL+)			+	
Prevotella spp (BL−)	+	+	+	
Bacteroides fragilis group (BL+)	+			+

Source: From Ref. 48.

found in the only three studies that employed methods for their isolation (41,49,56).

The predominant isolates in ethmoid rhinosinusitis were *S. aureus* (19%) and alpha-hemolytic streptococci (23%) in one study (52), and *S. epidermidis* and alpha-hemolytic streptococci in another (50). The most common organism in a study of children with allergies was *M. catarrhalis,* although a quarter of the patients had polymicrobial flora (58). *Streptococcus pneumoniae* and *H. influenzae* predominated in children with acute exacerbations of CRS (59).

Brook and Yocum (60) studied 40 children with CRS. The sinuses infected were the maxillary (15 cases), ethmoid (13), and frontal (7). A total of 121 isolates (97 anaerobic and 24 aerobic) were recovered. Anaerobes were isolated from all 37 culture-positive specimens, and in 14 cases they were mixed with aerobes. The predominant anaerobes were Gram-negative bacilli (36), anaerobic gram-positive cocci (28), and *Fusobacterium* spp. (13). The predominant aerobic isolates were alpha-hemolytic streptococci (7), *S. aureus* (7), and *Haemophilus* spp. (4).

Brook et al. (49) correlated the microbiology of concurrent chronic otitis media with effusion and chronic maxillary rhinosinusitis in 32 children. A bacterial etiology was present in two-third of the patients. The most common isolates were *H. influenzae* (nine isolates), *S. pneumoniae* (seven), *Prevotella* spp. (eight), and *Peptostreptococcus* spp. (six). A concordance in the microbiology between the ear and sinus was present in 22 (69%) of culture-positive patients.

Erkan et al. (56) evaluated 93 children with chronic maxillary rhinosinusitis. Anaerobes were recovered in 81 of 87 (93%) culture-positive specimens, were present alone in 61 (70%), and mixed with aerobic or facultative bacteria in 20 (23%). Aerobic or facultative bacteria were present alone in six cases (7%). A total of 261 isolates (3/specimen), 19 (2.4/specimen) anaerobes, and 69 (2.6/specimen) aerobes or facultatives were isolated. The main anaerobes were *Bacteroides* spp. and anaerobic cocci and the predominant aerobes or facultatives were *Streptococcus* spp. and *S. aureus.*

Studies in Adults

Anaerobic bacteria were isolated in CRS whenever appropriate methods for their recovery were used (39,61,62). The main isolates were pigmented *Prevotella, Fusobacterium,* and *Peptostreptococcus* spp. The predominant aerobic bacteria were *S. aureus, M. catarrhalis,* and *Haemophilus* spp. Aerobic and anaerobic BLPB were found in over 33% of these patients (36,39,40,43,62,63). These were *S. aureus*, and *Haemophilus, Prevotella, Porphyromonas,* and *Fusobacterium* spp.

Finegold et al. (42) found the recovery of anaerobes in CRS to be clinically significant. In a study of chronic maxillary rhinosinusitis in adults, recurrence of signs and symptoms was twice as frequent when cultures showed anaerobic bacterial counts over 10^3 colony-forming units per milliliter.

A summary of 17 studies of CRS that attempted to recover anaerobes and included 1758 patients (133 were children) is shown in Table 2 (41–43,64–76). Anaerobes were recovered in 12–93% of the patients. The variability in isolation rate may be due to differences in the methodologies used for transportation and cultivation, patient populations studied, geography, and previous antimicrobial treatments.

Brook and Frazier (77) correlated the microbiology with the history of previous sinus surgery in 108 adults with chronic maxillary rhinosinusitis. Those with past surgery had a higher rate of isolation of *P. aeruginosa* and other gram-negative bacilli while anaerobes were found significantly more frequently in patients who did not have prior surgery.

Brook studied the microbiology of 13 cases of chronic frontal (78), seven cases of chronic sphenoid (79), and 17 cases of chronic ethmoid sinusitis (80) (Table 1). Anaerobic bacteria were recovered in over two-thirds of the cases. The predominant ones included *Prevotella, Peptostreptococcus,* and *Fusobacterium* spp. The main aerobic organisms were Gram-negative bacilli (*H. influenzae, K. pneumoniae, E. coli,* and *P. aeruginosa*).

Gram-negative rods were also recovered more commonly by Nadel et al. (36) in patients who had previous surgery or those who had their sinuses irrigated. *Psendomonas aeruginosa* was isolated more often in individuals on systemic steroids. Other studies have also noted this shift toward Gram-negative organisms in patients who have been extensively and repeatedly treated (35,38,81). Their bacterial flora includes *Pseudomonas* spp., *Enterobacter* spp., methicillin-resistant *S. aureus, H. influenzae,* and *M. catarrhalis.*

Bacteriology of Acute Exacerbation of CRS

Acute exacerbation of chronic rhinosinusitis (AECS) is defined as a sudden worsening of CRS with either worsening of the baseline or new symptoms. We evaluated the microbiology of maxillary AECS by performing repeated endoscopic aspirations in seven patients over a period of 125–242 days (82). Organisms were isolated from all aspirates and the number of isolates varied between two and four. The aerobic isolates were *H. influenzae, S. pneumoniae, M. catarrhalis, S. aureus,* and *K. pneumoniae.* The anaerobes recovered were pigmented *Prevotella* and *Porphyromonas, Peptostreptococcus, Fusobacterium* spp., and *Propionibacterium acnes.* A change in the types of isolates was noted in all consecutive cultures obtained from the same patients, as different organisms emerged, and previously isolated bacteria were no longer found. An increase in antimicrobial resistance was noted in six instances. These findings illustrate the microbial dynamics of AECS and highlight the importance of obtaining cultures for guidance in selection of proper antimicrobial therapy.

The microbiology of maxillary AECS in 30 patients was compared with the microbiology of 32 patients with chronic maxillary rhinosinusitis (83). The predominant organisms were anaerobic bacteria, and polymicrobial infection was present in both conditions (2.5–3 isolates/sinus). However, aerobic organisms that are generally present in acute infections (e.g., *S. pneumoniae, H. influenzae*, and *M. catarrhalis)* emerged in some of the acute episodes.

Bacteriology of Nosocomial Rhinosinusitis

Nosocomial rhinosinusitis afflicts those that receive extended periods of intensive care that require prolonged endotracheal or nasogastric intubation (84). Nasotracheal intubation is especially associated with a high risk for nosocomial rhinosinusitis (85). The common pathogens are aerobic gram-negative bacilli (i.e., *P. aeruginosa, K. pneumoniae, Enterobacter* spp., *P. mirabilis*, and *Serratia marcescens)* and gram-positive cocci (occasionally streptococci and staphylococci). The pathogenicity of these bacteria is unclear as they may only represent colonization that is assisted by the impaired sinus mucociliary transport and the presence of a foreign body in the nose.

Anaerobic bacteria, always mixed with aerobic and facultatives, were found in six sinus aspirates, and only aerobic bacteria were found in three of nine children with neurologic impairment who had nosocomial rhinosinusitis (86). The main aerobic bacteria were *K. pneumoniae, E. coli, S. aureus, P. mirabilis, P. aeruginosa, H. influenzae, M. catarrhalis*, and *S. pneumoniae*. The predominant anaerobes were *Prevotella* spp., *Peptostreptococcus* spp., *F. nucleatum*, and *B. fragilis*. Organisms similar to those isolated from the sinuses were also recovered from the tracheostomy site and gastrostomy wound aspirates in five of seven patients. This study demonstrates that, in neurologically impaired children, facultative and anaerobic gram-negative organisms that can colonize other body sites are predominant in addition to the organisms known to cause chronic infection in normal children.

Osteitis Associated with CRS

Even though bacterial organisms have not yet been identified in the bone in either humans or animal models of CRS, there is clinical and experimental evidence to suggest that the bone underlying the diseased sinus mucosa is involved in the disease process. However, it is well known that in chronic osteomyelitis organisms are difficult to isolate.

Areas of increased bone density and thickening are often observed on computed tomography (CT) in areas of chronic inflammation and may be the result of the chronic inflammation itself. During the initial phases of a severe ethmoid CRS these bony changes manifest as rarefaction of the bony ethmoid partitions. Histologic evaluation of ethmoid bone in individuals with CRS has confirmed marked activity in chronic disease not seen in controls (86). Features identified included a marked increase in fibrosis, remodeling, and woven bone. Osteopenia was rarely seen while mixed or chronic inflammation with mast cells within the bone was typical even when the overlying mucosa was normal. Histomorphometric assessments indicate the presence of marked elevation of overall bone physiology with increased bone resorption along with marked neogenesis. These findings of bone resorption, neogenesis, and fibrosis are similar to the findings seen in osteomyelitis and suggest that the underlying ethmoid bone may serve as a nidus for CRS. Another study also illustrated that the ethmoid bone underwent rapid remodeling in CRS that was histologically identical to the remodeling seen in osteomyelitis (87).

Giacchi et al. (88) valuated decalcified ethmoid bone specimens from patients undergoing endoscopic sinus surgery for CRS and observed histopathologic changes consistent with varying grades of bone remodeling. The changes were in the extracellular matrix, and included bone resorption and osteoneogenesis associated with osteitis of the underlying ethmoid bone.

In experimentally induced rhinosinusitis with *P. aeruginosa* using an animal model, Bolger et al. (89) demonstrated bone changes as early as 4 days after infection of a maxillary sinus. These changes included a coordinated osteoclasis and appositional bone formation adjacent to the sinus, as well as subsequent intramembranous bone formation. A follow-up study revealed clear histologic evidence of bone involvement adjacent to the infected sinuses, and the bony changes extended to the noninfected side in all specimens (90).

Khalid et al. (91) evaluated and confirmed the histologic inflammatory changes that occur in bone and in the overlying mucosa in experimentally induced CRS due to *P. aeruginosa* and *S. aureus* in rabbits and evaluated the differences in the inflammatory patterns that may occur with different organisms. Histologic evidence of CRS in the inoculated sinus was demonstrated in 86% of animals (25 of 29). Evidence of chronic osteomyelitis in the noninfected side was seen in 15 of 29 animals (52%) overall, or 9 of 15 animals (60%) infected with *P. aeruginosa* and 6 of 14 (43%) animals infected with *S. aureus*. The study provides further evidence that bacterial rhinosinusitis can involve bone at a distance from the site of primary infection, thereby suggesting that infectious agents may spread through bony structures in the pathogenesis of CRS. These findings, if further confirmed in patients, may help to explain the recalcitrance of severe CRS to medical and surgical therapy, and the clinical observation of the tendency of the disease to persist in localized areas until the underlying bone is removed.

The finding of bone involvement in CRS may have significant implications for disease management and deserves further animal and clinical investigation (92). If osteitis is proved to have a significant role it would justify the use of antibiotics (initially intravenously and later orally) that penetrate well into the bone, the administration of the antibiotics for an extended period of time (for at least 4–6 weeks), and the selection of the antibiotics, whenever possible, based on direct culture results in samples from the infected site. Further surgical management may involve removal of the nidus of infection, implantation of antibiotic beads or pumps, hyperbaric oxygen therapy, or other modalities (92).

Biofilms and Intraepithelial Bacteria as Potential Causes of CRS

Recent attention has been given to the possibility that mucosal bacterial biofilm or intracellular staphylococci may contribute to the pathogenesis of CRS. Bacterial biofilm, which is known to form on inert surfaces, such as prosthetic heart valves, indwelling catheters, and tooth surfaces, is increasingly recognized as a potential source of chronic infection on mucosal surfaces, such as bladder epithelium in chronic urinary tract infection and respiratory epithelium in cystic fibrosis (93,94). The biofilm consists of clusters of bacteria held together by an extracellular glycocalyx with interspersed water channels. Using a combination of scanning electron microscopy to demonstrate biofilm and transmission electron microscopy to demonstrate bacteria on the mucosal surface, a recent study found evidence for bacterial biofilm with associated bacteria in 80% of a small population of CRS patients compared to none in healthy controls (95). A concern is whether incomplete eradication of chronic bacterial infection due to poor antibiotic tissue penetration or antibiotic resistance might promote the development of biofilm or an intracellular reservoir, particularly for *S. aureus* (96).

Antimicrobial Treatment of CRS

The majority of bacteria isolated from CRS resist penicillins through the production of the enzyme beta-lactamase (48). These include aerobic bacteria, including *S. aureus, H. influenzae,* and *M. catarrhalis,* and anaerobic bacteria, including *B. fragilis* and over half of the *Prevotella, Porphyromonas,* and *Fusobacterium* spp.

The superiority of therapy effective against both aerobic and anaerobic bacteria (amoxicillin-clavulanate or clindamycin) when compared with therapy effective only against aerobic bacteria was demonstrated in two retrospective studies of CRS (97,98).

The selected antimicrobial agent in CRS should cover the common pathogens in acute rhinosinusitis (e.g., *S. pneumoniae, H. influenzae,* and *M. catarrhalis*) as well as aerobic and anaerobic BLPB seen in CRS. Utilization of a broad-spectrum antibiotic that is beta-lactamase stable, effective against penicillin-resistant *S. pneumoniae,* and possesses anti-anaerobic coverage may be optimal for the treatment of CRS. The choices of agents include the combination of a penicillin (e.g., amoxicillin) and a beta-lactamase inhibitor (e.g., clavulanic acid), clindamycin, chloramphenicol, the combination of metronidazole and a macrolide, or a fluoroquinolone (only in adults) with minimal anti-anaerobic efficacy (e.g., levofloxacin, moxifloxacin, and gatifloxacin). A fluoroquinolone with adequate anti-anaerobic efficacy (e.g., trovafloxacin) can be administered as single agent therapy but is reserved for serious hospital-based infections owing to its potential to cause serious hepatic toxicity. These agents are available in oral and parenteral forms. Other agents that are only available in parenteral form include some of the second-generation cephalosporins (e.g., cefoxitin, cefotetan, and cefmetazole), combinations of a penicillin (e.g., ticarcillin, piperacillin, and ampicillin) and a beta-lactamase inhibitor (e.g., clavulanic acid, tazobactam, and sulbactam) and the carbapenems (i.e., imipenem, and meropenem). Extra coverage against aerobic gram-negative organisms, such as *P. aeruginosa,* can be provided by parenteral therapy with an aminoglycoside, a fourth-generation cephalosporin (ceftazidime or cefepime) or oral or parenteral treatment with a fluoroquinolone effective against this organism (e.g., ciprofloxacin). Coverage against *S. aureus* is attained by some of these agents (clindamycin is also effective against methicillin-resistant Staphylococcus—MRSA). However, specific MRSA coverage can also be attained by agents such as vancomycin or linezolid. A carbapenem (e.g., imipenem) provides coverage for both aerobic and anaerobic pathogens (99).

Clinicians should consider the anaerobic activity for the various antimicrobials before selecting an antibiotic agent for the empiric treatment of CRS. It is not recommended or generally necessary to perform a culture for anaerobic bacteria in these patients. However, these cultures should be considered in patients who have failed antimicrobial therapy or have developed serious infection, or complications.

The length of therapy of CRS is at least 21 days, and may be extended up to 12 weeks when necessary. Although there are no data to support this recommendation, it is based on the author's clinical experience. Even though antimicrobial blood levels may be therapeutic, the diminished vascularity of the chronically inflamed sinus membranes may not allow for proper permeability of the antibiotic into the infected tissues and sinus cavity. The reduction in the pH and oxygen tension within the inflamed sinus may also interfere with the activity of the antimicrobial agents, which can result in bacterial survival despite high antibiotic levels.

Several studies evaluated the use of intravenous antimicrobial therapy for patients with CRS who mostly had a recalcitrant infection resistant to oral antibiotics. One of the reasons for utilizing this approach was an attempt to treat the osteitis involved with CRS, following the approach used in treating osteomyelitis. The studies published so far have largely been uncontrolled, nonrandomized case series with a limited number of patients. The efficacy of treatment varied among the studies (29–89%), but the studies were uniform in their relatively high rate of complications (14–26%) (100,101). One study reported a relapse rate of 89% at a mean follow-up of 11.5 weeks (102). Complications ranged from the benign such as diarrhea, to the serious and life-threatening, including septic thrombophlebitis and neutropenia (103). Until more data are available, intravenous antibiotic use should be reserved for select cases in which orbital and/or intracranial complications arise, or in a chronic infection in which there are no other oral antibiotic alternatives.

Surgical drainage is often needed in CRS, especially in cases that do not respond to medical therapy. Impaired drainage can contribute to the development of CRS, and correction of an obstruction may alleviate the infection and prevent recurrence. Therefore, the utilization of antimicrobial therapy without surgical drainage of collected pus may fail to resolve the infection.

SUMMARY

Incomplete resolution of acute rhinosinusitis leading to CRS is associated with a corresponding change in the microbiology of the disease. The shift in microbiology from acute to CRS favors infection with *S. aureus*, *S. epidermidis*, anaerobic bacteria (including beta-lactamase-producing strains), and gram-negative bacteria. With the exception of *S. epidermidis*, there is substantial evidence supporting the role of these organisms in the pathogenesis of CRS. It is worth noting that not all CRS patients are chronically infected. In fact, other inflammatory factors in the disease may predominate in the clinical presentation. This creates a clinical conundrum in which it is difficult to ascertain whether bacteria are involved. In general, a chronic bacterial infection is more likely if there is: underlying immune deficiency, one or more opacified sinuses on sinus CT in the absence of polyps, the presence of frank purulence draining from one or more sinus cavities, or the presence of gram-negative or antibiotic-resistant organisms (e.g., MRSA) on sinus culture. For patients seen for the first time, the approach to antibiotic treatment is usually empiric, following the guidelines outlined in this chapter and directing treatment at both aerobic and anaerobic bacteria. Whenever possible, the choice of antibiotics should be guided by properly obtained sinus cultures. In cases where empiric antibiotics have failed, the need for bacterial cultures is even more critical to assure proper treatment and to minimize antibiotic side effects.

REFERENCES

1. Gwaltney JM. Acute community-acquired sinusitis. Clin Infect Dis 1996; 23:1209–25.
2. Berg O, Carenfelt C, Rystedt G, Anggard A. Occurrence of asymptomatic sinusitis in common cold and other acute ENT infections. Rhinology 1986; 24:223–5.
3. Socransky SS, Manganiello SD. The oral microflora of man from birth to senility. J Periodontol 1971; 42:485–96.
4. Gibbons RJ, Socransky SS, Dearaujo WC, et al. Studies of the predominant cultivable microbiota of dental plaque. Arch Oral Biol 1964; 9:365–70.

5. Valenti WM, Trudell RG, Bentley DW. Factors predisposing to oropharyngeal colonization with gram-negative bacilli in the aged. N Engl J Med 1978; 298:1108–10.
6. Brook I. Beta-lactamase producing bacteria in head and neck infection. Laryngoscope 1988; 98:428–31.
7. Brook I. The role of beta-lactamase-producing bacteria in the persistence of streptococcal tonsillar infection. Rev Infect Dis 1984; 6:601–7.
8. Brook I, Gober AE. Emergence of beta-lactamase-producing aerobic and anaerobic bacteria in the oropharynx of children following penicillin chemotherapy. Clin Pediatr 1984; 23:338–41.
9. Tuner K, Nord CE. Emergence of beta-lactamase-producing microorganisms in the tonsils during penicillin treatment. Eur J Clin Microbiol 1986; 5:399–404.
10. Mackowiak PA. The normal flora. N Engl J Med 1983; 307:83–93.
11. Sprunt K, Redman W. Evidence suggesting importance of role of interbacterial inhibition in maintaining balance of normal flora. Ann Intern Med 1968; 68:579–90.
12. Bernstein JM, Sagahtaheri-Altaie S, Dryjd DM, Vactawski-Wende J. Bacterial interference in nasopharyngeal bacterial flora of otitis-prone and non-otitis-prone children. Acta Otorhinolaryngol Belg 1994; 48:1–9.
13. Murray PR, Rosenblatt JE. Bacterial interference by oropharyngeal and clinical isolates of anaerobic bacteria. J Infect Dis 1976; 134:281–5.
14. Faden H, Zaz MJ, Bernstein JM, Brodsky L, Stamievich J, Ogru PL. Nasopharyngeal flora in the first three years of life in normal and otitis-prone children. Ann Otol Rhinol Laryngol 1991; 100:612–5.
15. Brook I, Gober A. Bacterial interference in the nasopharynx of otitis media prone and not otitis media prone children. Arch Otolaryngol Head Neck Surg 2000; 126:1011–3.
16. Brook I, Gober AE. Bacterial interference in the nasopharynx and nasal cavity of sinusitis prone and non-sinusitis prone children. Acta Otolaryngol 1999; 119:832–6.
17. Brook I, Gober AE. Bacterial interference in the nasopharynx following antimicrobial therapy of acute otitis media. J Antimicrob Chemother 1998; 41:489–92.
18. Brook I, Foote PA. Effect of antimicrobial therapy with amoxicillin and cefprozil on bacterial interference and beta-lactamase production in the adenoids. Ann Otol Rhinol Laryngol 2004; 113:902–5.
19. Brook I, Gober AE. Long-term effects on the nasopharyngeal flora of children following antimicrobial therapy of acute otitis media with cefdinir or amoxycillin-clavulanate. J Med Microbiol 2005; 54:553-6.
20. Gwaltney JM Jr, Sydnor A, Sande MA. Etiology and antimicrobial treatment of acute sinusitis. Ann Otol Rhinol Laryngol 1981; 90(Suppl. 84):68–71.
21. Brook I, Frazier EH, Foote PA. Microbiology of the transition from acute to chronic maxillary sinusitis. J Med Microbiol 1996; 45:372–5.
22. Carenfelt C, Lundberg C. Purulent and non-purulent maxillary sinus secretions with respect to Po_2, Pco_2 and pH. Acta Otolaryngol 1977; 84:138–44.
23. Brook I. Role of encapsulated anaerobic bacteria in synergistic infections. Crit Rev Microbiol 1987; 14:171–93.
24. Gwaltney JM Jr, Scheld WM, Sande MA, Sydnor A. The microbial etiology and antimicrobial therapy of adults with acute community-acquired sinusitis: a fifteen-year experience at the University of Virginia and review of other selected studies. J Allergy Clin Immunol 1992; 90:457–62.
25. Wald ER, Milmore GJ, Bowen AD, Ledema-Medina J, Salamon N, Bluestone CD. Acute maxillary sinusitis in children. N Engl J Med 1981; 304:749–54.
26. Wald ER, Guerra N, Byers C. Upper respiratory tract infections in young children: Duration of and frequency of complications. Pediatrics 1991; 87:129–33.
27. Lew D, Southwick FS, Montgomery WW, Weber AL, Baker AS. Sphenoid sinusitis. A review of 30 cases. N Engl J Med 1983; 309:1149–54.
28. Brook I, Frazier EH, Gher ME Jr. Microbiology of periapical abscesses and associated maxillary sinusitis. J Periodontal 1996; 67:608–10.
29. Brook I, Friedman EM. Intracranial complications of sinusitis in children. A sequela of periapical abscess. Ann Otol Rhinol Laryngol 1982; 91:41–3.

30. Shapiro ED, Milmoe GJ, Wald ER, et al. Bacteriology of the maxillary sinuses in patients with cystic fibrosis. J Infect Dis 1982; 146:589–93.
31. Wald E.R. Microbiology of acute and chronic sinusitis in children and adults. Am J Med Sci 1998; 316:13–20.
32. Biel MA, Brown CA, Levinson RM, et al. Evaluation of the microbiology of chronic maxillary sinusitis. Ann Otol Laryngol Rhinol 1998; 107:942–5.
33. Gordts F, Halewyck S, Pierard D, et al. Microbiology of the middle meatus: a comparison between normal adults and children. J Laryngol Otol 2000; 14:184–8.
34. Jiang RS, Hsu CY, Jang JW. Bacteriology of the maxillary and ethmoid sinuses in chronic sinusitis. J Laryngol Otol 1998; 112:845–8.
35. Hsu J, Lanza DC, Kennedy DW. Antimicrobial resistance in bacterial chronic sinusitis. Am J Rhinol 1998; 12:243–8.
36. Nadel DM, Lanza DC, Kennedy DW. Endoscopically guided cultures in chronic sinusitis. Am J Rhinol 1998; 12:233–41.
37. Bahattacharyya N, Kepnes LJ. The microbiology of recurrent rhinosinusitis after endoscopic sinus surgery. Arch Otolaryngol Head Neck Surg 1999; 125;1117–20.
38. Bolger WE. Gram negative sinusitis: emerging clinical entity. Am J Rhinol 1994; 8:279–83.
39. Nord CE. The role of anaerobic bacteria in recurrent episodes of sinusitis and tonsillitis. Clin Infect Dis 1995; 20:1512–24.
40. Brook I, Thompson D, Frazier E. Microbiology and management of chronic maxillary sinusitis. Arch Otolaryngol Head Neck Surg 1994; 120:1317–20.
41. Brook I. Bacteriologic features of chronic sinusitis in children. JAMA. 1981; 246:967–69.
42. Finegold SM, Flynn MJ, Rose FV, et al. Bacteriologic findings associated with chronic bacterial maxillary sinusitis in adults. Clin Infect Dis 2002; 35:428–33.
43. Brook I. Bacteriology of chronic maxillary sinusitis in adults. Ann Otol Rhinol Laryngol 1989; 98:426–8.
44. Brook I. Brain abscess in children: microbiology and management. Child Neurol 1995; 10:283–8.
45. Westrin KM, Stierna P, Carlsoo B, Hellstrom S. Mucosal fine structure in experimental sinusitis. Ann Otol Rhinol Laryngol 1993; 102(8 Pt 1):639–45.
46. Jyonouchi H, Sun S, Kennedy CA, et al. Localized sinus inflammation in a rabbit sinusitis model induced by *Bacteroides fragilis* is accompanied by rigorous immune responses. Otolaryngol Head Neck Surg 1999; 120:869–75.
47. Brook I, Yocum P. Immune response to *Fusobacterium nucleatum* and *Prevotella intermedia* in patients with chronic maxillary sinusitis. Ann Otol Rhinol Laryngol 1999; 108:293–5.
48. Brook I, Yocum P, Frazier EH. Bacteriology and beta-lactamase activity in acute and chronic maxillary sinusitis. Arch Otolaryngol Head Neck Surg 1996; 122:418–22.
49. Brook I, Yocum P, Shah K. Aerobic and anaerobic bacteriology of concurrent chronic otitis media with effusion and chronic sinusitis in children. Arch Otolaryngol Head Neck Surg 2000; 126:174–6.
50. Orobello PW, Jr. Park RI, Belcher L, et al. Microbiology of chronic sinusitis in children. Arch Otolaryngol Head Neck Surg 1991; 117:980–3.
51. Tinkleman DG, Silk HJ. Clinical and bacteriologic features of chronic sinusitis in children. Am J Dis Child 1989; 143:938–41.
52. Muntz HR, Lusk RP. Bacteriology of the ethmoid bullae in children with chronic sinusitis. Arch Otolaryngol Head Neck Surg 1991; 117:179–81.
53. Otten FWA, Grote JJ. Treatment of chronic maxillary sinusitis in children. Int J Pediatr Otorhinolaryngol 1988; 15:269–78.
54. Otten FWA. Conservative treatment of chronic maxillary sinusitis in children. Long term follow-up. Acta OtoRhinoLaryngologica Belg 1997; 51:173–5.
55. Don D, Yellon RF, Casselbrant M, Bluestone CD. Efficacy of stepwise protocol that includes intravenous antibiotic treatment for the management of chronic sinusitis in children and adolescents. Otolaryngol Head Neck Surg 2001; 127:1093–8.
56. Erkan M, Ozcan M, Arslan S, Soysal V, Bozdemir K, Haghighi N. Bacteriology of antrum in children with chronic maxillary sinusitis. Scand J Infect Dis 1996; 28:283–5.

57. Slack CL, Dahn KA, Abzug MJ, Chan KH. Antibiotic-resistant bacteria in pediatric chronic sinusitis. Pediatr Infect Dis J 2001; 20:247–50.

58. Goldenhersh MJ, Rachelefsky GS, Dudley J, et al. The microbiology of chronic sinus disease in children with respiratory allergy. J Allergy Clin Immunol 1998; 85:1030–9.

59. Wald ER, Byers C, Guerra N, et al. Subacute sinusitis in children. J Pediatr 1989; 115:28–32.

60. Brook I, Yocum P. Antimicrobial management of chronic sinusitis in children. J Laryngol Otol 1995; 109:1159–62.

61. Finegold SM. Anaerobic bacteria in human disease. Orlando, FL: Academic Press Inc, 1977.

62. Brook I. Pediatric Anaerobic Infections. 3rd ed. NY: Marcel Dekker Inc., 2002.

63. Mustafa E, Tahsin A, Mustafa Ö, Nedret K. Bacteriology of antrum in adults with chronic maxillary sinusitis. Laryngoscope 1994; 104:321–4.

64. Frederick J, Braude AI. Anaerobic infections of the paranasal sinuses. N Engl J Med 1974; 290:135–7.

65. Van Cauwenberge P, Verschraegen G, Van Renterghem L. Bacteriological findings in sinusitis (1963-1975). Scand J Infect Dis Suppl 1976; 9:72–7.

66. Karma P, Jokipii L, Sipila P, Luotonen J, Jokipii AM. Bacteria in chronic maxillary sinusitis. Arch Otolaryngol 1979; 105:386–90.

67. Berg O, Carenfelt C, Kronvall G. Bacteriology of maxillary sinusitis in relation to character of inflammation and prior treatment. Scand J Infect Dis 1988; 20:511–6.

68. Fiscella RG, Chow JM. Cefixime for the teatment of maxillary sinusitis. Am J Rhinol 1991; 5:193–7.

69. Sedallian AB, Bru JP, Gaillat J. Bacteriologic finding of chronic sinusitis. The 17th International Congress of the Management of Infection. Berlin, 1992. (Abstr No. P2.71).

70. Simoncelli C, Ricci G, Molini E, von Garrel C, Capolunghi B, Giommetti S. Bacteriology of chronic maxillary sinusitis. HNO 1992; 40:16–8.

71. Tabaqchali S. Anaerobic infections in the head and neck region. Scand J Infect Dis Suppl 1988; 57:24–34.

72. Hartog B, Degener JE, Van Benthem PP, Hordijk GJ. Microbiology of chronic maxillary sinusitis in adults: isolated aerobic and anaerobic bacteria and their susceptibility to twenty antibiotics. Acta Otolaryngol 1995; 115:672–7.

73. Ito K, Ito Y, Mizuta K, et al. Bacteriology of chronic otitis media, chronic sinusitis, and paranasal mucopyocele in Japan. Clin Infect Dis 1995; 20(Suppl. 2):S214–9.

74. Erkan M, Aslan T, Ozcan M, Koc N. Bacteriology of antrum in adults with chronic maxillary sinusitis. Laryngoscope 1994; 104(3 Pt 1):321–4.

75. Edelstein DR, Avner SE, Chow JM. et al. Once-a-day therapy for sinusitis: a comparison study of cefixime and amoxicillin. Laryngoscope 1993; 103:33–41.

76. Klossek JM, Dubreuil L, Richet H, Richet B, Beutter P. Bacteriology of chronic purulent secretions in chronic rhinosinusitis. J Laryngol Otol 1998; 112:1162–6.

77. Brook I, Frazier EH. Correlation between microbiology and previous sinus surgery in patients with chronic maxillary sinusitis. Ann Otol Rhinol Laryngol 2001; 110:148–51.

78. Brook I. Bacteriology of acute and chronic frontal sinusitis. Arch Otolaryngol Head Neck Surg 2002; 128:583–5.

79. Brook I. Bacteriology of acute and chronic sphenoid sinusitis. Ann Otol Rhinol Laryngol 2002; 111:1002–4.

80. Brook I. Bacteriology of acute and chronic ethmoid sinusitis. Abstract of the 103 General Meeting of the American Society for Medical Microbiology, Washington DC, 2003. (Absract #D-138).

81. Bhattacharyya N, Kepnes LJ. The microbiology of recurrent rhinosinusitis after endoscopic sinus surgery. Arch Otolaryngol Head Neck Surg 1999; 125:1117–20.

82. Brook I, Foote PA, Frazier EH. Microbiology of acute exacerbation of chronic sinusitis. Laryngoscope 2004; 114:129–31.

83. Brook I. Bacteriology of Chronic Sinusitis and Acute Exacerbation of Chronic Sinusitis. Arch Otolaryngol Head Neck Surg 2006; 132:1099–1101.

84. Arens JF, LeJeune FE Jr, Webre DR. Maxillary sinusitis, a complication of nasotracheal intubation. Anesthesiology 1974; 40:415–6.

85. Brook I, Shah K. Sinusitis in neurologically impaired children. Otolaryngol Head Neck Surg 1998; 119:357–60.
86. Kennedy DW, Senior BA, Gannon FH, Montone KT, Hwang P, Lanza DC. Histology and histomorphometry of ethmoid bone in chronic rhinosinusitis. Laryngoscope 1998; 108(4 Pt 1):502–7.
87. Hwang P, Montone KT, Gannon FH, et al. Applications of in situ hybridization techniques in the diagnosis of chronic sinusitis. Am J Rhinol 1999; 13:335–38.
88. Giacchi RJ, Lebowitz RA, Yee HT, Light JP, Jacobs JB. Histopathologic evaluation of the ethmoid bone in chronic sinusitis. Am J Rhinol 2001; 15:193–7.
89. Bolger WE, Leonard D, Dick EJ, et al. Gram negative sinusitis: a bacteriologic and histologic study in rabbits. Am J Rhinol 1997; 11:15–25.
90. Perloff JR, Gannon FH, Bolger WE, et al. Bone Involvement in Sinusitis: An apparent pathway for the spread of disease. Laryngoscope 2000; 110:2095–99.
91. Khalid AN, Hunt J, Perloff JR, Kennedy DW. The role of bone in chronic rhinosinusitis. Laryngoscope 2002; 112:1951–7.
92. Brook I. Joint and bone infections due to anaerobic bacteria in children. Pediatr Rehabil 2002; 5:11–9.
93. Anderson, GG, Palermo JJ, Schilling JD, Roth R, Heuser J, Hultgren SJ. Intracellular bacterial biofilm-like pods in urinary tract infections. Science 2003; 301:105–107.
94. Garcia-Medina R, Dunne WM, Singh PK, Brody SL. *Pseudomonas aeruginosa* acquires biofilm-like properties within airway epithelial cells. Infect Immun 2005; 73:8298–305.
95. Sanclement JA, Webster P, Thomas J, Ramadan HH. Bacterial biofilms in surgical specimens of patients with chronic rhinosinusitis. Laryngoscope 2005; 115:578–82.
96. Clement S, Vaudaux P, Francois P, et al. Evidence of an intracellular reservoir in the nasal mucosa of patients with recurrent Staphylococcus aureus rhinosinusitis. J Infect Dis 2005; 192:1023–8.
97. Brook I, Thompson DH, Frazier EH. Microbiology and management of chronic maxillary sinusitis. Arch Otolaryngol Head Neck Surg 1994; 120:1317–20.
98. Brook I, Yocum P. Management of chronic sinusitis in children. J Laryngol Otol 1995; 109:1159–62.
99. Sanders CV, Aldridge KE. Current antimicrobial therapy of anaerobic infections. Eur J Clin Microbiol 1992; 11:999–1011.
100. Don DM, Yellon FR, Casselbrant ML, et al. Efficacy of a stepwise protocol that includes intravenous antibiotic therapy for the management of chronic sinusitis in children and adolescents. Arch Otolaryngol Head Neck Surg 2001; 127:1093–8.
101. Gross ND, McInnes RJ, Hwang PH. Outpatient intravenous antibiotics for chronic rhinosinusitis. Laryngoscope 2002; 112:1758–61.
102. Fowler KC, Duncavage JA, Murray JJ, et al. Chronic sinusitis and intravenous antibiotic therapy: resolution, recurrent and adverse events. J Allergy Clin Immunol 2003; 111:S85.
103. Tanner SB, Fowler KC. Intravenous antibiotics for chronic rhinosinusitis: are they effective? Curr Opin Otolaryngol Head Neck Surg 2004; 12:3–8.

10 *Staphylococcus aureus* Enterotoxins as Immune Stimulants in Chronic Rhinosinusitis

Claus Bachert
Upper Airway Research Laboratory, ENT-Department, University Hospital Ghent, Ghent, Belgium

Nan Zhang
Upper Airway Research Laboratory, ENT-Department, University Hospital Ghent, Ghent, Belgium, and ENT-Department, Zhongshan City Peoples Hospital, Zhongshan, Guangdong Province, China

Thibaut van Zele, Philippe Gevaert, Joke Patou, and Paul van Cauwenberge
Upper Airway Research Laboratory, ENT-Department, University Hospital Ghent, Ghent, Belgium

INTRODUCTION

Recent evidence supports the view that chronic rhinosinusitis (CRS) with or without nasal polyps represents different disease entities, characterized by specific cytokine and mediator profiles. Nasal polyps in adults, characterized by abundant eosinophils, local overproduction of immunoglobulin E, and often associated with asthma, have been appreciated as an eosinophilic inflammation, potentially of allergic origin, but unrelated to a bacterial impact. Evidence accumulates, however, that *Staphylococcus aureus* colonizes CRS with polyps, but not without, with significantly increased prevalence. The bacteria release enterotoxins, which act as superantigens and induce a local multiclonal immunoglobulin (IgE) formation as well as a severe, possibly steroid-insensitive eosinophilic inflammation.

Recently, *S. aureus* was demonstrated to reside intraepithelially, and potentially to release superantigens into the tissue from within the epithelial cells. An immune defect, either in innate or adaptive immunity, might be responsible for this phenomenon. Follicle-like structures and lymphocyte accumulations, specifically binding enterotoxins, can be found within the polyp tissues, giving rise to local IgE formation.

The superantigen-induced immune response also leads to a modulation of the severity of the eosinophilic inflammation, and may be linked to lower airway co-morbidity in polyp patients. Interestingly, IgE antibodies to enterotoxins can be found in the majority of aspirin-sensitive polyp tissues, associated with a substantial increase in eosinophil cationic protein and interleukin-5. The possible role of *S. aureus* enterotoxins in polyp disease in Europe, the US and Asia has meanwhile been supported by several studies, demonstrating the presence of IgE antibodies to enterotoxins and inflammatory consequences in nasal polyp tissue.

First studies also point to an involvement of *Staphylococcus* derived enterotoxins in lower airway disease, such as severe asthma and exacerbated chronic obstructive pulmonary disease, clearly suggesting a clinical need for diagnosis and treatment of the germ and its related effects. Therapeutic approaches are so far empirical, and need further study, also serving to prove the clinical relevance of the concept.

Chronic rhinosinusitis represents a frequent, debilitating, inflammatory disease of the nose and the paranasal sinuses, characterized by symptoms such as blockage/congestion, reduction or loss of smell, anterior discharge/postnasal drip, and facial pain/pressure (1). Corresponding changes in either the sinus computed tomography (CT) scan or nasal endoscopy are needed to support the diagnosis. Nasal polyps (NP) in the middle meatus, which would be diagnosed by means of nasal endoscopy, would classify the patient into the "nasal polyp subgroup" according to recent position papers (1,2). The classification of all CRS disease in one single group is based on the lack of a clear differentiation of CRS from NP based on clinical symptoms or the CT scan.

However, recent evidence points to the possibility of differentiating chronic sinus disease groups based on the measurement of inflammatory cytokines, chemokines, and remodelling factors within the mucosal tissue (3). In NPs, we found significantly higher concentrations of eosinophilic markers, such as eotaxin, eosinophil cationic protein (ECP), and interleukin-5 (IL-5), and also immunoglobulin E (IgE), compared to CRS samples. In contrast, in CRS, we demonstrated significantly higher levels of interferon-γ (IFN-γ), transforming growth factor-β (TGF-β) and pro-inflammatory cytokines compared to NPs, pointing to different T-helper cell populations (Th2 vs. Th1) involved in the regulation of these inflammatory diseases. A set of markers could be selected for each disease entity, with a specificity and sensitivity above 60% for each of them. Based on these specific cytokine and mediator profiles, at least two distinct disease entities (CRS vs. NPs) within the large group of CRS disease have to be assumed (Fig. 1). As immune responses to staphylococcal enterotoxins so far only have been observed in NPs, but not in CRS (4); this chapter focuses on their contribution to NP disease.

Nasal polyps are characterized by abundant eosinophils, T-cell activation, overproduction of IgE, and originally were thought to represent an allergic disease (4–9). In Western countries, more than 70% of polyps show tissue eosinophilia, and increased concentrations of IL-5 and eotaxin, inducing eosinophil chemotaxis, migration, activation, and prolonged survival (6,7). Recent evidence accumulates, however, that *Staphylococcus aureus* enterotoxins (SE), acting as superantigens, induce a substantial inflammatory reaction in a large subgroup of NP, and strongly modify the disease (7).

We here summarize the evidence gathered so far, from our and other groups, on the impact of staphylococcus-derived superantigens and provide an outlook on the possible clinical implications for the management and therapy of nasal polyposis.

STAPHYLOCOCCAL ENTEROTOXINS CAN ACT AS SUPERANTIGENS

About 25% of the population are permanent carriers of *S. aureus* in the nostrils, and approximately 20% of all human staphylococcal infections are autogenous (10). Although the pathogenicity of *S. aureus* is closely correlated with the production of coagulase enzymes, these organisms also contain a number of cellular antigens and produce a variety of toxins with superantigenic properties (11,12). The classical SEs comprise SE A-E and TSST-1 (toxic shock syndrome toxin-1), however, other enterotoxins have been described recently, derived from the egc-gene

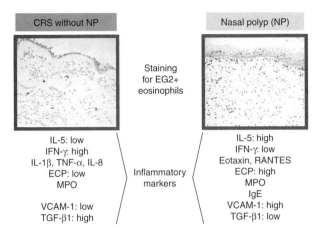

CRS without NP		Nasal polyp (NP)

| | Staining for EG2+ eosinophils | |

IL-5: low		IL-5: high
IFN-γ: high		IFN-γ: low
IL-1β, TNF-α, IL-8		Eotaxin, RANTES
ECP: low	Inflammatory	ECP: high
MPO	markers	MPO
		IgE
VCAM-1: low		VCAM-1: high
TGF-β1: high		TGF-β1: low

FIGURE 1 *(See color insert.)* Chronic rhinosinusitis versus nasal polyps (NPs) with respect to staining for EG2-positive eosinophils and the presence of other inflammatory markers in sinus tissue.

locus (13); these seem to be of relevance, as they frequently are produced by nasal *S. aureus*, and partially are unrelated to the production of classical enterotoxins (T. van Zele, unpublished data). SEs, as well as molecules derived from *Streptococcus pyogenes* (14) and some viruses (15,16), are able to activate T-cells via the T-cell receptor (TCR) major histo-compatibility complex (MHC) class II-complex independent of the antigen-specific groove by binding to the variable beta-chain of the TCR. The susceptibility of a T-cell to superantigens therefore is dependent on the usage of a specific beta-chain repertoire, possibly leading to the activation of abundant T-cells in a given tissue (vastly exceeding the percentage of T-cells that would be activated by a specific antigen). Another recently described possibility of modifying the response to superantigens is based on the finding that HLA-DQ polymorphisms may alter the binding of superantigens to the MHC class II complex (17). Thus, the resulting response of a T-cell population in a given tissue is dependent on many factors, such as production of and exposure to SEs, the intactness of the epithelial barrier, as well as the specific distribution of TCR and MHC class II molecules on immune cells. Once activated, T-cells would produce interleukins including IL-4, IL-5 and IL-13 and many other cytokines, which would lead to severe eosinophilic inflammation and local IgE production. Other direct actions of superantigens on B-cells, epithelial cells, eosinophils, etc., have been described, which are summarized in a recent review (18). All of these actions add to the enormous inflammatory potential of *S. aureus* derived superantigens (Fig. 2).

The finding of IgE antibodies to SEs SE A and SE B in nasal polyp tissue homogenates (7) for the first time indicated that these superantigens could be involved in the pathogenesis of nasal polyposis. Investigating tissue homogenates, we sought to determine the association between total and specific IgE to a variety of allergens in polyp and control samples, and to markers of eosinophilic inflammation. The concentrations of total IgE, IL-5, eotaxin, ECP, the cysteinyl leukotrienes (LT), and the soluble low-affinity IgE-receptor (CD23) were significantly higher in polyp tissue compared to controls. Total IgE was significantly correlated with IL-5, ECP, LTC4/D4/E4, and sCD23, and to the number of eosinophils.

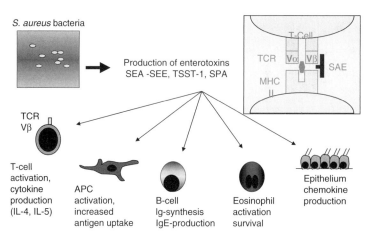

FIGURE 2 (*See color insert.*) Biological activities of *Staphylococcus aureus* enterotoxins.

An important subgroup of those polyp patients demonstrated a multiclonal IgE formation, including IgE to SEs, a high total IgE level, and a high prevalence of asthma. These studies suggested that bacterial superantigens could induce IgE synthesis in nasal polyps and impact the degree of eosinophilic inflammation (7,19).

IMMUNE RESPONSES TO STAPHYLOCOCCAL ENTEROTOXINS ARE INCREASED IN NASAL POLYPS

Staphylococcus aureus frequently colonizes the nostrils in healthy subjects, and can be found in acute and CRS (20). However, this germ has never been identified as a prominent player in chronic sinus disease without acute exacerbation, and studies in NP have not been performed. We recently reported an increased colonization rate of *S. aureus* in nasal polyps, but not in CRS without polyps (4), indicating that NP and CRS might be different disease entities with distinct underlying pathologic mechanisms. Colonization with *S. aureus* was present in 63.6% of subjects with polyps, with rates as high as 66.7% and 87.5% in the subgroups with asthma and aspirin sensitivity, which were significantly higher than in controls and subjects with CRS (33.3% and 27.3%, respectively). Furthermore, repeated swabbing of the middle meatus in eight subjects with polyps suggested long-term colonization with *S. aureus*. Using a combination of different enterotoxins in a screening assay, IgE antibodies to SEs were present in 27.8% in polyp samples, with rates as high as 53.8% and 80% in the subgroups with asthma and aspirin sensitivity, respectively, compared to 15% in controls and 6% in subjects with CRS. The concentration of ECP, reflecting the eosinophilic inflammation, was significantly increased in polyp samples with the presence of IgE antibodies to enterotoxins versus samples without IgE, suggesting a strong inflammatory effect of superantigens. In subjects with NPs and co-morbid asthma or aspirin sensitivity, rates of colonization and IgE response in nasal tissue homogenates were further increased, paralleled by increases in ECP and total IgE. These figures indicate that there is a strong relationship between staphylococcal colonization and tissue immune response to enterotoxins in nasal polyps, which may even be reflected in lower airway co-morbidity.

In line with these findings, only one-third of polyps collected within a defined time frame in a Chinese hospital were positive for enterotoxin-specific IgE: in a recent comparative study 10/27 samples in the polyp group versus 0/15 controls contained SAE-IgE (P < 0.01) (21). Furthermore, the number of EG2+ eosinophils was significantly lower in Chinese versus. Caucasian polyps, and asthma co-morbidity was negligible in Chinese polyp patients.

Comparable rates of colonization with *S. aureus* (71%) and IgE antibody formation (50%) to superantigens were found in another polyp study, with low rates in control subjects (25% and 0%, respectively), confirming our first results (22). Colonization rates always exceeded those of IgE immune response to SEs, indicating that colonization may not necessarily lead to the production or contact of superantigens with the immune system.

A NEW CONCEPT: INTRAEPITHELIAL GROWTH OF *S. AUREUS*

Until now, *S. aureus* has been regarded as a non invasive extracellular pathogen (23). However, recent findings demonstrate the ability of this germ to invade non phagocytic eukaryotic cells, and to possibly persist there for weeks. *Staphylococcus aureus* small-colony variants (SCV) are a naturally occurring slowly growing subpopulation which was recently related to chronic recurrent antibiotic-resistant infections such as cystic fibrosis (24,25). It has been demonstrated that *S. aureus* invades cultured cells of non professional phagocytes and cell lines (26,27), as well as human respiratory epithelial cells (28–30). Analysis of invaded cultured cells by electron microscopy revealed *S. aureus* in vacuoles within the airway epithelium (28,31). The interaction between *S. aureus* and epithelial cells has been proposed to occur through binding of fibronectin-binding proteins (FnBPs) on germs to fibronectin, β1-integrins and heat shock protein 60 (Hsp60) (29,32,33). The ability to be internalized and survive within host cells may explain the refractory nature of polyp disease to antibiotic treatment, which represents a hallmark of polyposis, as well as the chronicity of disease and recurrence, months and even years after apparently successful therapy. Antibiotics commonly used for the management of *S. aureus* infections appear to create a niche for invasive intracellular *S. aureus* (34,35).

We recently used immunohistochemistry to demonstrate the presence of *S. aureus* and production of SEB in samples from polyps (Fig. 3). Intraepithelial staining for *S. aureus* was found in a substantial subgroup of polyps, with affected and unaffected areas coexisting in the same samples (J. Patou, unpublished data). SEB could be co-localized to the intracellular *Staphylococcus*, indicating the potential of releasing this enterotoxin into the tissue. Further studies need to address the issues of germ survival and ongoing enterotoxin production in intraepithelial *S. aureus*. Apoptotic epithelial cells with their contents, and *S. aureus* which crosses the basal membrane, would be taken up by macrophages, which have been shown to be prevalent in increased numbers in nasal polyps versus controls (36). These macrophages in nasal polyp tissue have been characterized as CD 68[+], macrophage mannose receptor (MMR)+, CD 163+, RFD7+ phagocytosing macrophages, which characterize a mature phenotype of macrophages. Surprisingly, there was a significant lack of staining for *S. aureus* in macrophages in the lamina propria in polyp tissues compared to controls. These new data suggest a reduced capacity of

Staining for *Staphylococcus aureus*   Staining for SEB (enterotoxin B)

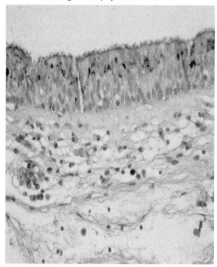 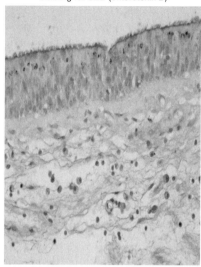

FIGURE 3 (*See color insert.*) Intraepithelial staining of *Staphylococcus aureus* bacteria and staphylococcal enterotoxin B (SEB) in nasal polyp epithelium.

these macrophages to phagocytose *S. aureus*, which needs further functional investigation. Of interest, the lack of defense against *S. aureus* seems to give rise to a local immune response to staphylococcal enterotoxins, as measured by increased IgE antibodies to enterotoxins, total IgE, ECP, and IL-5 versus controls in this patient group. In the skin, another possible deficiency in innate immunity, namely the lack of defensins, has been proposed (37), which we could not confirm in our studies on nasal polyps (38). Furthermore, a deficit in IgG$_2$ antibodies against enterotoxin C1 has been described recently, the clinical relevance of which is currently unclear (39) and has to also be studied in polyps. However, if confirmed, this finding could indicate a deficiency not only in the innate, but also in the adaptive immune regulation, which could predispose to the development of staphylococcal superantigen-driven disease.

ORGANIZATION OF SECONDARY LYMPHOID TISSUE AND EVIDENCE FOR LOCAL IgE FORMATION TO *S. AUREUS* ENTEROTOXINS

When nasal polyps were analyzed for T- and B-lymphocytes and IgE by immuno-histochemistry, follicular structures were found in 25% of the samples, and diffuse lymphoid accumulations were seen in all NP samples (22). Follicle-like structures are composed of T- and B-lymphocytes, and stain positive for IgE and the low affinity IgE receptor, whereas the high-affinity receptor is found outside the follicle only. Plasma cells expressing CD38 are prominent in the lymphoid accumulations, which also stain positive for IgE, CD3, and FcɛRI, but not for CD23. These lymphocyte accumulations therefore may be considered to develop from follicle-like structures, with B-cells maturing into IgE-producing plasma cells. Interest-ingly, we demonstrated binding of biotinylated SEA to follicular structures and lymphoid accumulations in polyp tissue (22). The specificity of the SE binding was confirmed by staining with an excess of non biotinylated SEA to biotinylated SEA, which completely blocked the signal. Furthermore, no follicular structures or SE staining were found in control tissue. These data suggest an organization of secondary lymphoid tissue with polyclonal B-cell activation in nasal polyps due to chronic microbial colonization and stimulation by enterotoxins, which is likely to be the cause of IgE switch and formation.

There is increasing evidence that SEs can directly affect the frequency and activation of the B cell repertoire. Functional studies in B-cells have shown that *S. aureus* protein A induces proliferation of these cells (40). Studies with TSST-1 indicated that staphylococcal superantigens may play an important role in the modulation of allergic disease, since they may augment isotype switching and synthesis of IgE, both in vitro (41) and in vivo, in a SCID mouse model (42). Although TSST-1-induced activation of B-cells in vitro is indirect and dependent on increased expression of CD40 ligand on T-cells, a more recent study has also provided evidence for a direct effect by demonstrating TSST-1-induced expression on B-cells of B7.2 (43), a molecule that has been shown to enhance Th2 responses and to be involved in IgE regulation. In mucosal tissues of hay fever and asthma patients, mRNA for the e-chain of IgE was found in a significant proportion of B cells using in situ hybridization (44–47), supporting the hypothesis of a truly local IgE synthesis in the airway mucosa. Pilot studies on the expression of co-stimulatory signals such as CD40/CD40 ligand and CD28/B7 in lymphocytes of nasal polyps support this notion (T. van Zele, unpublished data), and studies on local IgE switching events are currently being performed (48).

Nasal culture of the middle meatus demonstrated an increased staphylococcal colonization in polyp patients versus controls, as discussed before (4), associated with a significant increase in tissue concentrations of IgE, albumin, and eosinophil counts. Total IgE and IgE-antibody concentrations to enterotoxins were in all cases higher in tissue compared to serum, but SE-specific IgE antibodies may be detected in the serum of polyp patients (19), especially when asthma coexists. The IgE/albumin ratios in polyp tissue and in serum were dissociated, again indicating that tissue IgE is rather the result of a local IgE production than of extravasation. Furthermore, IgE antibodies in polyp tissue only showed a partial relation to IgE antibodies in serum and to skin prick test results. In a substantial subgroup of patients, the typical pattern of IgE expression in polyp tissue was found: a polyclonal type of IgE expression with IgE antibodies to common aeroallergens and a high level of total IgE. These findings resemble those in atopic dermatitis, where colonization of the inflamed skin with *S. aureus* clearly contributes to the high IgE levels in serum and to the severity of the disease (49).

THE RELATION OF SES TO ASPIRIN SENSITIVITY

From the first study in patients with local IgE against staphylococcal enterotoxins (7) it appeared that the highest IgE concentrations were obtained from samples of aspirin-sensitive subjects. We therefore extended our observations in this nonallergic, but severely inflamed subgroup of patients, who also suffered from asthma. Forty subjects with nasal polyps from Poland were classified as aspirin-sensitive (N = 13, ASNP) or aspirin-tolerant (N = 27, ATNP) based on a bronchial aspirin challenge test (50). Homogenates prepared from nasal polyp tissue and inferior nasal turbinates from healthy subjects were analyzed for concentrations of

IL-5, ECP, total IgE, and IgE to a mix of SEs (A, C, TSST-1), a screening test which was developed in cooperation with SGO Johansson (51).

A significant increase in IL-5 concentrations, total IgE and IgE antibodies to SEs was observed in samples from supernatants in NP patients compared to controls, with levels of IgE to SEs correlating with IL-5 and ECP levels. Patients were further analyzed in two groups, with or without aspirin sensitivity (ASNP and ATNP, respectively). Concentrations of total IgE and IgE antibodies to a mix of SEs (SEA, SEC, TSST-1) showed significantly higher levels in ASNP patients compared to ATNP and control groups as well. Moreover quantities of IL-5 and ECP were up-regulated in ASNP and differed significantly from ATNP and control subjects. These results confirmed that the immune response to SEs was linked to the up-regulation of eosinophilic inflammation, and suggested a possible link of SEs to aspirin sensitivity, which might be direct (SEs inducing superantigen) or indirect (via the severity of inflammation). Therefore, ASNP and ATNP patients were each divided in two subgroups, with and without SEs. Out of 13 patients with ASNP, 7 were SE(+) in comparison with 7 out of 27 in the ATNP group and none out of 12 subjects in the control group. Concentrations of inflammatory markers (IL-5 and ECP) did not differ between ASNP-SE(+) and SE(−) groups, but were up-regulated with respect to the control group. These observations rather suggested an indirect link between SEs and aspirin sensitivity.

Further investigations, comparing eicosanoid production and eosinophilic markers in CRS patients with and without nasal polyps, with nasal polyps and aspirin sensitivity, and finally in normal nasal mucosa from healthy subjects, showed that LTC_4S, 5-LO mRNA and $LTC_4/D_4/E_4$ concentrations increased with disease severity (per patient group) (52). Other metabolites such as COX-2 and prostaglandin E_2 (PGE_2) significantly decreased with disease severity. IL-5 and ECP were increased in both groups of nasal polyp tissues compared to controls and CRS, and correlated directly with $LTC_4/D_4/E_4$ and inversely with PGE_2 concentrations. These data confirmed the notion that changes of tissue eicosanoid metabolism do occur in CRS even in the absence of clinical aspirin sensitivity and appear to be related to severity of eosinophilic inflammation, with SEs being a strong modifier of local and systemic inflammation in nasal polyps.

Our findings were recently confirmed by Suh et al. (53), who studied IgE antibodies to SEs and eosinophilic markers in aspirin-sensitive and tolerant asthmatics with nasal polyps. These authors also found an increase in ECP, but not IL-5, between these groups, and significantly increased levels of IgE to SEs in aspirin-sensitive subjects. The authors also confirmed the relevance of the impact of SEs on nasal polyp disease in Korea, expanding on our European observations.

SES PROVIDING A LINK TO LOWER AIRWAY DISEASE

Until recently, there was only indirect evidence that SEs could possibly also impact lower airway disease unrelated to nasal polyposis, especially in poorly controlled asthma. By studying the TCR-Vbeta repertoire of broncho-alveolar lavage (BAL) cells and peripheral blood mononuclear cells (PBMCs) from subjects with poorly controlled asthma ($FEV_1 < 75\%$), subjects with well-controlled asthma, and control subjects, Hawk et al. found a significantly higher expression of Vbeta8(+) T cells in BAL fluid of poorly controlled asthmatics compared to the other groups. Increased Vbeta8(+) BAL T cells were present in the CD4(+) and CD8(+) subsets, suggesting activation by SEs (54).

Experiments in mice to delineate the type of immune response triggered by superantigen exposure to the airway mucosa showed that a low dose of SEB could trigger an inflammatory response characterized by mucosal and airway recruitment of lymphocytes, eosinophils, and neutrophils. These responses were associated with the development of increased airway responsiveness in SEB-treated mice, observed in IgE-high responder BALB/c as well as in IgE-low/intermediate responder C57BL/6 mice. These results suggested that the local immune response following mucosal superantigen administration triggers a unique inflammatory response in the airways in mice, resembling many features of "intrinsic asthma" (55). A similar experimental model is currently being used to further elucidate the interaction between lower and upper airway staphylococcal enterotoxin effects.

Evidence for a direct impact of enterotoxins on lower airway disease is also growing in humans. Based on our previous findings, we used a sensitive and highly specific screening tool, the SAE mix, to detect IgE to SAEs in serum of mild and severe asthmatics, classified by lung function and need for drug treatment, versus controls. IgE antibodies to SAE mix were found significantly more frequently in severe asthmatics (62%) versus controls (13%, $P = 0.01$), and were linked to concentrations of IgE antibodies in serum, severity of eosinophilic inflammation (ECP in serum), and corticosteroid dependence (56). Thirty-one out of the 55 asthma patients showed increased concentrations of total IgE in serum ($>100 kU/L$), and 21 of those had IgE antibodies to SAE mix. Consequently, 10 subjects had an increased total IgE, but no IgE antibodies to SAE mix. Twelve sera had a total IgE above $500 kU/L$, and of those nine were positive and three negative for IgE-antibodies to SAE. These data suggest that, in some patients, other superantigens than the ones tested here (for instance those derived from certain Streptococci) may also play a role. We therefore proposed a crucial role for SEs in the pathophysiology of upper and lower airway disease, linked to severity of eosinophilic inflammation, total IgE synthesis, but also clinical disease severity, to be confirmed in larger populations as well as in confirmatory treatment studies.

We also studied the expression of total IgE and IgE antibodies to SEs in chronic obstructive pulmonary disease (COPD) patients, smokers without COPD, and healthy controls (56). SE-IgE antibodies were found in 1/10 controls and 1/16 smokers, but in 7/18 patients with stable disease (38.9%) and 21/54 patients with exacerbated COPD (38.9%). The IgE concentrations of patients with stable or exacerbated COPD were significantly higher than those of smokers or controls. Furthermore, IgE to SEs decreased significantly in the exacerbated patients during hospitalization, going along with a significant increase in FEV_1. These data suggest a role for superantigens in exacerbated COPD similar to that in severe asthma.

CLINICAL IMPLICATIONS AND PERSPECTIVES

In summary, there is accumulating evidence that superantigens, primarily derived from *S. aureus*, but possibly also from other sources such as *Streptococcus*, fungi (AFS), or viruses (57), may have a major impact on upper and lower airway diseases such as nasal polyposis and asthma. Superantigens at least appear to modify, if not cause, severe airway disease (18,58). Staphylococcal enterotoxins may furthermore affect treatment possibilities, as it was shown that these compounds may alter steroid sensitivity and expression of glucocorticoid receptor beta (59).

Dexamethasone caused a 99% inhibition of phytohemaglutinin (PHA)-induced PBMC proliferation, but only a 19% inhibition of the proliferation induced by SEB, 26% inhibition of that induced by TSST-1, and 29% inhibition of that induced by SEE, demonstrating that superantigens can induce steroid insensitivity. At the same time, stimulation of normal PBMCs with SEB induced a significant increase in glucocorticoid receptor beta expression compared with PHA and unstimulated cells, a possible mechanism to induce glucocorticoid insensitivity. It has also recently been shown that *S. aureus* superantigens can induce a specific pattern of phosphorylation of the glucocorticoid receptor leading to glucocorticoid resistance (60). For diagnostic purposes, *S. aureus* can be detected in the middle nasal meatus by swabs, but would only poorly predict production of an immune response to its enterotoxins. The potential production of enterotoxins by these germs, once cultured, can be shown by polynerase chain reaction (PCR) or protein assays, but clinical studies showing the clinical relevance in an individual patient have not yet been performed. The ability to produce enterotoxins by a given germ may also vary due to varying conditions in the nasal environment or number of colonies present. In contrast, the presence of IgE antibodies to SEs indicates a former or present stimulation of the local immune system by the respective enterotoxin, and can be tested in tissue homogenates. A polyclonal IgE response, high total IgE, and increased eosinophilic mediators (ECP) would indicate the activity of the superantigens. Furthermore, *Staphylococcus* can now be stained intraepithelially by immuno-histochemistry, however, a positive staining would again not necessarily predict a specific immune response.

The potential therapeutic effect of a treatment to eradicate *S. aureus* in polyp disease or asthma has not yet been studied, but large-scale double-blind placebo-controlled studies are currently ongoing. From atopic dermatitis (AD), a disease sharing the modifying effects of staphylococcal superantigens on inflammation and disease severity, we can deduce therapeutic approaches. The skin of up to 100% of patients with AD is colonized with *S. aureus*, of which up to 65% have been shown to produce enterotoxins with superantigenic properties. Ten patients were treated orally with antibiotics, chlorhexidine ointment was applied to the skin, the anterior nares were treated with mupirocin ointment, and a bath containing potassium permanganate was taken daily (61). In addition, their partners were treated topically. The Severity Scoring in AD (SCORAD) score decreased in nine of ten patients who received antimicrobial treatment, and this effect was more pronounced in patients with a higher baseline SCORAD. Thus, antimicrobial treatment led to a significant, albeit temporary, improvement of AD in patients who were colonized with *S. aureus*. A similar effect may be anticipated for nasal polyps, however, this needs to be confirmed. Other approaches, such as long-term antibiotic treatment with intracellular activity in combination with corticosteroids to decrease the immune response and increase steroid sensitivity, antibiotic treatment with intracellularly active drugs, or vaccination therapy against the germs might be developed in the future for sustained treatment success.

ACKNOWLEDGMENTS

This work was supported by a grant to Claus Bachert from the Flemish Scientific Research Board, FWO, Nr. A12/5-K/V-K17, and by a grant to Nan Zhang from the University of Ghent, BOF VB0149.

REFERENCES

1. Fokkens W, Lund V, Bachert C, et al. EAACI Position Paper on Rhinosinusitis and Nasal Polyposis. Rhinology 2005; 18(Suppl.):1–87.
2. Meltzer EO, Hamilos DL, Hadley JA, et al. Rhinosinusitis: Establishing definitions for clinical research and patient care. J Allergy Clin Immunol 2004; 114(6 Suppl.):155–212.
3. Van Zele T, Claeys S, Gevaert P, Holtappels G, Van Cauwenberge P, Bachert C. Differentiation of chronic sinus diseases by measurement of inflammatory mediators. Allergy 2006; 61:1280–89.
4. Van Zele T, Gevaert P, Watelet JB, et al. *Staphylococcus aureus* colonization and IgE antibody formation to enterotoxins is increased in nasal polyposis. J Allergy Clin Immunol 2004; 114:981–3.
5. Park HS, Jung KS, Shute J, Robert K, Holgate ST, Djukanovic R. Allergen-induced release of GM-CSF and IL-8 in vitro by nasal polyp tissue from atopic subjects prolongs eosinophil survival. Eur Respir J 1997; 7:1476–82.
6. Simon HU, Yousefi S, Schranz C, Schapowal A, Bachert C, Blaser K. Direct demonstration of delayed eosinophil apoptosis as a mechanism causing tissue eosinophilia. J Immunol 1997; 158:3902–8.
7. Bachert C, Gevaert P, Holtappels G, Johansson SG, Van Cauwenberge P. Total and specific IgE in nasal polyps is related to local eosinophilic inflammation. J Allergy Clin Immunol 2001; 107:607–14.
8. Conley DB, Tripathi A, Ditto AM, Reid K, Grammer LC, Kern RC. Chronic sinusitis with nasal polyps: staphylococcal exotoxin immunoglobulin E and cellular inflammation. Am J Rhinol 2004; 18:273–8.
9. Caplin I, Haynes TJ, Spahn J. Are nasal polyps an allergic phenomenon? Ann Allergy 1971; 29:631–34.
10. Farthing MJH, Jeffries DJ, Anderson. J. Infectious diseases, tropical medicine and sexually transmitted diseases. In: Kumar P, Clark M, eds. Clinical Medicine. 3rd edn. London: Baillie`re Tindall, 1994:1–105.
11. Balaban N, Rasooly A. Staphylococcal enterotoxins. Int J Food Microbiol 2000; 61:1–103.
12. Yarwood JM, Mccormick JK, Schlievert PM. Identification of a novel two-component regulatory system that acts in global regulation of virulence factors of *Staphylococcus aureus*. J Bacteriol 2001; 183:1113–23.
13. Jarraud S, Peyrat MA, Lim A, et al. egc, a highly prevalent operon of enterotoxin gene, forms a putative nursery of superantigens in *Staphylococcus aureus*. J Immunol 2001; 166:669–77.
14. De Marzi MC, Fernandez MM, Sundberg EJ, et al. Cloning, expression and interaction of human T-cell receptors with the bacterial superantigen SSA. Eur J Biochem 2004; 271:4075–83.
15. Sutkowski N, Chen G, Calderon G, Huber BT. Epstein–Barr virus latent membrane protein LMP-2A is sufficient for transactivation of the human endogenous retrovirus HERV-K18 superantigen. J Virol 2004; 78:7852–60.
16. Pobezinskaya Y, Chervonsky AV, Golovkina TV. Initial stages of mammary tumor virus infection are superantigen independent. J Immunol 2004; 172:5582–7.
17. Llewelyn M, Sriskandan S, Peakman M, et al. HLA class II polymorphisms determine responses to bacterial superantigens. J Immunol 2004; 172:1719–26.
18. Bachert C, van Zele T, Gevaert P, De Schrijver L, Van Cauwenberge P. Superantigens and nasal polyps. Curr Allergy Asthma Rep 2003; 3:523–31.
19. Tripathi A, Conley DB, Grammer LC, et al. Immunoglobulin E to staphylococcal and streptococcal toxins in patients with chronic sinusitis/nasal polyposis. Laryngoscope 2004; 114:1822–6.
20. Gittelman P, Jacobs J, Lebowitz A, Tierno P. *Staphylococcus aureus* nasal carriage in patients with rhinosinusitis. Laryngoscope 1991; 101:733–7.
21. Zhang N, Holtappels G, Claeys C, Huang GQ, van Cauwenberge P, Bachert C. Pattern of inflammation and impact of Staphylococcs aureus enterotoxins in nasal polyposis from South of China. Am J Rhinol 2006; 20:445–50.

22. Gevaert P, Holtappels G, Johansson SG, Cuvelier C, Cauwenberge P, Bachert C. Organization of secondary lymphoid tissue and local IgE formation to *Staphylococcus aureus* enterotoxins in nasal polyp tissue. Allergy 2005; 60:71–9.
23. Alexander EH, Hudson MC. Factors influencing the internalization of *Staphylococcus aureus* and impacts on the course of infections in humans. Appl Microbiol Biotechnol 2001; 56:361–6.
24. von Eiff C, Proctor RA, Peters G. Small colony variants of staphylococci: a link to persistent infections. Berl Munch Tierarztl Wochenschr 2000; 113:321–5.
25. von Eiff C, Becker K, Metze D, et al. Intracellular persistence of *Staphylococcus aureus* small-colony variants within keratinocytes: a cause for antibiotic treatment failure in a patient with darier's disease. Clin Infect Dis 2001; 32:1643–7.
26. Jevon M, Guo C, Ma B, et al. Mechanisms of internalization of *Staphylococcus aureus* by cultured human osteoblasts. Infect Immun 1999; 67:2677–81.
27. Ellington JK, Reilly SS, Ramp WK, Smeltzer MS, Kellam JF, Hudson MC. Mechanisms of *Staphylococcus aureus* invasion of cultured osteoblasts. Microb Pathog 1999; 26:317–23.
28. Kahl BC, Goulian M, van Wamel W, et al. *Staphylococcus aureus* RN6390 replicates and induces apoptosis in a pulmonary epithelial cell line. Infect Immun 2000; 68:5385–92.
29. Jett BD, Gilmore MS. Internalization of *Staphylococcus aureus* by human corneal epithelial cells: role of bacterial fibronectin-binding protein and host cell factors. Infect Immun 2002; 70:4697–700.
30. Kintarak S, Whawell SA, Speight PM, Packer S, Nair SP. Internalization of *Staphylococcus aureus* by human keratinocytes. Infect Immun 2004; 72:5668–75.
31. da Silva MC, Zahm JM, Gras D, et al. Dynamic interaction between airway epithelial cells and *Staphylococcus aureus*. Am J Physiol Lung Cell Mol Physiol 2004; 287:L543–51.
32. Dziewanowska K, Carson AR, Patti JM, Deobald CF, Bayles KW, Bohach GA. Staphylococcal fibronectin binding protein interacts with heat shock protein 60 and integrins: role in internalization by epithelial cells. Infect Immun 2000; 68:6321–8.
33. Fowler T, Wann ER, Joh D, Johansson S, Foster TJ, Hook M. Cellular invasion by *Staphylococcus aureus* involves a fibronectin bridge between the bacterial fibronectin-binding MSCRAMMs and host cell beta1 integrins. Eur J Cell Biol 2000; 79:672–9.
34. Krut O, Sommer H, Kronke M. Antibiotic-induced persistence of cytotoxic *Staphylococcus aureus* in non-phagocytic cells. J Antimicrob Chemother 2004; 53:167–73.
35. Clement S, Vaudaux P, Francois P, et al. Evidence of an Intracellular Reservoir in the Nasal Mucosa of Patients with Recurrent *Staphylococcus aureus* Rhinosinusitis. J Infect Dis 2005; 192:1023–8.
36. Claeys S, Van Hoecke H, Holtappels G, et al. Nasal polyps in patients with and without cystic fibrosis: a differentiation by innate markers and inflammatory mediators. Clin Exp Allergy 2005; 35:467–72.
37. Ong PY, Ohtake T, Brandt C, et al. Endogenous antimicrobial peptides and skin infections in atopic dermatitis. N Engl J Med 2002; 347:1151–60
38. Claeys S, De Belder T, Holtappels G, et al. Macrophage mannose receptor in chronic sinus disease. Allergy 2004; 59:606–12.
39. Mrabet-Dahbi S, Breuer K, Klotz M, et al. Deficiency in immunoglobulin G2 antibodies against staphylococcal enterotoxin C1 defines a subgroup of patients with atopic dermatitis. Clin Exp Allergy 2005; 35:274–81.
40. Inganas M, Johansson SG, Bennich HH. Interaction of human polyclonal IgE and IgG from different species with protein A from *Staphylococcus aureus*: demonstration of protein-A-reactive sites located in the Fab'2 fragment of human IgG. Scand J Immunol 1980; 12:23–31.
41. Jabara HH, Geha RS. The superantigen toxic shock syndrome toxin-1 induces CD40 ligand expression and modulates IgE isotype switching. Int Immunol 1996; 8:1503–10.
42. Tumang JR, Zhou JL, Gietl D, Crow MK, Elkon KB, Friedman SM. T helper cell-dependent, microbial superantigen mediated B cell activation in vivo. Autoimmunity 1996; 24:247–55.
43. Hofer MF, Harbeck RJ, Schlievert PM, Leung DY. Staphylococcal toxins augment specific IgE responses by atopic patients exposed to allergen. J Invest Dermatol 1999; 112:171–6.

44. Ying S, Humbert M, Meng Q, et al. Local expression of epsilon germline gene transcripts and RNA for the epsilon heavy chain of IgE in the bronchial mucosa in atopic and nonatopic asthma. J Allergy Clin Immunol 2001; 107:686–92.
45. Kleinjan A, Vinke JG, Severijnen LW, Fokkens WJ. Local production and detection of (specific) IgE in nasal B-cells and plasma cells of allergic rhinitis patients. Eur Respir J 2000; 15:491–7.
46. Durham SR, Gould HJ, Thienes CP, et al. Expression of epsilon germ-line gene transcripts and mRNA for the epsilon heavy chain of IgE in nasal B cells and the effects of topical corticosteroid. Eur J Immunol 1997; 27:2899–906.
47. Smurthwaite L, Walker SN, Wilson DR, et al. Persistent IgE synthesis in the nasal mucosa of hay fever patients. Eur J Immunol 2001; 31:3422–31.
48. Coker HA, Durham SR, Gould HJ. Local somatic hypermutation and class switch recombination in the nasal mucosa of allergic rhinitis patients. J Immunol 2003; 171:5602–10.
49. Zollner TM, Wichelhaus TA, Hartung A, et al. Colonization with superantigen-producing *Staphylococcus aureus* is associated with increased severity of atopic dermatitis. Clin Exp Allergy 2000; 30:994–1000.
50. Perez-Novo CA, Kowalski ML, Kuna P, et al. Aspirin sensitivity and IgE antibodies to *Staphylococcus aureus* enterotoxins in nasal polyposis: studies on the relationship. Int Arch Allergy Immunol 2004; 133:255–60.
51. Bachert C, Gevaert P, Howarth P, Holtappels G, van Cauwenberge P, Johansson SG. IgE to *Staphylococcus aureus* enterotoxins in serum is related to severity of asthma. J Allergy Clin Immunol 2003; 111:1131–2.
52. Perez-Novo C, Watelet JB, Claeys C, van Cauwenberge P, Bachert C. Prostaglandin, leukotriene, and lipoxin balance in chronic rhinosinusitis with and without nasal polyposis. J Allergy Clin Immunol 2005; 115:1189–96.
53. Suh YJ, Yoon SH, Sampson AP, et al. Specific immunoglobulin E for staphylococcal enterotoxins in nasal polyps from patients with aspirin-intolerant asthma. Clin Exp Allergy 2004; 34:1270–5.
54. Hauk PJ, Wenzel SE, Trumble AE, Szefler SJ, Leung DY. Increased T-cell receptor vbeta8+ T cells in bronchoalveolar lavage fluid of subjects with poorly controlled asthma: a potential role for microbial superantigens. J Allergy Clin Immunol 1999; 104:37–45.
55. Herz U, Ruckert R, Wollenhaupt K, et al. Airway exposure to bacterial superantigen (SEB) induces lymphocyte-dependent airway inflammation associated with increased airway responsiveness—a model for non-allergic asthma. Eur J Immunol 1999; 29:1021–31.
56. Rohde G, Gevaert P, Holtappels G, et al. Increased IgE-antibodies to *Staphylococcus aureus* enterotoxins in patients with COPD. Respir Med 2004; 98:858–64.
57. Schubert MS. A superantigen hypothesis for the pathogenesis of chronic hypertrophic rhinosinusitis, allergic fungal sinusitis, and related disorders. Ann Allergy Asthma Immunol 2001; 87:181–8.
58. Bachert C, Gevaert P, van Cauwenberge P. *Staphylococcus aureus* enterotoxins: a key in airway disease? Allergy 2002; 57:480–7.
59. Hauk PJ, Hamid QA, Chrousos GP, Leung DY. Induction of corticosteroid insensitivity in human PBMCs by microbial superantigens. J Allergy Clin Immunol 2000; 105:782–7.
60. Li LB, Goleva E, Hall CF, Ou LS, Leung DY. Superantigen-induced corticosteroid resistance of human T cells occurs through activation of the mitogen-activated protein kinase kinase/extracellular signal-regulated kinase (MEK-ERK) pathway. J Allergy Clin Immunol 2004; 114:1059–69.
61. Breuer K, Häussler S, Kapp A, Werfel T. *Staphylococcus aureus*: colonizing features and influence of an antibacterial treatment in adults with atopic dermatitis. Br J Dermatol 2002; 147:55–61.

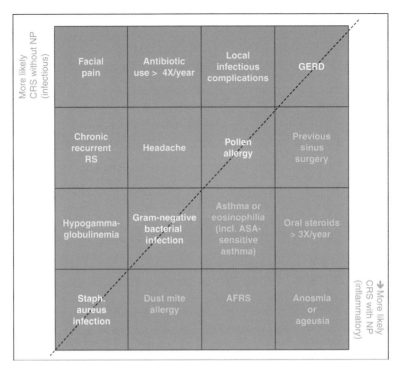

Facial pain	Antibiotic use > 4X/year	Local infectious complications	GERD
Chronic recurrent RS	Headache	Pollen allergy	Previous sinus surgery
Hypogamma-globulinemia	Gram-negative bacterial infection	Asthma or eosinophilia (incl. ASA-sensitive asthma)	Oral steroids > 3X/year
Staph. aureus infection	Dust mite allergy	AFRS	Anosmia or ageusia

More likely CRS without NP (infectious)

More likely CRS with NP (inflammatory)

FIGURE 1.3 Clinical/pathologic matrix of symptoms and clinical features associated with CRS without NP or CRS with NP. (*See p. 12.*)

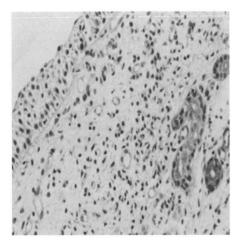

FIGURE 5.1 H&E staining showing inflammatory T cells and eosinophils in nasal mucosa in CRS.

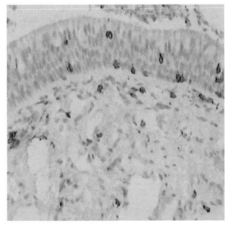

FIGURE 5.2 Immunostaining with CD4 antibody showing infiltration of the nasal mucosa and epithelium with T cells.

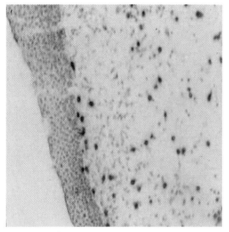

FIGURE 5.3 In-situ hybridization showing Th2-type cytokines produced by T cells.

FIGURE 5.4 MBP staining of eosinophils in the mucosa and epithelium in nasal tissue in CRS.

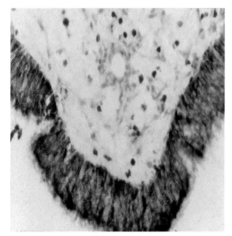

FIGURE 5.5 Eotaxin immunostaining in the epithelium in CRS.

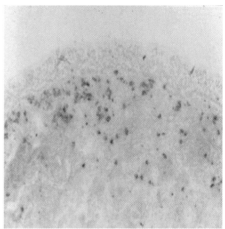

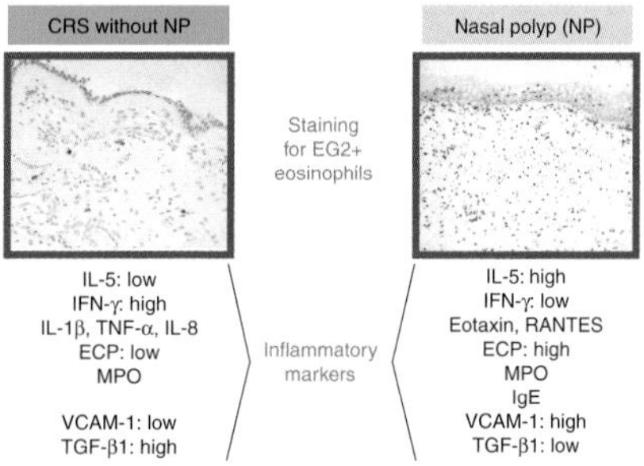

CRS without NP		Nasal polyp (NP)

Staining for EG2+ eosinophils

IL-5: low
IFN-γ: high
IL-1β, TNF-α, IL-8
ECP: low
MPO

VCAM-1: low
TGF-β1: high

Inflammatory markers

IL-5: high
IFN-γ: low
Eotaxin, RANTES
ECP: high
MPO
IgE
VCAM-1: high
TGF-β1: low

FIGURE 10.1 Chronic rhinosinusitis versus nasal polyps (NPs) with respect to staining for EG2-positive eosinophils and the presence of other inflammatory markers in sinus tissue.

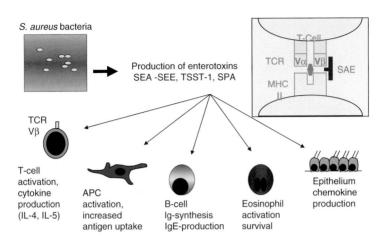

FIGURE 10.2 Biological activities of *Staphylococcus aureus* enterotoxins.

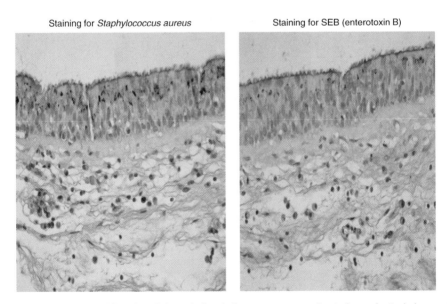

FIGURE 10.3 Intraepithelial staining of *Staphylococcus aureus* bacteria and staphylococcal enterotoxin B (SEB) in NP epithelium.

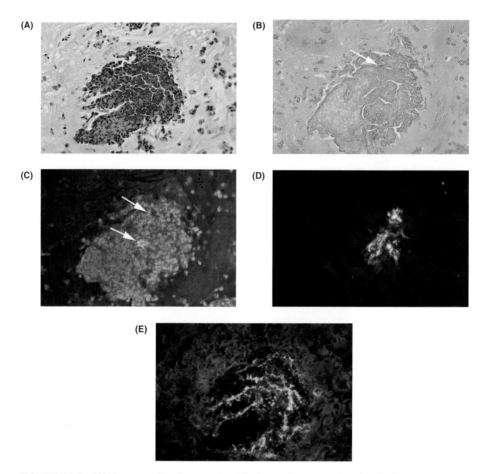

FIGURE 11.1 (**A**) An example of an eosinophil cluster in the mucin of a CRS patient, where eosinophils appear to target fungal organisms. This specimen was attached to sinus tissue and was removed during surgery. Due to the heterogeneous nature of the eosinophilia, where areas with and without eosinophils coexist, these clusters can be easily missed on examination (hematoxylin and eosin counterstain of the same section shown in **E**; magnification, ×800). (**B**) Serial section of the same cluster shown in (**A**), stained with Gomori's methamire silver. The white arrow identifies a fungal organism. Note that the larger organism visible with the chitinase and anti-*Alternaria* staining (**B** and **C**) is not visible using the GMS stain technique (magnification, ×800). (**C**) Serial section of the same cluster shown in (**A**) and (**B**) stained for chitinase by immunofluorescence. Fungal elements (white arrows) are evident within the eosinophil cluster (magnification, ×800). (**D**) Serial section of the same cluster shown in (**A–C**) stained for *Alternaria* by immunofluorescence. Staining occurs both within and around fungal organisms (magnification, ×800). (**E**) Same section as that shown in (**A**) stained for eosinophil granule major basic protein (MBP) by immunofluorescence. Extracellular deposition of the toxic eosinophil granule protein MBP is evident within the eosinophil cluster (magnification, ×800).

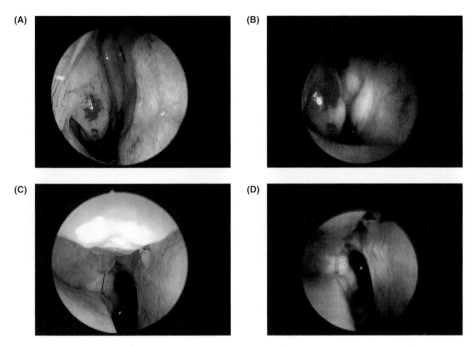

FIGURE 13.1 The anterior and posterior right nasal cavity is examined in the same patient with the same sized rigid (**A, C**) and flexible (**B, D**) endoscopes. Rigid scopes carry more light to the object and have superior optics resulting in a better image quality. Flexible scopes rely on bundles of optical fibers to transmit the image back to the examiner, thereby decreasing the optical quality and giving a more pixilated or grainy image.

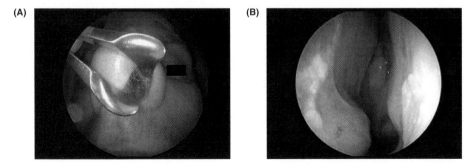

FIGURE 13.2 Anterior rhinoscopy should be performed in the native and decongested state. Excellent illumination is provided directly by a headlight or indirectly by a head mirror. A nasal speculum (**A**) increases visualization and allows for visualization of the anterior nasal cavity (**B**). Although polyps and purulence of the middle meatus may be visualized, anterior rhinoscopy is more adept in evaluating the nasal septum and inferior turbinate pathology, as is the case in this patient with a large septal spur running near the floor of the left nasal cavity.

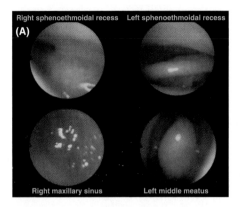
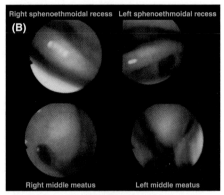

FIGURE 19.6 *Case study no. 1: CRS without NP.* The patient is a 36-year-old Caucasian female with a history of recurrent CRS that responded well to antibiotics. Her evaluation revealed no allergies or hypogammaglobulinemia. (*See p. 315.*)

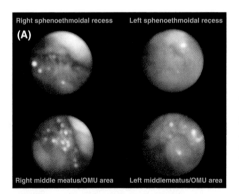
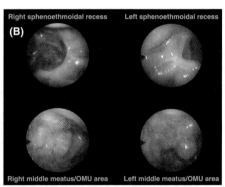

FIGURE 19.7 *Case study no. 2: CRS with NP.* The patient is a 65-year-old Caucasian male with CRS with NP. (*See p. 316.*)

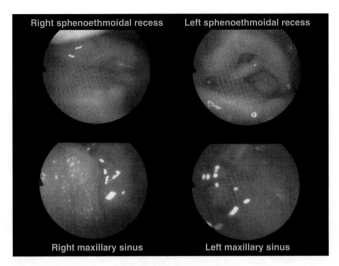

FIGURE 19.8 *Case study no. 3: Eosinophilic mucin in a patient with AFRS.* The patient is a 52-year-old Caucasian female with a history of AFRS. (*See p. 317.*)

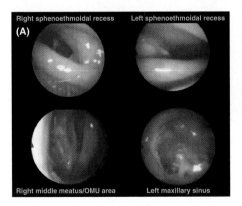
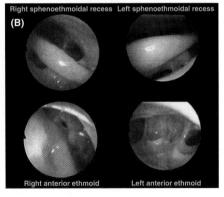

FIGURE 19.9 *Case study no. 4: AFRS.* A 42-year-old African-American male had a 1-year history of CRS with NP and repeated "infections" for which antibiotics were given. (*See p. 318.*)

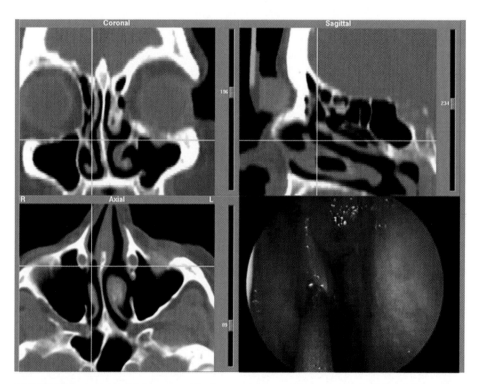

FIGURE 20.1 Image guided surgery. The bottom right panel is an endoscopic view of a patient's nostril during functional endoscopic sinus surgery with a suction tip that carries the sensor for image guidance. The position of the sensor is seen on the computed tomography scan that was obtained preoperatively and is available in the operating suite. Three views are delineated: coronal, sagittal, and axial.

11

The Role of Ubiquitous Airborne Fungi in Chronic Rhinosinusitis

Jens U. Ponikau and David A. Sherris
Department of Otorhinolaryngology, University at Buffalo, State University of New York, Buffalo, New York, U.S.A.

Hirohito Kita
Division of Allergic Diseases, Department of Internal Medicine, Mayo Clinic, Rochester, Minnesota, U.S.A.

INTRODUCTION

Chronic rhinosinusitis (CRS) is a confusing disease for both allergists and otorhinolaryngologists, partially due to its poorly understood pathophysiology and partially due to its limited treatment options. Several recent reports now provide evidence for a better understanding of the etiology and the relationship of CRS to airborne fungi, especially to *Alternaria*. First, the development of novel methods enables detection of certain fungi in mucus from the nasal and paranasal sinus cavities. Second, a nonimmunoglobulin E-mediated immunologic mechanism for reactivity of CRS patients to certain common fungi has been described. Third, these fungi are surrounded by eosinophils in vivo, suggesting that they are targeted by eosinophils. Fourth, the preliminary results of studies using antifungal agents to treat patients with CRS are promising. Overall, these recent discoveries provide a logical mechanism for the pathophysiology of CRS, and they also suggest promising avenues for treatment of CRS with antifungal agents.

A current report by the Centers for Disease Control and Prevention estimates that the prevalence of sinusitis is up to 14.1% (29.2 million) of the adult US population, and the fact that there is no US Food and Drug Administration (FDA)-approved treatment for this disorder emphasizes the profound impact of this disease (1,2). Patients with CRS suffer from long-term nasal congestion, thick mucus production, loss of sense of smell, and intermittent acute exacerbations secondary to bacterial infections (1,3). All of these symptoms can impair the patient's quality of life more severely than that of patients with congestive heart failure (4). In recent years, it has become clear that to understand CRS, one needs to examine the inflammation that exists within and outside the hyperplastic tissue.

UNDERSTANDING THE INFLAMMATION

Chronic rhinosinusitis is characterized histologically by an intense eosinophilic infiltration into the nasal mucosa (5–8). The study by Harlin et al. (7) was the first

Reprinted with permission of Current Science from Curr Rev Allergy Immunol 2005; 5:472–81. Supported by NIH grants AI 50494, AI 49235 and the Mayo Foundation.

to link the damage in CRS to the eosinophilic inflammation. This eosinophilic inflammation occurs with or without nasal polyposis, is independent of atopy, and is present neither in healthy controls nor in patients with acute bacterial or viral sinus infections. The inflammation can be easily overlooked if patients are given systemic steroids or other anti-inflammatory medication before harvesting the tissue for examination. This distinctive eosinophilic inflammation is also very heterogeneous (i.e., without eosinophilic infiltration in one area of a nasal mucosal tissue specimen, but with intense eosinophilic infiltration in another area of the same specimen) (9). Thus, reports in which only single biopsies are examined and in which it was unclear whether patients had received steroids before the biopsies were taken need to be interpreted carefully regarding the intensity of the eosinophilic infiltrate. In addition, granule proteins from the eosinophils, such as major basic protein (MBP), that are toxic to sinus epithelium have been co-localized with the epithelial damage found in CRS (7,10). Recent in vivo observations noted mostly intact eosinophils in the nasal tissues, but in the mucus the eosinophils formed clusters, degranulated, and released their MBP at estimated levels far exceeding those needed to damage the epithelium (11). These in vivo observations explain the patterns of damage in CRS, where only the outer layers of tissue are damaged, suggesting that the damage to the epithelium is inflicted from the outside (luminal side). This epithelial damage may predispose CRS patients to be susceptible for the secondary bacterial infections, leading to acute exacerbations, which are observed clinically. Because bacteria typically elicit a neutrophilic inflammation, these acute exacerbations of CRS are presumed to be of bacterial origin. However, the underlying eosinophilic inflammation that predominates in CRS is unlikely to be caused by bacterial infection, suggesting a nonbacterial etiologic mechanism for CRS.

Eosinophilic inflammation has been observed in tissues that contain large, nonphagocytosable parasites—e.g., helminthes (12). Earlier reports documented the accumulation of eosinophils and their subsequent degranulation on the surfaces of the parasites. The toxic proteins in the granule (including MBP) damage and kill the organisms. Recent observations of eosinophil clusters in mucus from CRS patients are reminiscent of the accumulations around parasites (11,13–15).

Two prospectively designed histologic studies of mucus obtained during CRS surgery used extra caution to preserve the mucus. Eosinophilic mucus with clusters of aggregated eosinophils was found in 96% (97/101) and 94% (35/37) of consecutive CRS patients (14,15). Another study demonstrated that eosinophils released their toxic MBP in the mucus within these clusters, and not in the tissue (11). Estimated concentrations of MBP within the clusters, based on digital analysis of the intensity of the MBP staining, were as high as 2 mM and exceeded those capable of mediating epithelial damage. Overall, the clusters of eosinophils and intense eosinophil degranulation in the mucus suggest that eosinophils move from tissue to mucus with the fungi as their targets (Fig. 1).

A key question is whether the eosinophils in CRS play a defensive role similar to the one they play against parasites in their accumulation around extramucosal fungi. Stated another way, are eosinophils recruited to target fungi in the mucus of the CRS patient? To answer this question, it is necessary to study whether certain fungi induce the recruitment, activation, survival, and degranulation of eosinophils from CRS patients, but not from healthy controls.

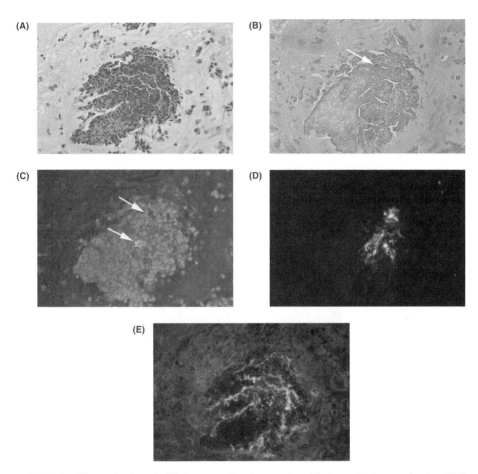

FIGURE 1 (*See color insert.*) (**A**) An example of an eosinophil cluster in the mucin of a CRS patient, where eosinophils appear to target fungal organisms. This specimen was attached to sinus tissue and was removed during surgery. Due to the heterogeneous nature of the eosinophilia, where areas with and without eosinophils coexist, these clusters can be easily missed on examination (hematoxylin and eosin counterstain of the same section shown in **E**; magnification, ×800). (**B**) Serial section of the same cluster shown in (**A**), stained with Gomori's methamire silver. The white arrow identifies a fungal organism. Note that the larger organism visible with the chitinase and anti-*Alternaria* staining (**B** and **C**) is not visible using the GMS stain technique (magnification, ×800). (**C**) Serial section of the same cluster shown in (**A**), stained for chitinase by immunofluorescence. Fungal elements (*white arrows*) are evident within the eosino- phil cluster (magnification, ×800). (**D**) Serial section of the same cluster shown in (**A–C**) stained for *Alternaria* by immunofluorescence. Staining occurs both within and around fungal organisms (magnification, ×800). (**E**) Same section as that shown in (**A**) stained for eosinophil granule major basic protein (MBP) by immunofluorescence. Extracellular deposition of the toxic eosinophil granule protein MBP is evident within the eosinophil cluster (magnification, ×800).

WHERE ARE FUNGI?

The role for fungi in CRS is noninvasive, and it is not a fungal infection. In fact, it needs to be differentiated from other forms of fungal sinusitis, such as fungus balls (noninvasive) and invasive fungal sinusitis (acute fulminant or chronic form).

The fungi in CRS patients are found only in the nasal mucus. Recently, striking progress has been made in the development of better techniques to detect fungi in the nasal secretions. To improve the sensitivity of fungal culture techniques, adequate amounts of mucus need to be harvested, and the disulfide bridges need to be chemically broken in the mucin to release the entrapped fungi (14,15). Using these novel culturing techniques, newer studies demonstrated the presence of fungi in 96% (N = 202) and 91.3% (N = 92) of mucus from unselected CRS patients (14,15). For the first time, these techniques revealed the presence of fungi in almost every healthy control; this is not surprising, given the ubiquity of fungi in the air. Finally, fungi have been found in nasal secretions of healthy infants (16). Immediately after birth, 20% of babies showed positive fungal cultures in their nasal secretions; at 5 days, 15% showed positive cultures; at 2 months, 72% showed positive cultures; and at 4 months, 94% showed positive cultures.

Increased awareness among pathologists and surgeons coupled with new techniques for mucus collection has resulted in higher detection rates of fungi on histology. An earlier comparison study showed a 47% failure rate in the demonstration of fungi and eosinophilic mucin in patients who were suspected for "allergic fungal sinusitis" (AFS) (17). More recently, with careful collection of nasal mucus specimens from CRS patients and with Gomori's methamine silver stain (GMS), 82% (N = 101) and 75% (N = 82) of CRS patients showed fungal elements in their mucus (14,15). With the use of a chitin-based immunofluorescence staining technique, it was found that 100% of nasal mucus specimens contained fungal elements (18). Overall, the newer techniques for fungal detection demonstrate increased specificity and sensitivity over old techniques in detecting the presence of fungi.

Other techniques have been used by researchers to further enhance the detection of fungi. Polymerase chain reaction (PCR) with specific fungal primers has been used to find fungal DNA in polypoid nasal tissues from 100% of CRS patients (N = 27) (19). The authors speculated that this might represent fungal DNA that is being processed for antigen presentation. Interestingly, *Alternaria*-specific DNA was present in tissues from CRS patients, but not in tissues from healthy controls. Immunoassays detected levels of *Alternaria* antigens (ALT-a1) and total *Alternaria* proteins in the mucus of 100% of CRS patients as well as in the mucus from all healthy controls (20,21). These results are not surprising in view of a new study from the National Institute of Environmental Health Science, which reports that virtually everyone is exposed to *Alternaria alternata* antigens at home (22).

Because of newer collection, extraction, and detection techniques, fungi, and specifically *Alternaria* species, are found to be present in the nasal secretions of both CRS patients and healthy controls. Thus, the mere presence of fungi in the nasal and paranasal secretions does not seem to induce a chronic eosinophilic inflammation, nor is the presence of fungi alone diagnostic of a disease. However, to understand the presence of these organisms or their products, it is necessary for one to hypothesize that the inflammation in CRS might be due to aberrant immune responses directed against certain fungi.

WHY DO EOSINOPHILS EXIST? THE IMMUNE RESPONSE TO FUNGI

Although some CRS patients produce specific immunoglobulin E (IgE) against fungi (23,24), there is no evidence that this IgE production directly results in the disease state of CRS. Furthermore, CRS develops in patients who both have or do not have IgE antibodies to fungi or other common aeroallergens. In contrast, IgE-mediated allergy and exposure to the relevant allergens leads to allergic rhinitis. Thus, patients with CRS may have IgE-mediated hypersensitivity to molds as a comorbid disease, but the underlying eosinophilic inflammation appears to be driven by a mechanism independent of an IgE-mediated one. If the human immune system in CRS patients recognizes these fungi as foreign and uses eosinophils to attack them, one could speculate that it should recruit and activate eosinophils by production of cytokines that regulate eosinophil inflammation. Tissue-bound lymphocytes have been found to be the main source of these cytokines in patients with CRS (25).

In addition, the expression of vascular cell adhesion molecule-1 (VCAM-1) has been identified in the vascular endothelium in CRS patients (26). This expression occurred independent of any IgE-mediated allergy and explains the presence of eosinophils in allergic as well as nonallergic patients with CRS (26). VCAM-1 is known to specifically bind to the very late-appearing antigen-4 (VLA-4) on eosinophils, thus causing selective adhesion and migration of eosinophils from the vasculature to the sinus tissue (26). Shin et al. (20) recently demonstrated that isolated peripheral blood mononuclear cells (PBMCs) from CRS patients, which contained lymphocytes and other cells that can serve as antigen-presenting cells, produced large amounts of interleukin (IL)-13 when exposed in vitro to certain mold extracts, especially from *Alternaria* species. This production of IL-13 in response to *Alternaria* may enhance expression of VCAM-1 by vascular endothelial cells (27).

Significantly elevated levels of IL-5, a cytokine that mediates eosinophil differentiation, survival, and activation, are present in tissue specimens of CRS patients and not in those of healthy controls (28–32,33). A majority of the IL-5 staining cells are lymphocytes (68%), followed by eosinophils (18%) and mast cells (14%) (33). PBMCs from 16 out of 18 CRS patients stimulated with *Alternaria* antigens in vitro showed increased production of IL-5, but PBMCs from 15 out of 15 healthy controls did not (20). Elevated levels of specific IgE for *Alternaria* were detected in only 28% of these CRS patients; the increased IgE levels did not correlate with increased levels of IL-5 (20). PBMCs from allergic and nonallergic CRS patients produced similar amounts of IL-5, indicating that this reaction is independent of an IgE-mediated allergic reaction (20). In addition, PBMCs from CRS patients stimulated with either *Cladosporium* (6/18) or *Aspergillus* (4/18) antigens also show increased production of IL-5; no response is seen with *Penicillium* antigen (20). Furthermore, production of interferon-γ (IFN-γ), which facilitates destruction of parasites by eosinophils, is 5.5 times higher in PBMCs from CRS patients stimulated with *Alternaria* antigen compared with production by healthy control PBMCs (20). These differences in cytokine production probably cannot be explained by differences in fungal contents in nasal mucus. When nasal secretions from nine healthy controls and nine CRS patients were examined, there were no differences in their levels of total *Alternaria* proteins (20).

However, there are differences between CRS patients and healthy controls in their immune responses to fungi. Mean serum IgG levels specific for Alternaria were increased about fivefold in the 18 CRS patients compared to the 15 healthy controls (20). Furthermore, serum IgG levels in the CRS patients directly correlated with the levels of IL-5 produced when patients' PBMCs were incubated with *Alternaria* (20). Given the general notion that the levels of IgG indicate the amount of immunologic exposure, these results suggest a direct correlation between the exposure to Alternaria antigens and the severity of the immune reaction as determined by the amount of IL-5 production. Other investigators also found an increase in nasal obstruction after challenge with *Alternaria* that was independent of an IgE-mediated hypersensitivity (34). In a recent study, eosinophils from healthy people that were incubated with *Alternaria* and *Penicillium* antigens released significant amounts of eosinophil-derived neurotoxin (EDN), a marker of eosinophil degranulation (35). When eosinophils from patients with asthma or allergies were used, they even released about 70% more EDN compared to the healthy controls. The fraction from *A. alternata*, which induced the degranulation, had a molecular weight of ≈60 kDa, was highly heat labile, and worked protease dependant through a G protein-coupled receptor (35). Other fungal antigens, including *Aspergillus*, *Cladosporium*, and *Candida*, did not induce eosinophil degranulation, nor did neutrophils respond to *Alternaria* extracts, suggesting the presence of a fungal species and cell type specific novel innate immune response to certain fungi in human. Thus, both innate and acquired immune responses to environmental fungi, such as *Alternaria* (independent of IgE antibodies to *Alternaria*) may increase production of the cytokines and provide cellular activation signals necessary for the robust eosinophilic inflammation in CRS patients.

ANTIFUNGAL TREATMENT OF CRS

Given the recent understanding of the association of numerous eosinophils with fungi in the mucus of CRS patients, it now appears that antifungal agents applied directly to the nasal mucus could be beneficial. By reducing the fungal burden, the eosinophilia and accompanying inflammation might also be attenuated.

In one open-label pilot study, topical intranasal treatment of 51 CRS patients, given as 20 mL of a 100 µg/mL amphotericin B solution per nostril, twice a day for average of 11.3 months (range 3–17 months), improved both symptoms and endoscopic staging in 75% of patients and reduced mucosal thickening on available computed tomography (CT) scans (36). Ricchetti et al. (37) reported disappearance of polyposis on endoscopy in 62% of mild and 42% of moderate patients with CRS when topical amphotericin B was used for 4 weeks. However, patients with severe CRS, who had polyps that filled the entire nasal cavity, showed no improvement (37). In this severe CRS group, failure might be due to the limited access of the topical medication, to the short duration of the therapy in the study, or both (38). Likewise, a trial with CRS patients, who also had severe nasal polyposis, used small volumes of amphotericin B, and found no benefit after 8 weeks (39). When a bulb syringe was used as a delivery vehicle, a double-blind, placebo-controlled trial of intranasal amphotericin B in an unselected CRS population found efficacy compared to placebo after 6 months (21). Reduced inflammatory mucosal thickening on CT scan and nasal endoscopy and decreased levels of intranasal cytokines and markers for eosinophilic inflammation in CRS patients could be demonstrated. Recently, a group of CRS patients was successfully treated with steroids and itraconazole in an open-label study, and no surgery was needed (40).

These results suggest that an antifungal treatment may reduce the fungal antigenic load in the nasal and paranasal cavities and subsequently decrease the eosinophilic response. Overall, topical antifungal treatments likely benefit patients with CRS; this treatment needs to be long term; and the dosage, formulation, and application methods still need further optimization, specifically in those with severely obstructed nasal and sinus passages.

A BROADER ROLE FOR FUNGI IN CRS

New data have been presented that highlight the importance of certain airborne fungi, in particular the *Alternaria* species, in the pathophysiology of CRS. Although newer detection techniques have demonstrated the presence of these fungi in virtually everyone, only patients with CRS may react to them with the production of cytokines, which are crucial for the eosinophilic inflammation. In addition, *Alternaria* extract induces a striking degranulation of eosinophils in vitro. Eosinophils apparently target fungi in vivo in the mucus of CRS patients, where they degranulate within clusters. This extramucosal release of cytotoxic proteins may explain the damage observed to the epithelium, which is inflicted from the outside (luminal side), and the susceptibility of CRS to secondary bacterial infection (acute exacerbations of CRS). Antifungal therapy, if used in the correct formulation, application form, and duration, may be effective in inhibiting the antigenic load with a subsequent reduction in intranasal cytokines and markers of eosinophilic inflammation.

REFERENCES

1. Benninger MS, Ferguson BJ, Hadley JA, et al. Adult chronic rhinosinusitis: definitions, diagnosis, epidemiology, and pathophysiology. Otolaryngol Head Neck Surg 2003; 129 (3Suppl.):S1–32.
2. Lethbridge-Çejku M, Schiller JS, Bernadel L. Summary health statistics for U.S. adults: National Health Interview Survey, 2002. National Center for Health Statistics. Vital Health Stat 10 2004; 222:1–151.
3. Atlas SJ, Metson RB, Singer DE, et al. Validity of a new health-related quality of life instrument for patients with chronic sinusitis. Laryngoscope 2005; 115:846–54.
4. Gliklich RE, Metson R. The health impact of chronic sinusitis in patients seeking otolaryngologic care. Otolaryngol Head Neck Surg 1995; 113:104–9.
5. Bryson JM, Tasca RA, Rowe-Jones JM. Local and systemic eosinophilia in patients undergoing endoscopic sinus surgery for chronic rhinosinusitis with and without polyposis. Clin Otolaryngol 2003; 28:55–8.
6. Bhattacharyya N. Chronic rhinosinusitis: is the nose really involved? Am J Rhinol 2001; 15:169–73.
7. Harlin SL, Ansel DG, Lane SR, et al. A clinical and pathologic study of chronic sinusitis: the role of the eosinophil. J Allergy Clin Immunol 1988; 81(5 Pt 1):867–75.
8. Stoop AE, van der Heijden HA, Biewenga J, van der Baan S. Eosinophils in nasal polyps and nasal mucosa: an immunohistochemical study. J Allergy Clin Immunol 1993; 91:616–22.
9. Ponikau JU, Sherris DA, Kephart GM, et al. Features of airway remodeling and eosinophilic inflammation in chronic rhinosinusitis: Is it the histopathology similar to asthma? J Allergy Clin Immunol 2003; 112:877–82.
10. Hisamatsu K, Ganbo T, Nakazawa T, et al. Cytotoxicity of human eosinophil granule major basic protein to human nasal sinus mucosa in vitro. J Allergy Clin Immunol 1990; 86:52–63.
11. Ponikau JU, Sherris DA, Kephart GM, et al. Striking deposition of toxic eosinophil major basic protein in mucus: implications for chronic rhinosinusitis. J Allergy Clin Immunol 2005; 116:362–9.
12. Kita H, Adolphson CR, Gleich GJ. Biology of eosinophils. In: Adkinson NF Jr, Bochner BS, Yunginger JW, eds. Middleton's Allergy Principles and Practice, 6th ed. Philadelphia, PA: Mosby, 2003:305–32.
13. Sasama J, Sherris DA, Shin SH, et al. New paradigm for the roles of fungi and eosinophils in chronic rhinosinusitis. Curr Opin Otolaryngol Head Neck Surg 2005; 13:2–8.
14. Ponikau JU, Sherris DA, Kern EB, et al. The diagnosis and incidence of allergic fungal sinusitis. Mayo Clin Proc 1999; 74:877–84.
15. Braun H, Buzina W, Freudenschuss K, et al. "Eosinophilic fungal rhinosinusitis": a common disorder in Europe? Laryngoscope 2003; 113:264–9.

16. Lackner A, Freudenschuss K, Buzina W, et al. Fungi: a normal content of human nasal mucus. Am J Rhinol 2005; 19:125–9.
17. Granville L, Chirala M, Cernoch P, et al. Fungal sinusitis: histologic spectrum and correlation with culture. Hum Pathol 2004; 35:474–81.
18. Taylor MJ, Ponikau JU, Sherris DA, et al. Detection of fungal organisms in eosinophilic mucin using a fluorescein-labeled chitin-specific binding protein. Otolaryngol Head Neck Surg 2002; 127:377–83.
19. Gosepath J, Brieger J, Vlachtsis K, Mann WJ. Fungal DNA is present in tissue specimens of patients with chronic rhinosinusitis. Am J Rhinol 2004; 18:9–13.
20. Shin S-H, Ponikau JU, Sherris DA, et al. Rhinosinusitis: an enhanced immune response to ubiquitous airborne fungi. J Allergy Clin Immunol 2004; 114:1369–75.
21. Ponikau JU, Sherris DA, Weaver A, Kita H. Treatment of chronic rhinosinusitis with intranasal amphotericin B: a randomized, placebo-controlled, double-blinded pilot trial. J Allergy Clin Immunol 2005; 115:125–31.
22. Salo PM, Yin M, Arbes SJ Jr, et al. Dustborne *Alternaria alternata* antigens in US homes: results from the National Survey of Lead and Allergens in Housing. J Allergy Clin Immunol 2005; 116:623-9.
23. Mabry RL, Manning S. Radioallergosorbent microscreen and total immunoglobulin E in allergic fungal sinusitis. Otolaryngol Head Neck Surg 1995; 113:721–3.
24. Feger TA, Rupp NT, Kuhn FA, et al. Local and systemic eosinophil activation in allergic fungal sinusitis. Ann Allergy Asthma Immunol 1997; 79:221–5.
25. Hamilos DL, Leung DY, Wood R, et al. Evidence for distinct cytokine expression in allergic versus nonallergic chronic sinusitis. J Allergy Clin Immunol 1995; 96:537–44.
26. Hamilos DL, Leung DY, Wood R, et al. Eosinophil infiltration in nonallergic chronic hyperplastic sinusitis with nasal polyposis (CHS/NP) is associated with endothelial VCAM-1 upregulation and expression of TNF-alpha. Am J Respir Cell Mol Biol 1996; 15:443–50.
27. al Ghamdi K, Ghaffar O, Small P, et al. IL-4 and IL-13 expression in chronic sinusitis: relationship with cellular infiltrate and effect of topical corticosteroid treatment. J Otolaryngol 1997; 26:160–6.
28. Hamilos DL, Leung DY, Wood R, et al. Evidence for distinct cytokine expression in allergic versus nonallergic chronic sinusitis. J Allergy Clin Immunol 1995; 96:537–44.
29. Durham SR, Ying S, Varney VA, et al. Cytokine messenger RNA expression for IL-3, IL-4, IL-5, and granulocyte/macrophage-colony-stimulating factor in the nasal mucosa after local allergen provocation: relationship to tissue eosinophilia. J Immunol 1992; 148:2390–4.
30. Lopez AF, Sanderson CJ, Gamble JR, et al. Recombinant human interleukin 5 is a selective activator of human eosinophil function. J Exp Med 1988; 167:219–24.
31. Simon HU, Yousefi S, Schranz C, et al. Direct demonstration of delayed eosinophil apoptosis as a mechanism causing tissue eosinophilia. J Immunol 1997; 158:3902–8.
32. Hamilos DL, Leung DY, Huston DP, et al. GM-CSF, IL-5 and RANTES immunoreactivity and mRNA expression in chronic hyperplastic sinusitis with nasal polyposis (NP). Clin Exp Allergy 1998; 28:1145–52.
33. Hamilos DL. Chronic sinusitis. J Allergy Clin Immunol 2000; 106:213–27.
34. Krouse JH, Shah AG, Kerswill K. Skin testing in predicting response to nasal provocation with alternaria. Laryngoscope 2004; 114:1389–93.
35. Inoue Y, Matsuzaki Y, Shin S-H, et al. Non-pathogenic, environmental fungi induce activation and degranulation of human eosinophils. J Immunol 2005; 175:5439–47.
36. Ponikau JU, Sherris DA, Kita H, Kern EB. Intranasal antifungal treatment in 51 patients with chronic rhinosinusitis. J Allergy Clin Immunol 2002; 110:862–826.
37. Ricchetti A, Landis BN, Maffioli A, et al. Effect of anti-fungal nasal lavage with amphotericin B on nasal polyposis. J Laryngol Otolaryngol 2002; 116:261–3.
38. Miller TR, Muntz HR, Gilbert ME, Orlandi RR. Comparison of topical medication delivery systems after sinus surgery. Laryngoscope 2004; 114:201–4.
39. Weschta M, Rimek D, Formanek M, et al. Topical antifungal treatment of chronic rhinosinusitis with nasal polyps: a randomized, double-blind clinical trial. J Allergy Clin Immunol 2004; 113:1122–8.
40. Rains BM III, Mineck CW. Treatment of allergic fungal sinusitis with high-dose itraconazole. Am J Rhinol 2003; 17:1–8.

12

Imaging of Paranasal Sinuses and Rhinosinusitis

Mahmood F. Mafee
Department of Radiology, University of California, San Diego, California, U.S.A.

PARANASAL SINUSES: EMBRYOLOGY AND DEVELOPMENT
Maxillary Sinuses

The paranasal sinuses develop as outgrowths of the walls of the primitive (fetal) nasal cavities (1,2). Maxillary and ethmoid sinuses develop during fetal life. Frontal and sphenoid sinuses are not present at birth, but develop during the early years of life (2,3). By 4–5 months after birth, the maxillary sinus can be readily identified particularly on computed tomography (CT) scans. After birth, growth of the maxillary sinus continues rapidly until about 3 years of age, and then slowly progress until the seventh year (3). At this time another acceleration in growth occurs until the age of 12 years. After the twelfth year much of the growth is related to an invasion of the alveolar process following the eruption of the secondary dentition (3).

Maxillary sinuses are the first to develop, around the 65th day of gestation (3). The size of the sinus at birth is about 6–8 cm^3. They can be seen on plain radiograph at 4–5 months of age. Rapid expansion occurs from 7–18 years, related to eruption of permanent teeth. Ethmoid and maxillary sinuses are the only sinuses that are large enough at birth to be clinically significant in rhinosinusitis. The maxillary sinuses are pyramidal cavities within the bodies of the maxillae and are the largest accessory air sinuses of the nose. The base of the pyramid is formed by the lateral wall of the nasal cavity; the apex extends into the zygomatic process of the maxilla and may reach the zygomatic bone itself. Its base faces medially and is the lateral wall of the nasal cavity and presents the maxillary hiatus in the disarticulated bone. In the articulated skull, this aperture hiatus is much reduced in size by the uncinate process of the ethmoid above, the maxillary process of the inferior nasal concha below, and the perpendicular plate of the palatine bone behind. The roof of the maxillary sinus is the orbital floor, which is ridged by the infraorbital canal that usually projects into the sinus. The floor is formed by the alveolar process of the maxilla. Several conical projections corresponding with the roots of the first and second molar teeth project into the floor. The floor is perforated sometimes by one or more of these roots. Occasionally the roots of the first and second premolars, the third molar, and at times the root of the canine, may also project into the sinus. The size of the maxillary sinus varies in different individuals, and even on the two sides of the same individual. The maxillary sinus communicates with the middle meatus of the nasal cavity, generally by two small apertures, one of which is usually closed by the mucous membrane in life (fontanell). The natural ostium of the maxillary sinus is located in the superior portion of its medial wall, usually posterior to the midpoint of the bulla ethmoidalis (4,5). The posterior extent of the uncinate process points to the position of the ostium and is an excellent imaging and endoscopic landmark for its localization.

Accessory ostia are present in 10–30% of cases, usually in the membranous medial aspect of the maxillary sinus where a double layer of mucosa with no intervening bone forms the nasoantral wall inferior to the uncinate process. The natural opening of the maxillary sinus is above the floor and poorly placed for natural drainage. The middle meatus is of such a form that pus running down from the frontal and anterior ethmoidal sinuses is directed by the hiatus semilunaris into the opening of the maxillary sinus, which may, in some cases, act as a secondary reservoir for pus discharged from these sinuses.

Ethmoid Sinuses

The anterior and middle ethmoid sinuses begin as evaginations of the lateral nasal wall in the region of the middle meatus in approximately the third month of fetal life (3). Shortly afterward, posterior ethmoid cells begin to evaginate the nasal mucosa in the superior meatus. The ethmoid sinuses progressively enlarge throughout fetal life. At birth the size of the anterior group is approximately 5 mm high, 2 mm long, and 2 mm wide, and the posterior group is 5 mm high, 4 mm long, and 2 mm wide (3). After birth or a few months later, the ethmoid air cells can be readily identified on CT scans. By the age of 12 years, the ethmoids have almost reached their adult size (24 mm high, 23 mm long, and 11 mm wide for the anterior group, and 21 mm high, 21 mm long, and 12 mm wide for the posterior group) (3). The anterior and middle groups are usually referred to as anterior air cells (two to eight cells), separated from the posterior compartment by the vertical portion of the basal lamella. Fundamentally, anterior ethmoid cells are defined as those whose ostia open in relation to the infundibulum and via the hiatus semilunaris superioris into the meatus (3,6,7). Bullar ethmoid cells are those opening either above, on, or under the bulla (3). Posterior ethmoid cells have their ostia in the superior meatus. The anterior ethmoidal air cells include: frontal recess air cells, infundibular (suprainfundibular) air cells, agger nasi air cells, terminal cells, ethmoid bulla, and concha bullosa (pneumatized anterior middle turbinate) (3). Although the limit of the ethmoid labyrinth is thought to be the ethmoid bone, ethmoid cells may encroach on any of the adjacent bones: the nasal and lacrimal bones anteriorly, the sphenoid bone posteriorly, the maxilla inferiorly, and the orbital plate of the frontal bone superiorly (3). Some air cells are not entirely enclosed by the ethmoid bone (extramural cells); instead, the ethmoid bone may be perforated so that the air cell mucosa extends upward against the ethmoidal notch of the frontal bone, anteriorly against the lacrimal and maxillary bones, and posteriorly against the sphenoid and palatine bones. The most anterior intramural ethmoidal air cells are the frontal recess air cells (cells developed in relation to and adjacent to the frontal recess), which extend toward the frontal bone anterosuperiorly. The frontal sinus arises from these cells, as do the supraorbital ethmoidal air cells (4,6). The next most anterior group is the infundibular cells. From these arise the most anterior extramural cells, the agger nasi cells, which pneumatize the lacrimal bone and frontal process of the maxilla (3,4,5,6). The agger nasi cells are located on the lateral nasal wall immediately anterior to the anterior end of the middle turbinate (8,9). These cells drain into the ethmoid infundibulum. The agger nasi cells are notable because they occur in about 80% of individuals (4). The agger nasi cells occupy the lateral nasal wall anterosuperiorly to the hiatus semilunaris and form an elevated area of bone in the anterior part of the middle meatus (4). The ostia of these cells open into the superior part of the infundibulum (4).

Frontal Sinuses

The frontal sinuses develop during the early years of life. Each frontal sinus begins in the ethmoid portion of the nasal capsule in the region of the frontal recess (3). At birth it is indistinguishable from the anterior ethmoid air cells (3). Postnatal growth is slow, and at 1 year the sinus is barely perceptible anatomically (3). At about the fourth year, the frontal sinus begins to invade the vertical plate of the frontal bone. By 7–8 years the sinuses are well developed but they increase progressively in size until the late teens (3). With advancing age, absorption of bone from the inner walls of the sinuses may occur as an atrophic change leading to further enlargement. Each extends backward into the medial part of the roof of the orbit. The part of the sinus extending upward in the frontal bone may be small and the orbital part large, or vice versa. Each frontal sinus opens into the anterior part of the corresponding middle meatus of the nose through the frontonasal duct (frontonasal recess), which traverses adjacent to the anterior part of the ethmoid labyrinth (1,4,5). Development of the frontal sinus is such that in 50% of cases the drainage of the frontal and anterior ethmoids into the middle meatus converges. In the other 50% of cases, the frontal sinus drains anteriorly to the anterior ethmoids. This explains why in some cases patients may have both ipsilateral frontal and anterior ethmoid disease and others do not.

Sphenoid Sinuses

The sphenoid sinuses originate during the third fetal month as an extension (evagination) of the developing nasal cavity. Although the sphenoid sinus can be identified as a tiny cavity in sections of the fetus at 4 months, at birth the sinus remains small and is little more than an evagination of the sphenoethmoid recess (3). After birth or many months later, the sphenoid sinuses cannot be identified on CT scans. At age 2 years, the sphenoid sinuses are barely identified on CT scans. After the fifth year, development of the sphenoid sinuses is more rapid, and by the age of 7, the sinuses have extended posteriorly to the level of the sella turcica (3). Further enlargement occurs after puberty. The sphenoid sinuses, like frontal sinuses, can vary considerably in size and shape. The intersphenoid septum is often deflected to one side; therefore, the sphenoid sinuses are rarely symmetrical. At times there may be lateral expansion (lateral recess) into the roots of the pterygoid processes or greater wings of the sphenoid, and it may invade the lesser wing and the basilar part of the occipital bone. At times there are gaps in the bony walls, and the mucous membrane may lie directly against the dura mater. Bony bridges, produced by the internal carotid artery and the pterygoid canal, may project into the sinuses from the lateral wall and floor, respectively (1,9). At times, a posterior ethmoidal sinus may extend into the body of the sphenoid and largely replace a sphenoidal sinus (1). Each sphenoid sinus drains into the nasal cavity via the sphenoethmoidal recess by an aperture in the upper part of its anterior wall. The sphenoid ostium is well above the floor of the sinus.

With advancing age, absorption of bone from the inner walls of the sinuses may occur as an atrophic change leading to further enlargement.

SPECIAL CONSIDERATIONS REGARDING ANATOMY OF THE SINUSES AND OSTIOMEATAL COMPLEX IN THE ADULT PATIENT
Ethmoid Sinuses

The advent of minimally invasive surgical tecnhiques (MIST), using powered instruments with real-time suction has further enhanced the knowledge base of the surgical anatomy of the paranasal sinuses. The ethmoid bone is a delicate and complex structure. It articulates with 13 other bones: the frontal, sphenoid, nasals, maxillae, lacrimals, palatines, inferior nasal conchae, and vomer (1,4). The ethmoid bone consists of four parts: a horizontal lamina, called the cribriform plate; a perpendicular plate; and two lateral masses, called the labyrinths (Fig. 1). Each ethmoidal labyrinth consists of thin-walled highly variable air cells arranged in three groups: anterior, middle, and posterior clusters (Fig. 1).

The medial surface of the ethmoidal labyrinth forms a part of the lateral wall of the corresponding half of the nasal cavity. Within the nasal cavity, scrolls of bone on the lateral walls, the conchae, project medially to divide the passageway into meatuses, or channels for air (Fig. 1) (1,4). The superior and middle conchae are parts of the ethmoid bone, but the inferior nasal conchae (a turbinate is a concha, plus a soft tissue complex) are a separate pair of bones. The superior, middle, and inferior meatuses (air channels), which are formed under the respective conchae, have increased contact with the nasal surfaces to permit more effective warming and moistening of inspired air (air conditioning) (4). The posterior ethmoidal air cells drain into the superior meatus. The middle meatus connects via various ostia and air passages with the anterior and middle ethmoidal air cells and the frontal and maxillary sinuses. The frontal sinuses communicate with the

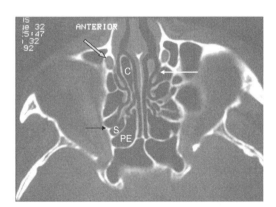

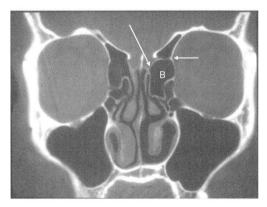

FIGURE 1   Normal sinonasal CT anatomy. Axial CT scan (*top*) showing nasolaracrimal duct (*gray arrow*), uncinate process (*long white arrow*), posterior ethmoid air cells (PE), sinus lateralis (S), attachment of basal lamella to the medial wall of the orbit (*black arrow*), concha bullosa (C). Coronal CT scan (*bottom*) showing ethmoid bulla (B), larteral lamela of cribriform plate (*long arrow*), and ethmoid artery canal (*short arrow*).

middle meatus of the corresponding half of the nasal cavity by means of a passage called the frontonasal canal (nasofrontal duct). This communication between the frontal sinus and the nasal cavity is not strictly a duct (10,11), but an internal channel positioned between the frontal sinus ostium and the anterior middle meatus referred to as the frontal recess. Just anterior to the anterior superior attachment of the middle turbinate and anterior to the frontal recess are the agger (ridge) nasi and agger nasi cells (3–5). This prominence on the lateral nasal wall represents the most anterior of the anterior ethmoidal cells. These cells (agger nasi cells) can invade the lacrimal bone or the ascending process of the maxilla. Because of their closeness to the frontal recess, they are excellent surgical landmarks. Opening these agger cells during external ethmoidectomy provides a good view of the nasofrontal duct.

Just posterior and inferior to the agger nasi cells lies the ethmoidal uncinate process, the starting point in an anterior-to-posterior endoscopic surgical procedures The uncinate process is a thin, curved bar of bone from the lateral side of the ethmoidal labyrinth that forms a portion of the lateral nasal wall (Fig. 1). It projects downward and backward and is subject to considerable variation in size. It ranges in height from 1 to 4 mm and is 14–22 mm long (8). Anteriorly it articulates with the lacrimal bone and ethmoidal process of the inferior nasal concha (Fig. 1). The superior edge of this process is free and forms the medial boundary of the hiatus semilunaris (Fig. 1) in the middle meatus of the nose (1). As it progresses posteroinferiorly, it forms the inferior border of the semilunar hiatus (Fig. 1) and the medial wall of the infundibulum (Fig. 1).

The exact drainage system of the frontal sinus depends on its embryologic development. The drainage usually occurs by way of rudimentary ethmoidal cells into the frontal recess (12). or directly into the frontal recess (4,5,8,9). Medial to the bulla ethmoidalis and the uncinate process is the middle turbinate. Anteriorly, it attaches to the medial wall of the agger nasi and the superoanterior edge of the uncinate process (11). Superiorly, it attaches to the cribriform plate. The attachment of the middle turbinate changes direction at its most posterior extent. Instead of running in an anteroposterior direction, it curves laterally, and the final lateral attachment of the middle turbinate is oriented in the frontal plane and is called the basal or ground lamella (Fig. 1) (9,11). The posterior ethmoidal air cells are between the basal lamella and the sphenoidal sinus. The basal lamella is an excellent landmark for separating the anterior and middle ethmoidal air cells from the posterior ethmoidal air cells (4,5).

Sinus Lateralis

An air space (cleft) is usually found between the ground lamella and the bulla ethmoidalis, which may extend superiorly to the bulla. This is called the sinus lateralis (Fig. 1). This sinus lateralis, unlike the anterior ethmoidal air cells that open into the infundibulum, may communicate with the frontal recess (4,5,11). or opens directly and independently into the middle meatus. Bogler et al. (13) found that a discrete retrobulbar recess was present in 93.8% of human cadavers they dissected by both gross and endoscopic techniques. A single, discrete, well-developed suprabullar recess was present in 70.9%. They found that the suprabullar recess did not communicate with the frontal recess. They recommended that the sinus lateralis more correctly be called the retrobullar and suprabullar recesses (13).

Sphenoid Sinuses

The sphenoid sinuses are contained within the body of the sphenoid bone. Sphenoid sinuses are related above to the pituitary gland (Fig. 1) and the optic chiasm, and on each side to the internal carotid artery and the cavernous sinuses.

OSTIOMEATAL COMPLEX (OSTIOMEATAL UNIT)—SPECIAL RELEVANCE TO FUNCTIONAL ENDOSCOPIC ENDONASAL SINUS SURGERY

Endoscopic sinus surgery has become an increasingly popular procedure since Messerklinger (14) and Wignad et al. (15) described the advantages of the intranasal endoscope and its surgical application. The concept of functional endoscopic sinus surgery (12) evolved from the work of Hilding (16,17), Proctor (18,19), and Messerklinger (20,21) investigating mucociliary clearance and air flow in the paranasal sinuses and the importance of establishing drainage and preserving the mucosa of the sinuses. Functional endoscopic sinus surgery is based on the hypothesis that the ostiomeatal complex (maxillary sinus ostium, anterior and middle ethmoid ostia, frontal recess, infundibulum, and middle meatal complex) is the key area in the pathogenesis of chronic sinus diseases (8,20,22). Minor pathologic changes in the nasal mucosa in the vicinity of the ostiomeatal complex (OMC), also referred to as the "ostiomeatal unit," may interfere with mucociliary clearance and ventilation of the maxillary, ethmoidal, and frontal sinuses. Ultrastructural changes in the respiratory mucosa can result from acute and chronic infections. Mucociliary transport plays an important role in the defense mechanism of the respiratory tract. Mucociliary transport depends to a large extent on the activity of cilia and the properties of the mucus layer.

The OMC is the key anatomic channel providing air flow and mucociliary clearance for the maxillary sinus and the anterior and middle ethmoidal air cells and occasionally for the frontal sinuses (4,5,9,11,12). The term OMC has been variously used to refer to the maxillary sinus ostium, anterior and middle ethmoidal air cells ostia, frontonasal duct (frontal recess), infundibulum, or the middle meatal complex. In addition, in some otolaryngologic communications, the anterior and middle ethmoidal air cells have been collectively referred to as anterior ethmoidal air cells. Recognition of the importance and complexity of the ostiomeatal complex has given the radiologist an important role in the assessment of patients scheduled for functional endoscopic sinus surgery. The radiologist should also be familiar with the principles of endonasal endoscopic operation, and make a careful evaluation of the paranasal sinuses, in particular, the ethmoid bone and the middle meatus region of the nasal cavity.

Certain anatomic variations are observed most commonly. These are as follows:

1. *Low position of fovea ethmoidalis (the roof of the ethmoid labyrinth)*. A low position of the cribriform plate, fovea ethmoidalis, and lateral lamella (thin bone between the cribriform plate and fovea ethmoidalis) is a potentially dangerous anatomic variation, because it can be penetrated easily unless the surgeon is aware of the finding (Fig. 2). The attachment of the middle turbinate to the cribriform plate is at the junction of the cribriform plate and its lateral lamella (Figs. 1 and 2). The anterior ethmoid artery canal is at the junction of the fovea ethmoidalis with the lateral lamella of the cribriform plate (Fig. 1).
2. *Bulging of the optic canal into the posterior ethmoidal complex.* An important observation is extensive lateral pneumatization of the posterior ethmoidal air

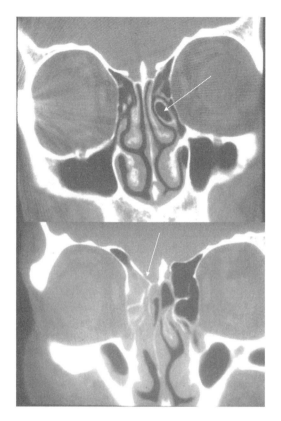

FIGURE 2 Anatomical variations. Coronal CT scan (*top*) showing pneumatized uncinate process (*arrow*). Coronal CT scan (*bottom*) showing low lying fovea ethmoidalis (*arrow*).

cells, which can increase the vulnerability of the optic nerve. In rare instances, the internal carotid artery may be exposed in the posterior ethmoidal sinus. In addition, identification of an asymmetric intersphenoid septum is important because the posterior extension of this partition usually marks the location of the internal carotid artery.

3. *Deviation of the uncinate process.* The superior edge of the uncinate process may deviate medially to obstruct the middle meatus or, more importantly, may deviate laterally to obstruct the infundibulum. Marked lateral deviation or even fusion of the uncinate process to the medial orbital wall may endanger the orbit and, hence, the optic nerve, during an uncinectomy performed during anterior endoscopic sinus surgery.

4. *Haller cells.* These are ethmoidal air cells extending along the medial floor of the orbit (infraorbital air cells) (Fig. 3), which may cause narrowing of the infundibulum.

5. *Onodi cells.* These are posterior ethmoid air cells encroaching into the anterior aspect of sphenoid sinus. In 1995, an attempt was made to standardize the definition of Onodi cell. The Anatomic Terminology Group (23) defined the Onodi cell as the most posterior ethmoid cell that "pneumatizes laterally and superiorly to the sphenoid sinus and is intimately associated with the optic nerve" (23). Given this definition, the incidence of the Onodi cell has been estimated to range from 8% to 14% in the population (24). Extensive

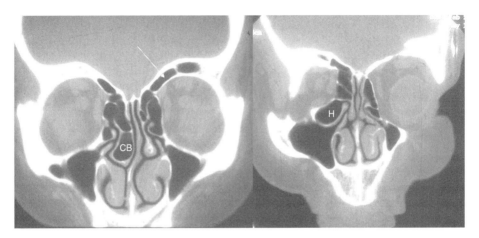

FIGURE 3 Anatomical variations. Coronal CT scans showing concha bullosa (CB), supraorbital ethmoid air cells (*arrow*), and Haller cell (H).

pneumatization of the sphenoid sinus may result in pneumatization of the medial aspect of the lesser wing, including the anterior clinoid. This has been called "pneumosinus dilatans" (24). The surgical significance of the presence of the Onodi cell makes its identification paramount (24). The presence of Onodi cell can increase the risk of orbital complications of endoscopic and other surgical approaches to the sphenoid and posterior ethmoid sinuses. During endoscopic sinus surgery, the Onodi cell may be mistaken for the sphenoid sinus, causing a distorted spatial perception for the surgeon (24). The presence of the Onodi cell and pneumatized anterior clinoid may possibly contribute to an increase in the risk of injury to the optic nerve and to the internal carotid artery.

Other Important Structures

There are several other structures of relevance to functional endoscopic sinus surgery. The reader is referred to Stammberger and Kennedy (23) for additional information about these structures.

IMAGING OF THE SINONASAL CAVITIES FOR ACUTE AND CHRONIC RHINOSINUSITIS AND ALLERGIC FUNGAL RHINOSINUSITIS
Overview of Radiologic Imaging

Conventional plain film radiography can be used as a screening method for acute and chronic rhinosinusitis (25). This will provide orientation and direction to further examinations that are indicated such as Ultrasound (US), CT, and magnetic resonance imaging (MRI) (25–27). Although a plain film sinus series can be of much value in acute and CRS and other sinonasal diseases, significant discrepancies are noted between a sinus series and a CT scan (49). Chronic rhinosinusitis associated with inspissated mucus has a characteristic CT appearance. This characteristic CT finding may be very hard to appreciate on plain film and could be totally missed or misinterpreted on MRI (27–29).

In order to maximize information obtained from CT, correct imaging strategies must be obtained (5,30,31). It is important to use thin sections (3–5 mm) so that small polyps or abscess cavities are not missed. Scans in both coronal and axial planes are useful whenever possible. The axial sections are taken parallel to the orbitomeatal line or parallel to the hard palate (27,30).

The coronal sections are obtained with the patient prone or supine, the head hyper-extended, and the gantry tilted to a plane as close to 90° to the canthomeatal line as possible. Thinner sections (2.5–3.75 mm) are used to identify small lesions and evaluate the ostiomeatal complex (25–28,32). In terms of filming or viewing on a PACS (picture archiving and communications system) monitor, some authors recommend an intermediate window width/level (W/L) technique (28,32). We prefer CT images to be viewed or filmed for routine soft tissue setting and bone setting; with extended window width-window level bone technique (4000/700–800 W/L) (5,27,30,31).

In addition to infectious processes, inflammatory and immunologic (cellular and molecular) responses play a role in the pathophysiology of soft tissue and hard tissue of the sinonasal cavities (mucosal, osteoblastic and osteoclastic, response). Soft tissue changes are better evaluated on CT viewed with soft tissue setting. Osteolysis, pressure atrophy of the sinus walls such as in long-standing sinonasal polyps, and osteoblastic changes are best evaluated on CT scans viewed with extended window width-window level bone technique. With mucosal thickening and air fluid level in the sinus cavity, there may be air bubbles scattered within the fluid or thick mucus in the sinus. These changes are better seen with soft tissue setting technique. Subperiosteal edema/fluid is also best seen on CT scans viewed with soft tissue technique.

Computed tomography scanning remains the study of choice for the imaging evaluation of acute and chronic inflammatory diseases of the sinonasal cavities, osseous lesions, chondrogenic lesions, fibro-osseus lesions, such as ossifying fibroma, and developmental disorders, such as fibrous dysplasia and craniofacial synostosis. Although CT scan can be more specific in the diagnosis of osteogenic and chondrogenic sarcomas, MRI is more sensitive in showing the extent of their soft tissue components, as well as the presence of subtle or obvious intracranial spread (33). MRI is superior to CT in differentiating inflammatory conditions from neoplastic processes (28,34,35). Most inflammatory lesions are quite hyperintense on T2-weighted (T2W) MR scans as opposed to most malignant tumors, lymphoreticular proliferative, myeloproliferative, and chronic granulomatous disorders (28,33). Most tumors of the sinonasal cavities are not as hyperintense as the surrounding inflammation and retained secretions; therefore, MRI plays an important role in the mapping and staging of these tumors. Sinogenic intracranial complications are best evaluated using MRI. The intraorbital complications of sinus surgery are also often best evaluated using MRI.

Computed tomography has proved to be the best preoperative evaluation for endoscopic sinus surgery (30,31,33,35–38). The complex anatomy of the ethmoid bone and the ostiomeatal unit can be visualized on CT scans with exquisite detail (36).

Risk of Radiation from Sinus Imaging

The risk of radiation from the sinus series or screening sinus CT is small (37). Approximately 0.3 cG is given per each film view obtained during plain X-ray sinus series (26,33). The organs most likely to be affected by a cumulative radiation dose are the lens, thyroid gland, and gonads. The dose to the lens of the eye is small if Waters and Caldwell views are obtained posterior-inferior as they should be (37). With the combination of high-speed film and a posterior-inferior projection, the dose to the eye in a sinus series should be on the order of 0.0001 Gy (0.01 cGy) to 0.005 Gy (0.5 cGy) (33,37). The radiation dose to the lens of the eye from a CT examination of the head may range from 3 to 6 cGy (25,33). The radiation from a CT scan of the sinuses to the lens, cornea, and other organs included in the CT sections can be significantly reduced by decreasing mAs (140–200 mAs), without significantly sacrificing details (38). The imaging plane also can be chosen to avoid scanning directly through the lens of the eye.

Techniques

Optimal imaging protocols for preoperative CT scanning of the paranasal sinuses, including preparation of the patient, CT technique, and data display (filming), have been reported by many authors (26,28,31,38–40). In CRS, treatment with appropriate medical therapy and adequately preparing patients enables the best CT assessment of mucosal disease of the sinonasal cavities (25,26,39). Three-millimeter section, direct coronal CT scanning with the patient preferably in the prone position and the head hyperextended currently affords the best preoperative evaluation for endoscopic sinus surgery (22,26,28,34,41,42). A complete CT study of the paranasal sinuses should include axial and coronal views (24,33). however, in most cases the coronal views provide sufficient information for evaluating the OMC (26). However, the combination of coronal and axial CT scans allows the surgeon to assess more easily the three-dimensional aspects of the OMC (22). Coronal scanning should extend from the frontal sinus anteriorly to the sphenoidal sinus posteriorly.

Axial CT scan should be included whenever coronal CT scans show a mass or mucosal disease, associated with expansion of the sinuses (22). Erosion of the posterior table of the frontal sinus, the sphenoethmoidal bony plate, basal lamella, pterygomaxillary fissure, and pterygopalatine fossa is best evaluated in axial and sagittal CT scans (43,44). The introduction of spiral and helical CT has a great impact in cross-sectional imaging. The speed with which studies can be carried out allows much faster patient throughput. With spiral CT, the quality of reformatted images has significantly improved. For children and agitated patients, spiral CT is extremely useful to provide acceptable diagnostic information in a matter of a few seconds. Contrast-enhanced CT should not be part of preoperative CT for endoscopic sinus surgery. Contrast material is used only when the preliminary evaluation of CT scans suggests a mass. In addition, contrast material should be given whenever orbital and intracranial complications of sinonasal infections or tumors are suspected. Three-dimensional reconstruction CT imaging has been most useful for studying facial deformity and for planning surgery (45,46). For sinonasal tumors, the combination of CT and MRI provide the maximum diagnostic imaging information. Our protocol for MRI of sinonasal disease, using a head coil include 5-mm-thick sections, sagittal TIW localization, axial T2W fast spin echo (SE) single echo or standard spin echo (SE), long time of repetition (TR), double echoes (2500, 80–100 ms TR/time of echo (TE)), and TIW (600–800, 25 ms TR/TE) coronal sections. Following IV administration of gadolinium-based contrast material, post-contrast TIW axial, coronal, and sagittal views are obtained. We prefer to obtain one of the postcontrast TlW pulse sequences with fat suppression. The magnetic susceptibility artifacts as well as those related to dental fillings are more pronounced on fat suppression pulse sequences.

Imaging of Acute Rhinosinusitis

In patients with viral rhinosinusitis, sinus CT scans may reveal mucosal thickening of nasal passages, along with mucosal thickening and air fluid level in the paranasal sinuses. There may be air bubbles scattered within the fluid (transudate or exudates) in the sinuses. After resolution of common colds, sinus CT scans will demonstrate complete resolution of mucosal changes as well as clearing of the fluid in the sinuses. Subperiosteal edema and bony changes (osteolysis, demineralization) are not seen unless there is associated superimposed bacterial or fungal infections.

An acutely infected sinus due to bacterial or fungal infection may show thickening of the mucosa (reflecting edematous tissue of the paranasal sinuses), an air fluid level, or both, and one or more of the sinus cavities may be completely opacified. Conventional radiography is adequate for the diagnosis of clinically uncomplicated acute sinusitis (25,34). Bacterial and invasive fungal infection of the paranasal sinuses can extend through the cortical bone resulting in a collection of edema or purulence between the bone and the periorbita or epidural space (31). The subperiosteal edema and abscess can be best evaluated on enhanced CT scans. The abscess will be depicted as a low-density region surrounded by an enhancing abscess wall. The MRI including diffusion-weighted imaging (DWI) is equally useful for the evaluation of subperiosteal effusion and abscess formation (42). The orbital involvement from acute bacterial and fungal sinusitis includes inflammatory eyelid edema (preseptal edema), subperiosteal edema (orbital periostitis), subperiosteal cellular induration (phlegmon), subperiosteal abscess (organized abscess), orbital cellulitis, and orbital abscess. Should the infection spread from the sinuses into the cranial cavity, one or more of the following complications may ensue: cavernous sinus thrombosis, meningitis, and epidural, subdural, or brain abscess. Periostitis and osteomyelitis of the frontal sinus severe enough to involve the orbit may also extend through the posterior plate of the frontal sinus to involve the anterior cranial fossa. Intracranial complications of sinusitis can be best evaluated by MRI including contrast enhancement, DWI, MR angiography, and MR venography (Figs. 5–14) (34,42). Acute mycotic infections of the sinonasal cavities and craniofacial structures (rhinocerebral mycosis) are also best evaluated by MRI (Figs. 13 and 14).

Acute sinusitis is usually evident on clinical examination, confirmed by plain film studies and followed by CT study as needed (Fig. 4). Complications of sinusitis are an indication for CT and/or MRI (34,35,41,42). CT scanning is preferable for identifying bone destruction and osteomyelitis. MRI shows to better advantage the orbital and intracranial sinogenic complications (Figs. 5–14) (31,32).

Imaging of CRS

CRS Without NP

Acute sinus infections cause demineralization (rarefaction) of the wall of the sinus and subsequently, when the process becomes chronic, results in reactive sclerosis of the sinus walls (34,39). These changes in the wall of the sinus often indicate the presence of osteitis, which further raises the question as to whether it is a focus of persistent infection (39). CRS on CT scans appears as mucosal thickening which

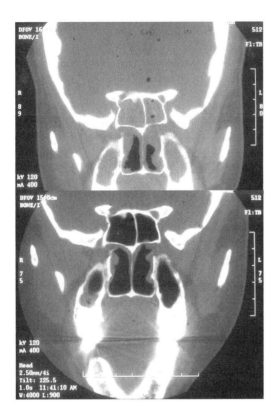

FIGURE 4 Acute sphenoid sinusitis. Coronal CT scan (*top*) showing complete opacification of sphenoid sinuses. Coronal CT scan (*bottom*) showing resolution of acute sinusitis.

may be associated with sclerosis of the wall of the sinus and bony septae. Complete opacification of one or more anterior ethmoid air cells is commonly seen and may represent the underlying focus of persistent symptoms (Fig. 15). Less commonly, other sinus cavities or posterior ethmoid air cells may be completely opacified.

Variable degrees of sinus ostial obstruction are also common in CRS. Obstruction of the OMU has been given special significance (individual "weighting") in some CRS staging systems, such as the Lund and Mackay system (47) based on the presumption that obstruction of this critical drainage pathway is more likely to cause persistent symptoms. However, most studies have found a lack of correlation between a single sinus CT severity score and patient's CRS symptoms. Similarly, sinus CT scoring has not been found to correlate particularly well with clinical response to medical or surgical intervention or relapses after sinus surgery. In one study, relapses after medical treatment were most closely related to a history of polyposis rather than persistence of sinus ostial obstruction after medical treatment (48). These observations raise a question as to whether ostial obstruction should receive separate weighting in sinus CT scoring systems, and in fact one recently developed scoring system grades sinus ostial obstruction independently of mucosal disease (49).

Sinus opacification in CRS without NP raises the question of persistent bacterial infection, mucus inspissation, or possibly focal polypoid thickening, or even a focus of allergic mucin due to allergic fungal rhinosinusitis (AFRS).

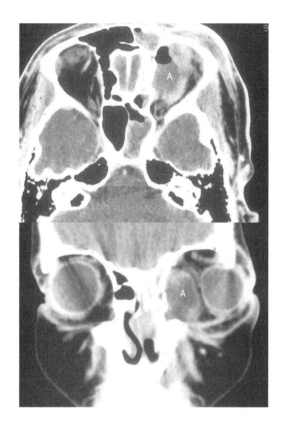

FIGURE 5 Acute sinusitis with subperiosteal abscess. Axial-enhanced CT scan (*top*), showing opacification of left frontal and sphenoid sinuses. Note a large subperiosteal abcess with air fluid level (A). Coronal-enhanced CT scan (*bottom*) in another patient with acute ethmoid sinusitis showing a large subperiosteal orbital abscess (A).

However, the latter is rarely seen in patients without a history of nasal polyposis. In contrast, sinus opacification in CRS with NP is commonly seen in the absence of gross infection.

CRS with NP

Mucosal thickening and/or sinus opacification are typically more pronounced in CRS with NP than CRS without NP (Fig. 16). Polyps are seen on CT scans as mucosal protrusions into the nasal cavity (Fig. 17). Polyps in the nasal cavity are a marker of extensive chronic sinonasal inflammatory disease. The CT density of polyps cannot be differentiated from nonpolypoid mucosal thickening. When the mucosal thickening appears polypoid in configuration, we use CT appearance in favor of polyp or polyps. The combination of CT and MRI including enhanced CT and MRI provide an imaging appearance that highly favors the presence of polyps.

A solitary polyp may not be distinguished from a retention cyst on unenhanced CT and MRI. Unlike cysts, polyps demonstrate moderate to marked contrast enhancement. When multiple polyps are present, sinus secretions become entrapped with the crevices between the polyps, as well as on their surfaces. On CT scans, polyps show soft tissue attenuation values (density); however, depending on the concentration of the entrapped mucosal secretions, the CT attenuation values rise, and the chronic sinonasal polyposis may show mixed CT attenuation values with areas of increased density, simulating focal or diffuse dystrophic calcifications.

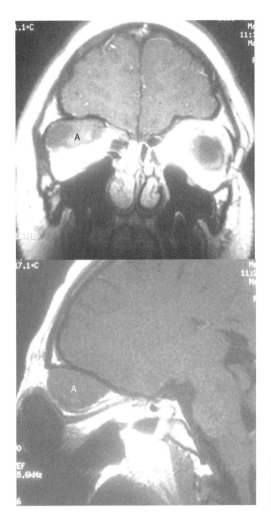

FIGURE 6 Sinogenic acute subperiosteal abscess. Coronal-enhanced T1W (*top*) and sagittal T1W (*bottom*) MR scans showing a large subperiosteal abscess (A).

These findings are highly suggestive that the CRS with NP is complicated further by the presence of AFRS. In aggressive long-standing polyposis, there may be significant expansion of the sinuses as well as bone erosion. Again, these findings are highly suggestive of the presence of AFRS. Polyps tend to have various signal intensities on MR pulse sequences. The MRI characteristics of polyps reflect the various stages of polyps (edematous, glandular, cystic, and fibrous), as well as various stages of desiccation of the entrapped mucosal secretions within the crevices between the polyps and on the surfaces of the polyps (33).

Imaging of Allergic Fungal Rhinosinusitis

Most patients with this condition have sinonasal polyposis, and therefore the imaging appearance may be indistinguishable from that of CRS with NP, although certain radiologic features are highly suggestive of AFRS. The sinuses most often involved are the maxillary, ethmoid, and sphenoid sinuses. CT scan is the study of

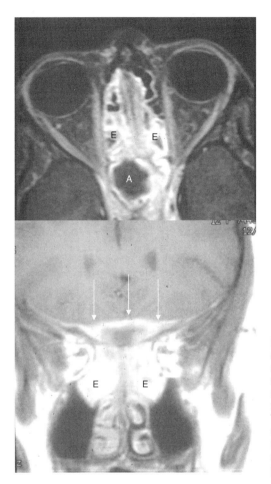

FIGURE 7 Acute sphenoid and ethmoid sinusitis with epidural abscess. Axial-enhanced T1W (*top*) MR scan, showing marked enhancement of inflammatory tissue in the ethmoid air cells (E) and a sphenoid sinus abscess (A). Coronal-enhanced T1W MR scan (*bottom*) showing marked enhancement of posterior ethmoid air cells (E), inflammatory mucosal thickening, and a large epidural abscess (*arrows*). The patient lost vision in her left eye.

choice. The CT findings include foci of increased density within the opacified sinuses (described below). Areas of focal hyperattenuation vary in size. At times they may form a cast of increased density within the sinus. As these materials accumulate, bony demineralization of the sinus walls ensues secondary to the release of inflammatory mediators and pressure, resulting in expansion of the sinus and possibly mucocele formation (28). True bone erosion is much less common, occurring in 20% of cases in the series of Nussenbaum et al. (50).

Allergic mucin has areas of high protein content and low water concentration that give rise to characteristic radiographic appearance on CT and MR images. These areas typically appear "hyperdense" on sinus CT but "hypointense" on corresponding T2W MR images. The increased CT density in AFRS is frequently seen centrally more than peripherally. It may be a confluent area of increased density like a cast or scattered and linearly oriented increased density. Desiccation of mucin contributes to the hyperdense areas on CT more than accumulations of heavy metals (e.g., iron and manganese). The argument we use is the appearance of lens of the infant on CT scan which appears as a hyperdense image related to high protein content of the lens which is also the least hydrated organ in the body.

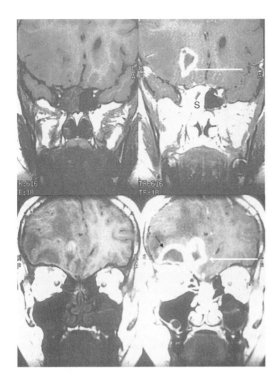

FIGURE 8 Sinogenic epidural and brain abcesses. Coronal precontrast and postcontrast T1W MR scans showing marked enhancement of inflammatory mucosal thickening of right sphenoid sinus (S). Note large epidural abscess (*short arrow*), a frontal lobe abscess (*long arrow*), and marked edema of the right frontal lobe.

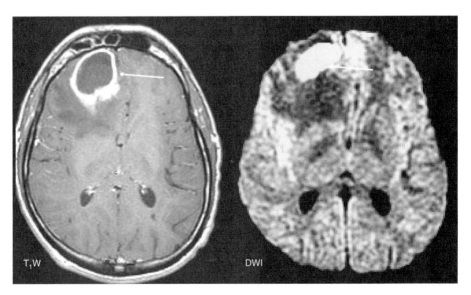

FIGURE 9 Sinogenic brain abscess. Axial-enhanced T1W MR scan showing marked enhancement of the capsule of the right frontal lobe abscess (*arrow*). Note abnormal enhancement of right frontal sinus thickened mucosal lining. Note marked edema of the right frontal lobe adjacent to the abscess. Axial diffusion-weighted MR imaging (DWI) showing marked hyperintensity of the frontal lobe abscess (*arrow*), indicative of diffusion restriction. Note that the surrounding vasogenic edema shows no diffusion restriction.

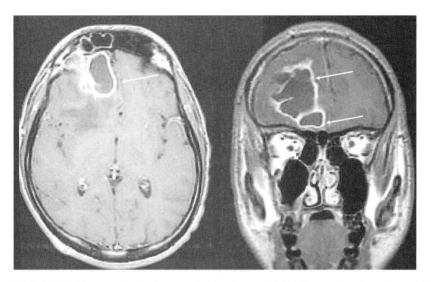

FIGURE 10 Sinogenic brain abscess. Axial-enhanced T1W MR scan showing a large right frontal lobe abscess (*single arrow*). This was related to infection of the right frontal sinus, which shows abnormal enhancement as well as focal bone defect along its posterior plate. Coronal-enhanced T1W MR scan showing the frontal lobe abscess (*double arrows*).

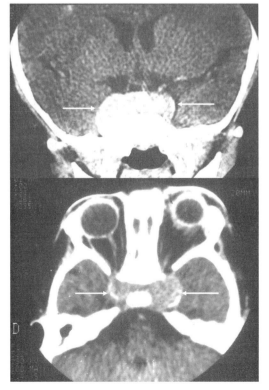

FIGURE 11 Mycotic aneurysm of internal carotid arteries. Enhanced coronal (*top*) and axial (*bottom*) CT scans showing enlargement of both cavernous sinuses related to mycotic aneurysm of the internal carotid arteries (*arrows*).

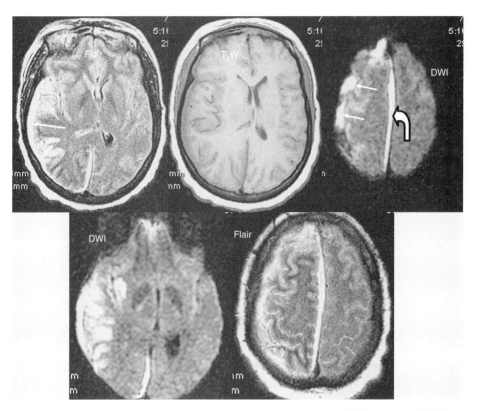

FIGURE 12 Sinogenic subdural empyema. Axial flair, axial-unenhanced T1W and axial DWI (*top*) axial DWI, and axial Flair (*bottom*) MR scans showing a right temporal (*straight arrows*) and an interhemispheric (*curve arrow*) subdural empyema. Note marked hyperintensity of empyema on DWI scans.

Both mucus accumulation and mucosal thickening contribute significantly to sinus opacification in this condition and are difficult to differentiate with sinus CT imaging. Assuming that more precise estimates of mucus accumulation and mucosal thickening are desired in the setting of clinical research, MRI imaging will be necessary. T1W imaging may show peripheral enhancement of involved paranasal sinus on postgadolinium MR images indicative of thickened mucosal lining. In addition, the involved paranasal sinus and nasal cavity demonstrate variable but predominantly hypointense signal intensity. In contrast, T2W imaging weighted is best for identification of allergic fungal mucin. This effect is more pronounced on T2W images as a result of shortened magnetic field relaxation times. The high protein and low water concentration of allergic fungal mucin, coupled with the high water content within the surrounding edematous paranasal sinus mucosa gives rise to rather specific magnetic resonance characteristics. The allergic fungal mucin appears markedly hypointense (dark) while the edematous, thickened mucosal lining appears markedly hyperintense (bright).

The combined CT and MRI findings provide an imaging appearance that is highly suggestive if not pathognomonic of AFRS. However, such classic findings are not present in all cases. In AFRS, the postcontrast (gadolinium-based contrast)

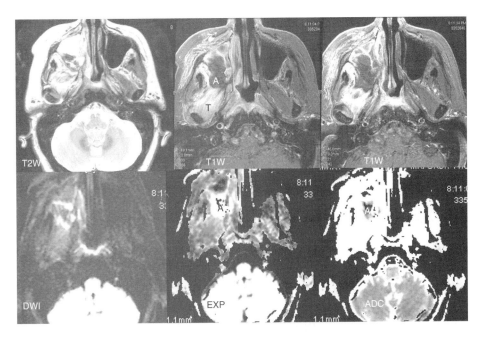

FIGURE 13 Mucormycosis. Axial T2W and enhanced T1W (*top*), and axial DWI, axial exponential (EXP), and apparent diffusion coefficient (ADC) mapping (*bottom*). Note hyperintensity of the right maxillary sinus on T2W MR scan, abscess along the posterior aspect of the right maxillary sinus (A), abnormal enhancement of the right temporal fossa (T), fluid in the right temporomandibular joint, and edema of the right face. The abscess (A) appears hyperintense on DWI and hypointense on ADC map.

T1W MR images will demonstrate a rim of contrast enhancement around the heterogeneous but predominantly hypointensive desiccated fungal allergic mucin.

Zinreich et al. (29). reported 25 patients with allergic fungal rhinosinusitis. Of these, 22 had areas of focal hyperattenuation on CT scans in sizes ranging from 4 mm in diameter to nearly forming a cast of the maxillary sinus. The presence of areas of increased densities in the paranasal sinuses correlated well with fungal rhinosinusitis in the study of Zinreich et al. (29). However, since pus, desiccated mucosal secretions, dystrophic calcifications (concretions, antrolith), and acute hemorrhage are also dense on CT scans; CT findings alone are not conclusive within a partially or totally opacified sinus. Therefore, the finding should serve as a high index of suspicion for allergic fungal rhinosinusitis, especially that caused by aspergillosis. The increased central density, with or without calcifications, reflects the extramucosal saprophytic growth of fungi in retained secretions. The presence of highly proteinaceous inspissated mucus creates areas of very high attenuation values on CT images (51). The presence of diffuse increased attenuation within the paranasal sinuses and nasal cavity should be considered as AFRS or chronic hyperplastic rhinosinusitis and polyposis associated with desiccated retained mucosal secretions (concretions) (Figs. 19–20). As these materials accumulate within the sinus, bony demineralization of the sinus walls ensues secondary to the release of inflammatory mediators and pressure, resulting in expansion of the sinus and mucocele formation (51).

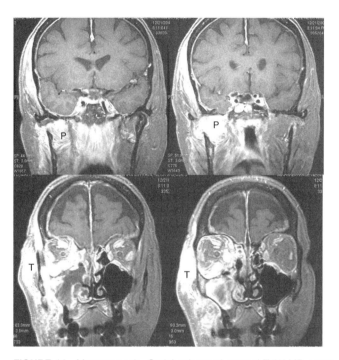

FIGURE 14 Mucormycosis. Serial-enhanced coronal T1W MR scans showing marked inflammatory changes in the right maxillary and ethmoid sinuses. Note abnormal enhancement of the right periorbita with enlargement of the right inferior and medial rectus muscles. Note abnormal enhancement of the right temporal fossa (T) and pterygoid muscles (P).

The MRI characteristics of fungal rhinosinusitis depend on the stage of the disease. In acute invasive fungal rhinosinusitis, regardless of the offending organism, there will be significant inflammatory edema and cellular infiltrate, resulting in marked hyperintensity in proton-weighted (PW) and particularly in T2W MR images. The process appears relatively hypointense in T1W MR images (Fig. 21). In allergic fungal rhinosinusitis, the presence of concretions and desiccated mucosal secretions results in low signal on T1W and marked hypointensity on T2W MR images. The reactive granulations or associated subacute or acute rhinosinusitis will demonstrate hyperintense signal on T2W MR images. There will be enhancement only of mucosal rim on enhanced MR images. All fungal concretions in the study of Zinreich et al. (30). stained positively for calcium. Decreased signal intensity on T1- and very decreased signal intensity on T2-weighted MR images were thought by Zinreich et al. (30). to be due to calcium as well as iron and manganese found in fungal rhinosinusitis. It is now, however, known that the presence of inspissated mucosal secretions within the sinus cavity or along the crevices of polyps result in a markedly hypointense T2W signal (28,51). In fact it seems that in practice, the majority of sinus cases with hypointense T2W signal are related to desiccated retained mucosal secretion without the presence of the fungus. Chronic noninvasive aspergillus rhinosinusitis and allergic fungal rhinosinusitis may have the same MR appearance as chronic hyperplastic sinonasal polyposis with inspissation of the retained secretion. The highly proteinaceous

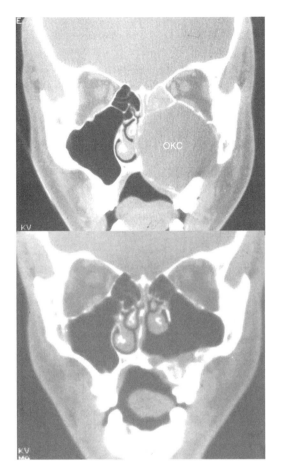

FIGURE 15 Odontogenic keratocyst and associated ethmoid sinusitis. Coronal CT scan (*top*) showing a large odontogenic keratocyst (OKC). Notice opacified left ethmoid sinus. Coronal CT scan (*bottom*), obtained following marsupialization of the OKC, showing resolution of ethmoid opacification related to relief of ostial obstruction/blockage.

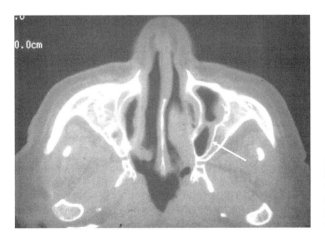

FIGURE 16 Chronic osteoblastic maxillary sinusitis. Axial CT scan showing marked osteoblastic reaction (*arrow*), resulting in contraction of both maxillary sinuses.

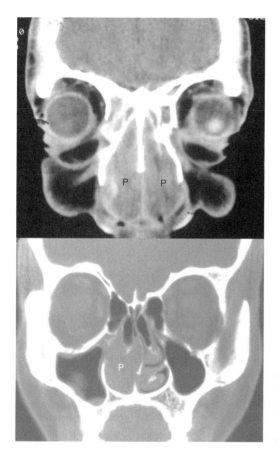

FIGURE 17 Nasal polyps. Coronal-enhanced CT scan (*top*) showing expansion of nasal cavities due to bilateral nasal polyps. Coronal CT scan (*bottom*) shows a right nasal cavity polyp (P) displacing inferior turbinate laterally.

central mucin (inspissated mucus) in allergic fungal rhinosinusitis corresponds to areas of high attenuation on CT images and corresponding areas of low-signal on both T1W and T2W MR images (Fig. 20).

Computed Tomography Technique

The CT scan is an excellent imaging modality to evaluate the sinonasal cavities. It provides an accurate assessment of the paranasal sinuses and craniofacial bones as well as the extent of pneumatization of the paranasal sinuses. Five-millimeter sections are often adequate for evaluation of most of the sinonasal and skull base structures. The axial sections are taken parallel to the orbitomeatal line or parallel to the hard palate. The coronal sections are obtained with the patient supine or prone, the head hyperextended, and the gantry tilted to a plane as close to 90° to the canthomeatal line as possible. Thinner sections (3 mm) are used to identify small lesions and evaluate the ostiomeatal unit. In terms of filming, some authors recommend an intermediate window width/level (W/L) technique (2500/250, W/L) (29,38).

We prefer CT images to be viewed or filmed with extended window width-window level bone technique (4000/700–800 W/L). In case that the study is

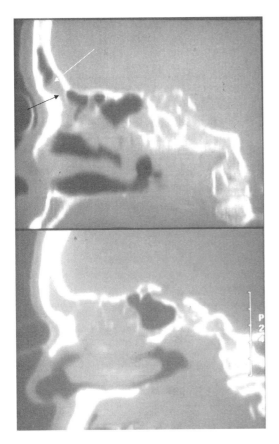

FIGURE 18 Chronic sinusitis. Sagittal reformatted CT scan showing mucosal thickening of the frontal sinus (*white arrow*). Note obliteration of the frontal sinus ostium (*black arrow*). Sagittal reformatted CT scan (*bottom*) showing marked inflammatory muscosal diseases of the frontal and ethmoid sinuses.

interpreted on hard copy films, we recommend that the technicians provide the copies using soft tissue window technique. The soft tissue technique allows better evaluation of inspissated mucosal debris and microcalcifications. Reformatted coronal images are routinely obtained when direct coronal sections cannot be performed. Reformatted sagittal images are obtained for image-guided surgery and evaluation of frontal recess and lesions that are better seen in sagittal plane.

Magnetic Resonance Imaging Technique

An opinion one frequently hears with regard to sinonasal imaging is that MRI is often not very helpful compared with CT scanning. This may be true for a few specific entities such as fibro-osseous lesions, however, for benign and malignant tumors, MRI is superior to CT scans to differentiate tumor from surrounding associated inflammatory disease and retained secretions. The marked hyperintensity on T2W MR images of the inflammatory mucosal disease as well as marked enhancement of inflammatory mucosal thickening on enhanced T1W MR images often allow the radiologist to differentiate tumors from surrounding inflammatory disease. Intracranial tumor extension and intracranial complications of sinonasal infections are better evaluated by MRI than CT scanning. In general, the combination of MR and CT imaging will allow for better evaluation of the disease and, at

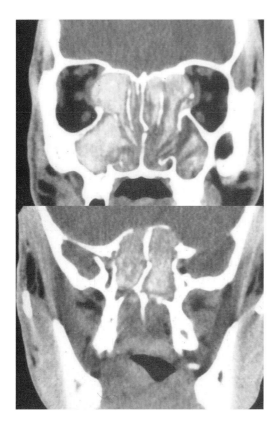

FIGURE 19 Allergic fungal rhinosinusitis. Coronal CT scans showing opacified nasal cavities and paranasal sinuses. Note cast of increased density within the sinuses as well as focal and linear areas of increased density within the nasal cavities. Note expansion of right ethmoid due to mucocele formation.

times, for making a more specific diagnosis. The radiologist should always be consulted in determining the most appropriate imaging study(ies) for each individual case. In the evaluation of suspected sinonasal disease processes, a typical MRI protocol consists of short TR/TE sagittal localization, unenhanced short TR short TE and long TR long TE axial sequences, followed by a contrast-enhanced short TR short TE axial, coronal, and sagittal pulse sequences.

Image-Guided Endoscopic Surgery

Image guidance systems are available that provide otolaryngologists with precise anatomic localization during head and neck surgery (52–54). The use of optical-based and electromagnetic-based image guidance systems has proved valuable in providing anatomic localization with an accuracy of 2 mm or better at the start of surgery (54). In one study, the accuracy had deteriorated by the conclusion of surgery by an average of 0.89 mm because of anatomical drift (54). Our CT protocol for image-guided endoscopic surgery includes 2.5 mm axial sections and reformatted sagittal and coronal views. The video display from the optical-based image guidance system during surgery will demonstrate the tip of the surgical instrument and corresponding position on axial, coronal, sagittal, and 3-dimensional images of the patient's preoperative CT scan. The use of the image-guidance system was found to increase the mean total operating time by 17.4 minutes per case (53,54).

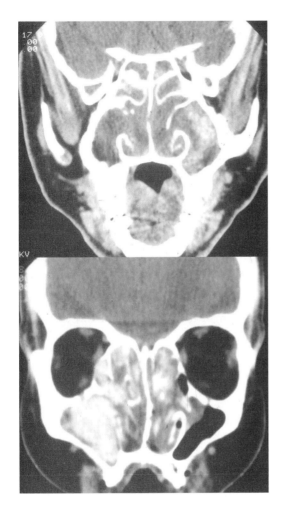

FIGURE 20 Allergic fungal rhinosinusitis. Coronal CT scans showing
changes characteristic of allergic fungal
rhinosinusitis.

INFLAMMATORY DISEASES OF SINONASAL CAVITIES
Acute Sinusitis

Mucosal thickening, the most common finding on imaging studies, usually indicates the presence of chronic sinusitis, but at times may be seen in acute rhinosinusitis. Postoperative scarring and periostial reaction after a sinus surgery such as Caldwell-Luc operation may result in loss of normal aeration of the sinuses. These changes may be permanent, even in the absence of any sinus disease (55). Although the lack of sclerosis and periostial reaction speaks against chronic sinusitis, it does not at all rule out a chronic infection. Bilaterality and absence of erosion weigh in favor of an inflammatory rather than neoplastic process.

Diffuse thickening of the mucosa and submucosa lining of the paranasal sinuses is a common finding on plain films, CT, and MR scans. Indeed, 20–40% of patients undergoing MRI of the head are found to have edematous tissue of the paranasal sinuses as an incidental finding. Sinusitis may accompany a viral infection, but is also seen in patients with allergies. An acutely infected sinus that is producing symptoms may show thickening of the mucosa, an air-fluid level, or both.

Sinus Infections and Their Complications

Osteomyelitis of the frontal bone may be accompanied by doughy edema overlapping the affected sinus and/or a subgaleal abscess, causing a mass effect termed a "Pott's puffy tumor." Acute, subacute, or CRS that has not responded to appropriate antibiotic and other medical treatments should be biopsied to rule out the presence of any underlying tumor, particularly if infection is limited to a single sinus. In the case of maxillary sinus, an underlying dental cause has to be excluded. A persistent air fluid level following dental extraction may indicate an oral-antral fistula (55). Orbital and intracranial complications resulting from acute or CRS can be best evaluated with combination of CT and MRI (Figs. 5–12).

The most common complications of rhinosinusitis in children occur in the orbit. These complications include the following in order of increasing severity: orbital edema, orbital cellulitis, subperiosteal orbital abscess, intraorbital abscess, thrombosis of superior ophthalmic vein and cavernous sinuses. Inflammatory orbital edema due to rhinosinusitis is edema of the eyelid which is often misdiagnosed as orbital or periorbital cellulitis. The infection in this early stage is actually still confined to the sinus (56,57). A CT or MRI scan at this stage will demonstrate the edema of the eyelids and conjunctivae and inflammatory changes of the infected sinus or sinuses. As the reaction of the orbital periostium begins and gradually advances, the edema of the eyelids and conjunctivae becomes more generalized and the eye begins to protrude. Inflammatory tissue collects beneath the periosteum to form a subperiosteal edema or phlegmon (Figs. 5 and 6); subsequently, pus may form to represent a subperiosteal abscess (Fig. 7). As the disease progresses, bacteria may infiltrate the periorbital and retro-orbital fat, giving rise to true orbital cellulitis and abscess. These two conditions frequently coexist. At this stage, extraocular mobility is progressively impaired. With severe involvement, visual disturbances can result from optic neuritis, ischemia (compression), or both. Abscess formation in the orbit may result from extension of a subperiosteal abscess through the periosteum or from localization of orbital and facial cellulitis (55,57). Usually, ethmoid sinus infection is responsible for orbital swelling, subperiosteal abscess, and orbital cellulitis, which extends from the ethmoid through the lamina papyracea. CT is an excellent radiologic method for evaluating acute ethmoiditis. The information obtained from the CT scan and MRI together with clinical findings (proptosis, limitation of extraocular muscle movement, and decreased visual acuity) may be the best guidelines for clinical management.

INTRACRANIAL COMPLICATIONS OF RHINOSINUSITIS

Although intracranial complications of rhinosinusitis are relatively rare, their prompt recognition is important to prevent permanent neurologic deficit or fatality (57,58). Intracranial complications of sinus infection derive from either indirect extension, via retrograde thrombophlebitis of valveless emissary veins, or directly, through bony contiguity associated with septic erosion, trauma, or structural abnormality (57). These complications include osteomyelitis, epidural empyema, subdural empyema (SDE), meningitis, cerebritis, brain abscess, sinodural thrombosis (cavernous sinus, superior sagittal sinus thrombosis) (58), infarct, and tension pneumocephalus, related to ruptured intracranial abscess into the ventricles, while in continuity with the sinonasal cavities.

SDE is thought to be the most common intracranial complication of sinus infections (58,59). Similarly, sinus infection is the most common cause of SDE (59). With the timely intervention, mortality rates associated with SDE range from 10% to 20% but may be as high as 70% under certain circumstances (58). SDE is a neurosurgical emergency that requires drainage to avert a rapidly evolving and fulminant clinical course. Inoculation of the subdural space most often occurs indirectly via thrombophlebitis of valveless emissary veins (58). The triad of fever, rhinosinusitis, and neurologic deficits is suggestive of intracranial spread of infection. In SDE, the infection lies adjacent to the leptomeninges; therefore, patients with SDE may present with meningeal signs, hemiparesis, seizure, or mental status changes. CT with contrast is usually sufficiently sensitive to detect an SDE, which is appreciated on the scan as a low-density extra-axial fluid collection in the setting of marked cortical swelling (56). There may be increased vascular enhancement related to generalized increased permability of the vasculature caused by the inflammatory response. A small interhemispheric subdural collection may be difficult to detect by CT scanning. MRI is superior to CT scanning for detection of subdural collection and pyogenic lesions. SDE is most commonly seen in young men and frequently associated with *Streptococcus anginosus* (58). Mental status changes in a patient with rhinosinusitis should be treated aggressively, and the diagnosis of SDE should be pursued with MRI, including DWI and a contrast study. Small SDE may not be detected by CT scan including contrast enhancement (58). MRI is the imaging study of choice for the diagnosis of SDE as well as other sinogenic intracranial complications (58,59). Early recognition and treatment are essential to reduce any subsequent morbidity or mortality (59). In addition to CT scanning, it is prudent to obtain an MRI of the sinuses, orbits, and brain whenever extensive or multiple complications of rhinosinusitis are suspected (60).

Acute Mycotic Sinonasal Diseases

Mycotic infection of the nasal and paranasal sinuses and craniofacial structures is a serious disease that requires prompt surgery and medical therapy to decrease its high morbidity rate (55,57,61). This type of infection is usually seen in immunocompromised individuals, such as AIDS patients or patients who have undergone therapy with immunosuppressive drugs or antimetabolites (55,57,62,63). Rhino-orbito-cerebral mucormycosis is typically seen in debilitated patients, patients with diabetic ketoacidosis, and patients who are severely immunocompromised. Leukemia and dialysis have also been reported to predispose patients to this infection (28,117,118). Recently, cases of rhino-orbito-cerebral mucormycosis have been described in patients with iron overload. Rhinocerebral myotic infection may be caused by the members of the family Mucoraceae (mucormycosis), which belongs to the class of Phycomycetes, and *Aspergillus* (aspergillosis) (61). The fungi responsible for mucormycosis are ubiquitous and normally saprophytic in humans; they rarely produce severe disease, except in those with predisposing conditions (57). The infection usually begins in the nose and spreads to the paranasal sinuses; then it extends into the orbit and cavernous sinuses (55,61,62). Orbital involvement results in such orbital signs as ophthalmoplegia, proptosis, loss of vision, and orbital cellulitis. At times orbital cellulitis may be associated with rapid and sudden loss of vision due to occlusion of the central retinal artery or vein. The inflammatory process soon extends along the intracranial and infra-orbital fissure and into the infratemporal fossa (Figs. 13 and 14). Black necrosis of a turbinate is a diagnostic clinical sign in mucormycosis, but it may not be present until late in the course of the disease (61). The radiographic findings of mucormycosis of the sinuses were first described by Green et al. (62), who noted three signs: nodular mucosal thickening, absence of fluid levels, and spotty destruction of bony walls. None of these signs can be considered pathognomonic for the diagnosis of fungal rhinosinusitis; however, a CT scan or MRI study may be very helpful and sometimes characteristic for the diagnosis of mucormycosis (57,61). The main contribution of CT or MRI scanning to the diagnosis of mucormycosis is its clear demonstration of the relationship between nasal, sinus, and orbital disease, a relationship so typical of mucormycosis that this diagnosis should be considered whenever combined nasal, sinus, and orbital diseases are encountered. Invasion of the medial orbit by the infecting organism results in phlegmon of the periorbital region and, therefore, elevation of the medial rectus, which later on becomes involved via direct invasion by hyphae. Effacement and edema of the fascial planes outside the involved sinus, bone destruction of the sinus walls, and, in particular, periosteal irregularity and cortical bony rarefaction indicative of periostitis and osteitis are common. In an appropriate clinical setting, CT and MRI scans usually help to differentiate the overall picture from that of a sinonasal malignant process (Figs. 13 and 14). Amphotericin B with aggressive debridement remains the mainstay of treatment of rhino-orbito-cerebral mucormycosis (63).

Aspergillosis

Aspergillosis is a ubiquitous mold found primarily in agricultural dust. It may produce rhinocerebral infection and orbital involvement similar to mucormycosis, although hematogenous spread from the lungs to the brain is more common (61,62). This fungus also has a well-known propensity for invading blood vessels, including the internal carotid artery. The combination of orbital and sinus involvement is not pathognomonic of rhinocerebral mucormycosis or aspergillosis; however, awareness of its possibility, particularly when any of the predisposing factors are present, would help in making an early diagnosis and facilitating treatment of this aggressive and fatal disease. In our practice, CT and MR scanning have been the most effective imaging modalities for making the correct diagnosis. It is important to include the nasal cavity, nasopharynx, and base of the skull and the brain when performing CT or MRI in a patient with a potential or tentative diagnosis of mucormycosis or aspergillosis or other opportunistic infections of the sinonasal tracts.

Chronic Fungal (Mycotic) Rhinosinusitis and Classic Allergic Fungal Rhinosinusitis

Fungal sinus disease is often diagnosed because an apparently routine infection fails to respond to a commonly used antibiotic regimen (61). In immunocompetent patients, fungal sinus disease may first be recognized as a slowly progressing extramucosal fungus ball, a noninvasive disease (64). In immunocompromised patients, however, fungal sinus diseases of the sinonasal cavities are more typically invasive conditions, such as fulminant mucormycosis and aspergillosis. The benign extramucosal fungal disease has been attributed to the *Aspergillus* species (64). However, appraisal of the aggressiveness of the fungal disease on the basis of the organism alone may not always be valid (65–70). Extramucosal fungal rhinosinusitis develops as a saprophytic growth in retained secretions in a sinus cavity (i.e., a "fungus ball"). This disorder is usually benign and is rarely associated with mucosal invasion. The treatment of extramucosal fungal disease entails removing the fungal ball, and restoring mucocilliary drainage and sinus ventilation. A biopsy should be obtained from the mucosa to rule out mucosal invasion (71).

Imaging Diagnosis of Chronic Mycotic Rhinosinusitis

The imaging manifestations of mycotic rhinosinusitis may be nonspecific or highly suggestive of the presence of fungal infection. The most often involved sinuses are the maxillary, ethmoid, and sphenoid sinuses. The findings on plain radiography may vary from those of nonspecific mucosal disease without any bone involvement to an opacified sinus with a polypoid mass with a central or peripheral hyperdense (calcified) mass (fungal ball, occasionally referred to as a sinus "mycetoma") (61,64,71).[a] A fungal ball may appear as either a homogeneous soft tissue mass or in some cases as a well-defined mass with a density similar to that seen with calcium or bone (64). The increased density within the polypoid sinus mass in cases of chronic mycotic rhinosinusitis is believed to be due to calcium phosphate and calcium sulfate deposits within necrotic areas of the mycelium (71,72). CT is superior to plain radiography and complex motion tomography in detecting fungal concretions.

Chronic Sinonasal Inflammation Secondary to Nasal Cocaine Abuse

Intranasal cocaine abuse can cause a variety of otolaryngologic complications secondary to its potent vasoconstricting and direct irritating effects on the nasal mucosa (73). Repeated intranasal "snorting" or "sniffing" of cocaine can lead to ischemia and necrosis of the nasal septum, resulting in septal perforation, synechia, and CRS (73). Other complications of cocaine abuse include osteolytic rhinosinusitis, nasolacrimal duct obstruction, hypertensive crisis, vasculitis, ventricular arrhythmia, cardiopulmonary arrest, clonic–tonic seizures, and hyperpyrexia (73).

SILENT SINUS SYNDROME

Silent sinus syndrome has been described as spontaneous enophthalmos with chronic maxillary rhinosinusitis, associated with maxillary sinus atelectasis. Nasal endoscopy will commonly show retraction of the uncinate shelf and obliteration of the infundibulum (74–76). There are three theories regarding the pathogenesis of silent sinus syndrome. The most popular theory describes the obstruction of the outflow tract of the maxillary sinus, resulting in hypoventilation of the sinus, negative antral pressure, and subsequent atelectasis of sinus walls. The second theory suggests that inflammatory disease induces erosion of the floor of the orbit, and the third theory describes rhinosinusitis in a hypoplastic sinus (74). Radiologic findings include obstruction of the OMC at the maxillary infundibulum, atelectatic uncinate process, contracted maxillary component of antrum, opacification of maxillary sinus, inferior bowing of antral roof (floor of orbit), lateral bowing of the

---

[a]The term mycetoma can also refer to a cutaneous fungal condition distinct from a "fungus ball." See: http://www.doctorfungus.org/mycoses/human/other/mycetoma.htm.

medial wall, and anterior bowing of the posterior maxillary sinus. The maxillary walls may be thickened (chronic osteitis), thinned, or partially dehiscent.

Rhinolith

Foreign bodies within the nose and paranasal sinuses tend to become encrusted and calcified when retained for a long period of time and are thus known as rhinoliths and sinoliths, respectively. These calcareous bodies may be endogenous or exogenous in origin. Teeth, sequestra, and dried blood clots are considered endogenous (77). Exogenous material includes fruit seeds, beads, buttons, pieces of dirt and pebbles, and the remains of gauze tampon (77). A nidus of purulent exudate, deposits of blood products, cellular debris, and mineral salts, such as calcium phosphate and carbonate may form a rough surface. A rhinolith may produce nasal obstruction, a malodorous nasal discharge with local pain, and epistaxis. They may even project into the maxillary sinus by pressure necrosis of the nasoantral wall. Foreign bodies within the nose may be self-induced, due to dental root canal fillings, bullets, shrapnel, or buckshot. A calcified nasal mass on CT scan is characteristic of rhinolith. The calcification appears as a cast surrounded by soft tissue related to inflammatory reaction associated with rhinolithiasis. A sinolith appears similar to rhinolith, and is most commonly seen in the maxillary antrum.

Granulomatous Diseases

Sinonasal granulomas have an extensive differential diagnosis (Table 1) (78–99). The list includes: sarcoidosis, fungal infections, tuberculosis, syphilis, leprosy, rhinoscleroma, Wegener's granulomatosis, allergic granulomatosis and angiitis (Churg-Strauss syndrome), lymphoplasmatoid granuloma (pseudotumor), lymphoma, lymphomatoid granulomatosis, cholesterol granulomas, foreign body granulomas such as lipogranuloma due to oil drops, injected corticosteroids and

TABLE 1 Differential Diagnosis of Granulomatous
Lesions of the Sinonasal Cavities

Fungal infections
Sarcoidosis
Tuberculosis
Leprosy
Syphilis
Rhinoscleroma
Allergic granuloma and hypersensitivity angiitis
Polyarteritis nodosa and systemic lupus
Granuloma gravidum
Angiitis (Churg-Straus syndrome)
Foreign body granuloma (lipogranuloma, paraffinoma)
Cholesterol granuloma
Pyogenic granuloma
Idiopathic granuloma (destructive or nondestructive)
Nonspecific granuloma in nasal polyps
Wegener's granulomatosis
Lymphomatoid granulomatosis (T-cell lymphoma formerly referred to as pseudotumor or midline reticulosis)

Source: From Ref. 27.

paraffin, and unknown causes. Advances in immunocytochemical phenotyping and molecular genetics have revealed that the majority of the sinonasal destructive lesions referred to as midline destructive lesions can be classified into two distinct pathologic groups: Wegener's granulomatosis and various types of non-Hodgkin's lymphoma. Terms used to refer to such lesions include lethal midline granuloma, nonhealing midline granuloma (Stewart's Syndrome), idiopathic midline destructive disease, polymorphic reticulosis, lymphomatoid granulomatosis, pseudolymphoma, and others. It is now clearly established that polymorphic reticulosis is a non-Hodgkin's lymphoma (96). and midline destructive granuloma is linked to T-cell lymphoma (78). Sinonasal lymphoma is one of the rarest forms of extranodal lymphoma in western populations (78). This contrasts with the prevalence in some Asian countries, in which sinonasal lymphoma is the second most common type of extranodal lymphoma (78). In this geographic group, over 90% of cases have T-cell markers, and Epstein–Barr virus has been consistently demonstrated in the cell genome (78). Wegener's granulomatosis and lymphoma are not the main causes of destructive lesions of the sinonasal tract. There are other more common etiologies that should be excluded (Table 2).

TABLE 2   Differential Diagnosis of Destructive Lesions of the Sinonasal Cavities

Trauma
   Accidental
   Iatrogenic (post surgical)
   Self-induced (rhinotillexomania)
Infection
   Bacterial: Mycobacteria, syphilis, rhinoscleroma, leprosy, actinomycosis
   Fungal: Aspergillosis, mucormycosis, other mycotic rhinosinusitis
Toxic
   Cocaine abuse
   Chromium salts
Inflammatory
   Sarcoidosis
   Foreign body granuloma
   Wegener's granulomatosis
   Polyarteritis nodosa
   Systemic lupus
   Allergic hypersensitivity angiitis
Neoplastic
   Basal cell carcinoma
   Squamous cell carcinoma
   Adenocarcinoma
   Hemangiopericytoma
   Esthesioneuroblastoma
   Lymphoma
   Melanoma
   Rhabdomyosarcoma
   Kaposi sarcoma
   Post transplant lymphoproliferative disease
   Osteo-chondrogenic sarcoma
   Metastasis

Source: Modified from Ref. 78.

CYSTS
Mucoceles

The otolaryngologist and ophthalmologist should constantly be on the lookout for orbital complications of sinus disease. Most of these are readily apparent from their clinical manifestations. Others, however, such as mucocele and inflammatory polyps, have a slow insidious onset, which makes the diagnosis quite difficult (57,57). The slow and silent expansion of a mucocele may be unsuspected until bone is eroded and the cyst impinges on other structures (61). The etiology of mucocele (collection of mucus) is debatable. Most otorhinolaryngologists believe that mucoceles are secondary to obstruction of the main ostium of the sinus (100). This obstruction may be the result of inflammation, trauma, osteoma, fibrous dysplasia, or repeated surgery in and around the nasal cavity (55,57,61). A minority of investigators believes that mucoceles arise as small cysts within the mucous membrane and by continued growth, finally obstruct the ostium of the sinus. Similarly, inflammation, trauma, and surgery may contribute to the initial cyst, or it may arise de novo (57,61). Isolated fungal rhinosinusitis of the sphenoid sinus is a rare but well-documented phenomenon (100). *Aspergillus* is the organism most commonly involved in those cases, with the formation of fungus balls being the predominant pathologic process as opposed to other types of fungal rhinosinusitis, i.e. allergic, chronic invasive, and acute fulminant (100). Chronic noninvasive fungal sphenoid rhinosinusitis may result in the formation of sphenoid sinus mucoceles (100). All these theories differ only as to whether the cyst is the primary cause or the effect of obstruction. It is possible that both circumstances prevail. Irrespective of the pathogenesis and cause of the obstruction, mucoceles are cyst-like lesions that most commonly produce bone destruction within the paranasal sinuses (57,61). They are expanding cystic lesions covered by mucous membrane, which result from the continued accumulation of secretion and desquamation within an obstructed sinus cavity (55–57). Bilateral mucoceles are rare. The degree of inflammatory changes that either initiate or accompany the mucocele determines the amount of chronic inflammatory reaction in the covering wall of the mucous membrane (61). Their secretion is usually clear, thick (mucoid), and tenacious unless the mucocele has been converted to a pyocele by the invasion of bacteria (61). In pyoceles, the cyst contains a thick, viscid green or yellow material. Mucoceles are frequently discussed from the standpoint of sinus of origin. There is a definite predilection for the frontal and ethmoidal sinuses, presumably because of the dependent position of their ostia. Approximately two-thirds of all mucoceles involve the frontal sinuses (Fig. 21); the majority of the remainder involve the ethmoidal labyrinth. Maxillary and sphenoid mucoceles are rare. The sinus of origin, of course, is most important for treatment planning. The persistent expansion of the mucocele causes erosion of surrounding bone, with frequent exit into the adjacent orbit (Fig. 21). If the cyst continues to expand within the orbital cavity, the mass may mimic the behavior of many benign growths. In these circumstances, the tumor is of concern to the ophthalmologist because displacement of the eye may be the initial symptom of an otherwise insidious lesion. Proptosis or displacement of the eye, puffiness of the upper eyelid, a mild ophthalmoplegia, some degree of visual disturbance, and a palpable mass are clinical features encountered with an orbital mucocele. The mucocele usually enters the more anterior portion of the orbital cavity (usually from the frontal and ethmoid sinuses) in the upper nasal quadrant (Fig. 21); this results in a peculiar droopy appearance, and the puffy soft tissue of the upper eyelid and a mass will be

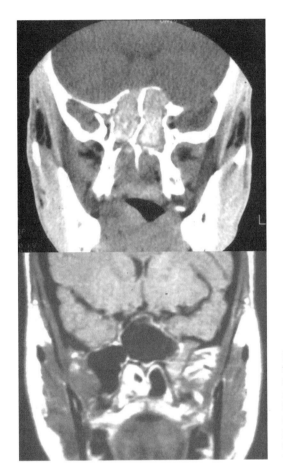

FIGURE 21   Allergic fungal rhinosinusitis (AFRS). Coronal CT scan (*top*), and enhanced coronal T1W MR scan (*bottom*) in another patient with AFRS. Note that the sphenoid sinus on MR appears apparently aerated, while it was completely opacified on CT scan. Note enhancement of peripheral mucosal thickening seen in MR scan.

palpable beneath and slightly behind the superior orbital rim. In a large frontal sinus mucocele, if bone erosion occurs along the orbital roof, it may imitate signs of other tumors of the posterior orbit and sphenoid. The sphenoidal mucocele may cause serious neurologic symptoms by intracranial extension. There may be destruction of the floor of the sella and encroachment of the pituitary gland. An orbital apex syndrome with loss of vision or constriction of the visual field may occur. A mucocele of the maxillary sinus, although infrequent, may result in upward displacement of the orbital contents and exophthalmos caused by elevation of the roof of the antrum.

Imaging Diagnosis of Mucocele
Computed tomography and MRI should be considered the radiologic method of choice for the diagnosis and management of mucocele. The radiographic characteristics of mucoceles have been well described (57,61). A large mucocele produces a classic roentgenographic appearance of an enlarged distorted sinus with a large bony defect representing a breakthrough into the adjacent structures (Fig. 21). Not all mucoceles are so classic, and there are many with subtle bone erosion. Cases

with minimal bone defects pose the greatest difficulty in diagnosis. The gradual pressure atrophy and erosion of the bone by the enlarging soft tissue mass of mucocele produces the expansible appearance on CT scanning (Fig. 21), with no enhancement after contrast infusion (except around the inflamed capsule and peripheral induration), and occasional peripheral calcification. The location, the intraorbital and intracranial extensions, and the surrounding inflammatory changes of a mucocele and the extent of the bone erosion can be best evaluated by combined axial and coronal CT scans. Occasionally, a large frontal sinus inflammatory polyp, if bone erosion occurs along the orbital roof, may imitate the CT scan appearance of a mucocele (Fig. 21) or other tumors of the orbit. Mucoceles are typically seen on MRI as hypointense or less frequently as hyperintense images on TlW and hyperintense on T2W MR scans (Fig. 21). Because of variable protein content within long standing mucoceles, signal intensity can be highly variable on both T1W and T2W MRI sequences. Some mucoceles contain thick inspissated mucus secretions that may be hypointense on T2W MR scans. The increased signal intensity of mucocele on T1W MR images is related to the proteinaceous content of mucosal secretion. Therefore, depending on the protein content, a mucocele may be slightly or markedly hyperintense on T1W MR images. On MRI, chronic fungal rhinosinusitis (both fungal balls and allergic fungal rhinosinusitis) and fungal mucoceles demonstrate a low or intermediate signal on both T1W and T2W MR images (100), with expansion of affected sinuses as well as peripheral rim enhancement on enhanced MR images. MRI may also demonstrate neoplastic or inflammatory disease obstructing the sinus ostium, the cause of mucocele formation. The traditional teaching has emphasized the need for complete removal of the mucocele lining to achieve a cure (101). However, simple drainage and marsupiallization of mucoceles has been performed with good long-term results (101). With the introduction of endoscopic techniques, there has been a trend toward transnasal endoscopic management of sinus mucoceles (101).

Nasal Polyps

Nasal polyps (NPs) are the most common mass lesion in the nose (102). They are benign mucosal protrusions into the nasal cavity of multifactorial origin and characterized by chronic mucosal inflammation (103) (see further discussion of nasal polyp pathogenesis in Chapters 1 and 5.) Chronic sinus inflammation most commonly results from repeated episodes of acute or subacute diseases of the sinonasal cavities. The sinus mucosa reflects these pathologic alterations as a combination of areas of hypertrophic, polypoids, atrophic, and fibrotic changes intermixed with regions of acute or chronic inflammation that are of either an infectious or an allergic origin. Chronic infections and allergies have both been regarded as possible factors involved in the pathogenesis of NPs.

Imaging Study of Polyps

A solitary polyp may not be distinguished from a retention cyst on an unenhanced CT and MRI. Unlike cysts, polyps demonstrate moderate to marked contrast enhancement. When multiple polyps are present, sinus secretions become entrapped within the crevices between the polyps, as well as on the surfaces of the polyps. On CT scans, they show soft tissue attenuation; however, depending on the concentration of the entrapped mucosal secretions, the CT attenuation rises,

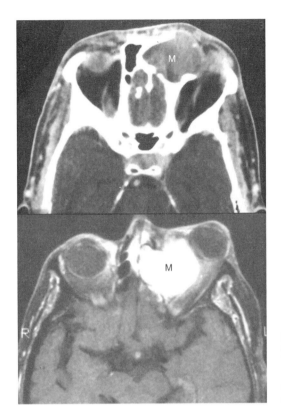

FIGURE 22 Mucocele. Axial-enhanced CT scan (*top*) and axial enhanced T1W MR scan (*bottom*) showing a frontoethmoid mucocele (M). The hyperintensity on MR scan is due to increased protein content of the mucocele.

and the chronic sinonasal polyposis may show mixed CT attenuation with areas of increased density, simulating focal or diffuse dystrophic calcifications (Fig. 22). One important observation on CT or MRI of NPs is the smooth expansion of nasal fossae (Figs. 19 and 22) and pressure atrophy of the adjacent bony wall of the sinonasal cavities. Bone erosion is not common with polyps. However, in aggressive, long-standing polyposis, there may be significant expansion of the sinuses, as well as bone erosion. Polyps tend to have various signal intensities on MR pulse sequences. The MRI characteristics of polyps reflect the various stages of polyps (edematous, glandular, cystic, and fibrous), as well as various stages of desiccation of the entrapped mucosal secretions within the crevices between the polyps and on the surfaces of the polyps. This appearance distinguishes them from tumors that do not have variable signal intensity in each MRI sequence. Polyps may coexist with mucoceles. At times it may be impossible to distinguish between mucoceles and multiple polyps (104).

Retention Cysts and Choanal Polyp

Intramural maxillary sinus cysts, defined by Lindsay as nonsecreting cysts (105) are a common incidental finding in sinus roentgenograms, CT, and MRI of the sinuses. They are estimated to be present in about 10% of the healthy adult populations (106). These cysts result from the obstruction of the ducts of mucosal serous and/or mucinous glands, and the cysts are usually small; rarely, however, they can enlarge sufficiently to fill a sinus cavity. The maxillary sinuses are the largest of the paranasal sinuses, they are the most commonly found to harbor intramural retention cysts. The sphenoid sinuses are the second to harbor retention cysts. These retention cysts are usually asymptomatic, but may become clinically important when they cause obstruction of the maxillary sinus outflow tract, or when they occur in the setting of symptoms compatible with CRS (107). These retention cysts originate from the mucosa of the sinuses due to obstruction of the submucosal gland drainage site. These cysts make up one of the most common incidental findings within the paranasal sinuses on CT or MRI scans (108). The incidence may range from 4.3% to 12.4% (107). The pathogenesis of maxillary retention cysts remains unclear. Some studies propose a postobstructive or allergic cause (109). Other reports (110). have included barotrauma in the formation of these cysts. It is likely that the initial event leading to the formation of a sinus retention cyst is inflammatory process as well as inflammatory obstruction of the OMC. These cysts are seen as a smoothly marginated, convex configuration (dome shaped) of water or soft tissue density on CT scans (109–113). Most commonly they are seen in the floor of the maxillary sinuses. The second most common location is along the floor of the sphenoid sinuses. The MRI appearance of retention cysts reflects an image with long T1 and long T2 characteristics. These are seen as therefore low signal intensity on T1W and high-signal intensity on T2W MR images. Mucous retention types as opposed to serous types may show slightly higher signal intensity on T1W MR images, related to their increased protein content. Retention cysts do not show contrast enhancement on enhanced CT and MR scans.

Choanal Polyp

The choanal polyp develops from an expanding intramural cyst that protrudes through the maxillary antrum ostium and into the nasal cavity (112). The close relationship between choanal polyps and the maxillary sinus was first described by Killian in 1906 (114) when he traced the polyps from the nasopharynx to the region of the ostium of the maxillary sinus, but not into the maxillary sinus cavity. Other authors found choanal polyps to be attached to the lateral wall of the maxillary sinus with a fibrous or polypoid pedicle (115). Mill (116) suggested that the antrochoanal polyps arise from blocked and ruptured mucous glands during the healing process of bacterial rhinosinusitis. Berg et al. (112), using the Preservative technique used in surgical antral exploration, were able to show the intrasinusoidal choanal polyps. An antral part of the polyp was recognized without exception. The polyps continued into the maxillary sinus with a thin walled cyst that, in most cases, completely filled the cavity (Fig. 23). The cyst wall was separated from the regular sinus mucosa. The histopathologic picture of the nasal part of the choanal polyps shows a central cavity surrounded by monomorphic edematous stroma in which only a few cells are seen (112). The external surface is covered by normal respiratory epithelium; the antral part of the choanal polyps demonstrates the same histologic appearances but the cyst wall may be thinner and less organized. Berg et al. (112), were not able to distinguish microscopically any portion of the choanal polyps from the structures observed in the intramural cysts. The cyst fluid aspirated from the choanal polyps revealed a similar distribution and concentration of proteins to that found in intramural cysts (112).

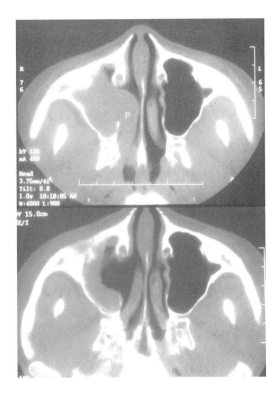

FIGURE 23 Antrochoanal polyp. Axial CT scan (*top*) showing an antrochoanal polyp (P). Axial CT scan (*bottom*) showing postoperative changes following removal of the polyp.

ACKNOWLEDGMENTS

Author is grateful to Mariam Mafee for helpful literature research and artwork and technical support, and Aura Smith for secretarial assistance.

REFERENCES

1. Warwick R, Williams PL, eds. Gray's Anatomy. Philadelphia: Saunders 1973; 300–2.
2. Wenig BM. Atlas of Head and Neck Pathology. Philadelphia, PA: W.B. Saunders, 1993.
3. Graney DO, Rice DH. Paranasal sinuses—anatomy. In: Cummings CW, Fredrickson JM, Harker LA, Krause CJ, Schuller DE, eds. Otolaryngology Head and Neck Surgery. St. Louis, MD: Mosby Year Book, 1993:901–6.
4. Mafee MF. Endoscopic sinus surgery: role of the radiologist. AJNR Am J Neuroradiol 1991; 12:855–60.
5. Mafee MF, Chow JM, Meyers R. Functional endoscopic sinus surgery: Anatomy, CT Screening, indications, and complications. Am J Roentgenol 1993; 160:735–44.
6. Daniels DL, Mafee MF, Smith MM, et al. The frontal sinus drainage pathway and related structures. AJNR Am J Neuroradiol 2003; 24:1618–27.
7. Van Ayela OE. Ethmoid labyrinth: anatomic study with consideration of the clinical significance of its structural characteristics. Arch Otolaryngol 1939; 39:881–902.
8. Rice DH. Endoscopic sinus surgery: anterior approach. Operative Techniques in Otolaryngol Head Neck Surg 1990; 1:99–103.
9. Zinreich SJ, Kenney DW, Rosenbaum AE, Gayer BW, Kumar AJ, Stammberger H. Paranasal sinuses: CT imaging requirements for endoscopic surgery. Radiology 1987; 163:709–75.

10. Kasper KA. Nasofrontal connections: a study based on one hundred consecutive dissections. Arch Otolaryngol 1936; 23:322–43.
11. Zinreich SJ, Abidin M, Kennedy DW. Cross-sectional imaging of the nasal cavity and paranasal sinuses. Operative Techniques in Otolaryngol Head Neck Surg 1990; 1:94–98.
12. Kennedy DW, Zenrich J, Rosenbaum AE, Johns ME. Functional endoscopic sinus surgery: theory and diagnostic evaluation. Arch Otolaryngol 1985; 111:576–82.
13. Bogler WE, Mawn CB. Analysis of the Suprabullar and retrobullar recesses for endoscopic sinus surgery. Ann Otol Rhinol Parymgol Suppl 2002; 186:3–14.
14. Messerklinger W. Endoscopy of the Nose. Baltimore, MD: Urban and Schwarzenberg, 1978.
15. Wignad ME, Steiner W, Jaumann MP. Endonasal sinus surgery with endoscopical control: from radical operation to rehabilitation of the mucosa. Endoscopy 1978; 10:255–60.
16. Hilding AC. The physiology of drainage of nasal mucus. IV. Drainage of the accesory sinuses in man. Otolaryngol Rhinol Laryngol 1944; 53:34–41.
17. Hilding AC. Physiologic basis of nasal operations. Calif Med 1950; 72:103–7.
18. Proctor DF. The nose, paranasal sinuses and pharynx. In: Waters W, ed. Lewis-Walters practice of surgery. Vol. 4. Haerstown, MD: Prior, 1966:1–37.
19. Proctor DF. The mucociliary system. In: Proctor DF, Anderson IHP, eds. The Nose: Upper Airway Physiology and Atmospheric Environment. New York: Elsevier, 1982.
20. Messerklinger W. On the drainage of the normal frontal sinus of man. Acta Otolaryngol 1967; 673:176–81.
21. Messerklinger W. Uber die Drainage der menschlichen Nasennebenhohlen unter normalen and pathologischen Bedingungen. II. Mitteilung: Die Stirnhohle und ihr Ausfuhrungssystem. Monatsschr Ohrenheilkd 1967; 101:313.
22. Chow JM, Mafee MF. Radiologic assessment preoperative to endoscopic sinus surgery. Otolaryngol Clin North Am 1989; 22:691–701.
23. Stammberger HR, Kennedy DW. Paranasal sinuses: anatomic terminology and nomenclature. The Anatomic Terminology Group. Ann Otal Rhinol Laryngol Suppl 1995; 167:7–16.
24. Allmond L, Murr AH. Opacified Onodi cell. Arch Otolaryngol Head Neck Surg 2002; 128:598–599.
25. Mafee MF. Imaging of paranasal sinuses and nasal cavity. In English GM, ed. Diseases of the Nose and Sinuses. Vol. 2. Lippincott-Raven, 1995:1–42.
26. Mafee MF. Imaging methods for sinusitis. JAMA 1993; 269:2808.
27. Mafee, MF, Vavlassori GE, Becker M, eds. Imaging of the Head and Neck. 2nd ed. Stutgart, Germany: Thieme, 2005.
28. Som PM, Curtin HD. Chronic inflammatory sinonasal diseases including fungal infections; the role of imaging. Radiol Clin North Am 1993; 31:33–4.
29. Zinreich SJ, Kennedy DW, Malat J, et al. Fungal sinusitis: diagnosis with CT and MR Imaging. Radiology 1988; 169:439–44.
30. Mafee MF. Endoscopic sinus surgery: role of the radiologist. AJNR Am J Neuroradiol 1991; 12:855–60.
31. Mafee ME. Preoperative imaging anatomy of nasal-ethmoid complex for functional endoscopic sinus surgery. Radiol Clin North Am 1993; 31:1–20.
32. Zinreich SJ, Albayrams S, Benson ML, Oliverio PJ. The ostiomeatal complex and functional endoscopic surgery. In: Som PM, Curtin HD, eds. Head and Neck Imaging. Vol. 1, 3rd ed. St. Louis, MD: Mosby 2003:149–73.
33. Mafee MF. Modern imaging of paranasal sinuses and role of limited sinus CT scanning consideration of time, cost and radiation. J Ear Nose and Throat 1994; 13:532–46.
34. Mafee MF. Imaging of the nasal cavities, paranasal sinuses, nasopharynx, orbits, inframtemporal fossa, pterygomaxillary fissure, parapharyngeal space, and base of skull. In: Ballenger JJ, Show JB, eds. Ballenger's Otorhinolaryngology Head and Neck Surgery. 16th ed. Canada: BC Decker, Inc., 2002.
35. Mafee MF. Nonepithelial tumors of the paranasal sinuses and nasal cavity: role of CT and MR imaging. Radiol Clin North Am 1993; 31:75–90.

36. Mafee MF, Chow JM, Meyers R. Functional endoscopic sinus surgery: anatomy, CT screening, indications, and complications. AJR Am J Roentgenol 1993; 160:735–44.
37. Poznanski AK. Do sinus roentgenograms in children pose a radiation risk? JAMA 1989; 262:3058.
38. Som PM, Brandwein M. Sinonasal cavities: inflammatory disease, tumors, fractures, and postoperative findings. In: Som PM, Curtin HD, eds. Head and Neck Imaging. Vol 1, 3rd. St. Louis, MO: Mosby, 1996:126–85.
39. Rice DH. Basic surgical techniques and variations of endoscopic sinus surgery. Otolaryngol Clin North Am 1989; 22:713–26.
40. Carter BL. Paranasal sinuses, nasal cavity, pterygoid fossa, nasopharynx, and infra-temporal fossa. In: Valvassori GE, Buckingham RA, Carter BL, Hanafee WN, Mafee MF, eds. Head and Neck Imaging. Stuttgart: Thieme, 1988:192–250.
41. Zinreich SJ, Kennedy DW, Rosenbaum AE, et al. Paranasal sinuses: CT imaging requirements for endoscopic survey. Radiology 1987; 31:709–75.
42. Kennedy DW, Zinrich J, Rosenbaum AE, et al. Functional endoscopic sinus surgery: theory and diagnostic evaluation. Arch Otolaryngol 1985; 111:576–82.
43. Mafee MF, Kumar A, Tahmoressi CN, et al. Direct sagittal CT in the evaluation of temporal bone disease. AJNR Am J Neuroradiol 1988; 9:371–8.
44. Ball JB JR, Towbin RB, Staton RE, Cowdrey K. Direct sagittal computed tomography of the head. Radiology 1985; 155:822.
45. Friedmann M, Mafee M, Ray C, et al. Three-dimensional imaging for evaluation of head and neck tumors. Arch Gynecol Head Neck Surg 1993; 119:601–7.
46. Ray CE, Mafee MF, Friedmann M, Tahmoressi CN. Applications of three-dimensional CT imaging in head and neck pathology. Radiol Clin North Am 1993; 31:181–94.
47. Lund VJ, Mackay IS. Staging in rhinosinusitis. Rhinology 31:183–4.
48. Subramanian HN, Schechtman KB, Hamilos DL. A retrospective analysis of treatment outcomes and time to relapse after intensive medical treatment for chronic sinusitis. Am J Rhinol 2002 Nov-Dec; 16(6):303–313.
49. Kennedy DW, Kuhn FA, Hamilos DL, et al. Treatment of chronic rhinosinusitis with high-dose oral terbinafine: a double blind, placebo-controlled study. Laryngoscope 2005 Oct; 115(10):1793-9.
50. Nussenbaum B, Marple BF, Schwade ND. Characteristics of bony erosion in allergic fungal rhinosinusitis. Otolaryngol Head Neck Surg 2001; 124:150–4.
51. Mukherji SK, Figueroa RE, Ginsberg LE, et al. Allergic fungal sinusitis: CT findings. Radiology 1998; 207:417–22.
52. Zinreich SJ, Tebos, Long DL, et al. Frameless stereotaxic integration of CT imaging data accuracy and initial applications. Radiology 1993; 188:735–42.
53. Fried MP, Kleefield J, Gopal H, et al. Image-guided endoscopic surgery: results of accuracy and performance in a multicenter clinical study using an electromagnetic tracking system. Laryngoscope 1997; 107:594–601.
54. Metson R, Coseza M, Gliklich RE, Montgomery WW. The role of image-guidance systems for head and neck surgery. Arch Otolaryngol Head Neck Surg 1999; 125:1100–4.
55. Salmon SD, Graeme-Cook F. Case records of the Massachusetts General Hospital. N Engl J Med 1990; 322:116–23.
56. Eustis HS, Mafee MF, Walton C, Mondonca J. MR Imaging and CT of orbital infections and complications in acute rhinosinusitis. Radiol Clin N Am 1998; 36:1165–83.
57. Mafee MF. Eye and Orbit. In: Som PM, Curtin HD, eds. Head and Neck Imaging. St. Louis, MO: Mosby, 1996:1009–1128.
58. Hutchin ME, Shores CG, Bauer MS, Yarbrough WG. Sinogenic subdural empyema and *Streptococcus anginosus*. Arch Otolaryngol Head Neck Surg 1999; 125:1262–6.
59. Jones NS, Walker JL, Bassi S, et al. The intracranial complications of rhinosinusitis: can they be prevented? Laryngoscope 2002; 112:59–63.
60. Younis RT, Anand VK, Davidson B. The role of computed tomography and magnetic resonance imaging in patients with sinusitis with complications. Laryngoscope 2002; 112:224–9.

61. Mafee MF. Orbital and intraocular lesions. In Edelman RR, Hesselink JR, Zlatkin MG, eds. Clinical Magnetic Resonance Imaging. Philadelphia, PA: WB Saunders, 1995: 985–1020.
62. Green WH, Goldberg HI, Wohl GT. Mucormycosis infection of the craniofacial structures. AJR Am J Roentgenol 1967; 101:802–6.
63. Talmi YP, Reouven AG, Bakon M, et al. Rhino-orbital and rhino-oribito-cerebral mucormycosis. Otolaryngol Head Neck Surg 2002; 127:22–31.
64. Zinreich SJ, Kennedy DW, Malat J, et al. Fungal sinusitis: diagnosis with CT and MR imaging. Radiology 1988; 169:439–44.
65. Pillsbury HC, Fischer ND. Rhinocerebral mucormycosis. Arch Otolaryngol 1977; 103:600–4.
66. Young RC, Bennett JE, Vogel CL, et al. Aspergillosis: the spectrum of disease in 98 patients. Medicine 1970; 49:147–73.
67. Meikle D, Yarington CT Jr, Winterbauer RH. Aspergillosis of the maxillary sinuses in other healthy patients. Laryngoscope 1985; 95:776–9.
68. McGill TJ, Simpson G, Nealy GB. Fulminant aspergillosis of nose and paranasal sinuses: a new clinical entity. Laryngoscope 1980; 90:748–54.
69. Beck-Mannagetta J, Necek K, Grasserbauer M. Solitary aspergillosis of maxillary sinus: a complication of dental treatment. Lancet 1983; 2:1260.
70. Terry D. Blastomycosis of the paranasal sinuses. Presented at the American Rhinologic Society, April 17–18, 1993, Los Angeles, CA.
71. Stammberger H. Endoscopic surgery for mycotic and chronic recurrent sinusitis. 11. Ann Otorhinolaryngol 1985; (Suppl.)119:3–10.
72. Kopp W, Fotter R, Steiner H, et al. Aspergillosis of the paranasal sinuses. Radiology 1985; 156:715–6.
73. Ayala C, Watkins L, Deschler DG. Tension orbital pneumocele secondary to nasal obstruction from cocaine abuse: a case report. Otolaryngol Head Neck 2002; 127:572–4.
74. Kim SA, Mathog RH. Radiology quiz case 2; Silent Sinus Syndrome: maxillary sinus atelectasis with enophthalmos. Arch Otolaryngol Head Neck Surg 2002; 128:81–3.
75. Boyd JH, Yaffee K, Holds J. Maxillary sinus atelectasis with enophthalmos. Ann Otal Rhinol Laryngol 1998; 107:34–9.
76. Gillman GS, Schaitkin BM, May M. Asymptomatic enophthalmos: the Silent Sinus Syndrome. Am J Rhinol 1999; 13:459–62.
77. Hadi U, Ghossaini S, Zaytoun G. Rhinolithiasis: A forgotten entity. Otolaryngology Head Neck Surg 2002; 126:48–51.
78. Borges A, Fink J, Villablanca P, et al. Midline destructive lesions of the sinonasal tract: Simplified terminology based on histopathologic criteria. AJNR Am J Neuroradiol 2000; 21:331–6.
79. Coup AJ, Hooper IP. Granulomatous lesions in nasal biopsies. Histopathology 1980; 4:293–308.
80. Krishna I, Balakrishnan K, Kumar N. Quiz Case 4; Nasal granuloma gravidum. Arch Otolaryngol Head Neck Surg 2000; 126:1156–60.
81. Neville E, Mills RG, James DG. Sarcoidosis of the upper respiratory tract and its relation to lupus pernio. Ann N Y Acad Sci 1976; 278:416–26.
82. McCaffrey TV, McDonald TJ. Sarcoidosis of the nose and paranasal sinuses. Laryngoscope 1983; 93:1281–94.
83. Thompson LDR. Rhinoscleroma. Ear Nose Throat J 2002; 81:506
84. Loh KS, Chong SM, Pang YT, Soh K. Rhinosporidiasis: differential diagnosis of a large nasal mass. Otolaryngol Head Neck Surg 2001; 124:121–2.
85. Lindsay JR, Perlman HB. Sarcoidosis of the upper respiratory tract. Ann Otol Rhinol Laryngol 1951; 60:549–66.
86. McDonald TJ, DeRemee RA, Kern FB, Harrison EG Jr. Nasal manifestations of Wegener's granulatosis. Laryngoscope 1974; 84:2102–12.
87. Hoffman GS, Kerr GS, Leavitt RY, et al. Wegener's granulomatosis: An analysis of 158 patients. Ann Intern Med 1992; 116:458–98.

88. Davies DJ, Moran JE, Neall JF, Ryan GB. Segmental necrotizing glomerulonephritis with antineutrophil antibody: possible arbovirus aetiology? BMJ 1982; 285:606.
89. Jennette JC, Charles LA, Falk RJ. Antineutrophil cytoplasmic autoantibodies: disease associations, molecular biology, and pathophysiology. Int Rev Exp Pathol 1991; 32:193–221.
90. Fanburg BL, Niles JL, Mark BJ. Case records of the Massachusetts General Hospital. N Engl J Med 1993; 329:2019–26.
91. van der Woude FJ, Rasmussen N, Lobatto S, et al. Autoantibodies against neutrophils and monocytes: tool for diagnosis and marker of disease activity in Wegener's granulomatosis. Lancet 1985; 1:425–9.
92. Jayne DRW, Marshall PD, Jones SJ, Lockwood CM. Autoantibodies to GBM and neutrophil cytoplasm in rapidly progressive glomerulonephritis. Kidney Int 1990; 37:965–70.
93. Weinberger LM, Cohen ML, Remler BF, Naheedy MH, Leigh RJ. Intracranial Wegener's granulomatosis. Neurology 1993; 43:1831–4.
94. Marsot-Dupuch K, Clement DeGivry S, Quayoun M. Wegener granulomatosis involving the pterygopalatine fossa: an unusual case of trigeminal neuropathy. AJNR Am J Neuroradiol 2002; 23:312–5.
95. McDonald TJ, Deremee RA, Harrison EG Jr, Facer GW, Devine KD. The protean clinical features of polymorphic reticulosis (lethal midline granulomatosis). Laryngoscope 1976; 86:936–45.
96. Weymuller EA, Rice DH. Surgical management of infections and inflammatory diseases. In: Cummings CW, Fredrickson JM, Harker LA, Krause EJ, Schuller DE, eds. Otolaryngology Head and Neck Surgery. Chapter 54, Vol 1. Mosby Year Book 1993:955–64.
97. Churg J, Strauss L. Allergic granulomatosis, allergic angiitis, and periarteritis nodosa. Am J Pathol 1951; 27:277–301.
98. Keefe MA, Bloom DC, Keefe KS, Killian PJ. Orbital paraffinoma as a complication of endoscopic sinus surgery. Otolaryngol Head Neck Surg 2002; 127:575–7.
99. Aferzon M, Millman B, O'Donell T, Gilroy PA. Cholesterol granuloma of the frontal bone. Otolaryngol Head Neck Surg 2002; 127:578–81.
100. Lee JT, Bhuta S, Lufkin R, Calcaterra TC. Fungal mucoceles of the sphenoid sinus. Laryngoscope 2002; 112:779–83.
101. Har-EL G. Endoscopic management of 108 sinus mucoceles. Laryngoscope 2001; 111:2131–4.
102. Ming CM, Hong CY, Shun CT, et al. Inducible cyclooxygenase and interleukin 6 gene expressions in nasal polyp fibroblasts. Arch Otolaryngol Head Neck Surg 2002; 128:945–51.
103. Hirschberg A, Darvas AJZ, Almay K, et al. The pathogenesis of nasal polyposis by immunoglobulin E and interleukin–5 is completed by transforming growth factor b1. Laryngoscope 2003; 113:120–4.
104. Som PM, Dillon WP, Sze G, et al. Benign and malignant sinonasal lesions with intracranial extension: their MR differentiation. Radiology 1989; 172:763–6.
105. Lindsay JR. Nonsecreting cysts of the maxillary sinus mucosa. Laryngoscope 1942; 52:84–100.
106. Hanna HH. Asymptomatic sinus disease in air-crew members. Clin Aviation Aerospace Med 1974; 45:77–81.
107. Bhattacharyya N. Do maxillary sinus retention cysts reflect obstructive sinus phenomena? Arch Otolaryngol Head Neck Surg 2002; 126:1369–71.
108. Cooke LD, Hadley DM. MRI of the paranasal sinuses: incidental abnormalities and their relationship to symptoms. J Laryngol Otol 1991; 105:278–81.
109. Berg O, Carenfelt C, Sobin A. On the diagnosis and pathogenesis of intramural maxillary cysts. Acta Otolaryngol 1989; 108:464–8.
110. Garges LM. Maxillary sinus barotrauma. Aviat Space Environ Med 1985; 56:796–802.
111. Fisher EW, Whittet HB, Croft CB. Symptomatic mucosal cysts of the maxillary sinus: antroscopic treatment. J Laryngol Otol 1989; 103:1184–6.

112. Berg O, Carenfelt C, Silfversward C, Sobin A. Origin of the choanal polyp. Arch Otolaryngol Head Neck Surg 1988; 114:1270–1.
113. Mafee MF. Imaging of the head and neck: computed tomography, magnetic resonance. In: Ballenger JJ, Snow JB, eds. Otorhinolaryngology Head and Neck Surgery. 15th ed., Baltimore, MD: Williams and Wilkins, 1996:699–797.
114. Killian G. The origin of choanal polypi. Lancet 1906; 2:81–2.
115. Van Alyea OE. Management of non-malignant growths in the maxillary sinus. Ann Otolaryngol 1951; 65:714–22.
116. Mills CE. Secretory cysts of the maxillary antrum and their relation to the development of antrochoanal polyp. J Laryngol Otol 1959; 73:324–34.
117. Bienfang DC, Karluk D. Mucormycosis, rhino-orbital. Case records of the Massachusetts General Hospital. N Engl J Med 2002; 346:924–9.
118. Mafee MF, Tran BH, Chapa AR. Imaging of Rhinosinusitis and its complications in plain film, CT, and MRI. Clinical Reviews in Allergy and Immunology 2006; 38: 165–185.

13 The Role of Nasal Endoscopy in the Diagnosis and Medical Management of Chronic Rhinosinusitis

Christopher T. Melroy
Georgia Nasal and Sinus Center, Savannah, Georgia, U.S.A.

Marc G. Dubin
Department of Otolaryngology–Head and Neck Surgery, Johns Hopkins University School of Medicine, Greater Baltimore Medical Center, Baltimore, Maryland, U.S.A.

Brent A. Senior
Department of Otolaryngology–Head and Neck Surgery, University of North Carolina Hospitals, Chapel Hill, North Carolina, U.S.A.

INTRODUCTION

Rhinosinusitis is characterized by inflammatory changes to the mucous membranes, the bone, or the fluid contents of the paranasal sinuses. Although the definition, diagnosis, and management of chronic rhinosinusitis (CRS) has been under debate and scrutiny over the past several years, there is a central, innate fact regarding this disease that is unequivocal: adequate visualization of the nasal cavity and paranasal sinuses is, at best, difficult for the majority of physicians who treat this disease. A more complete assessment and understanding of the area of pathology—the mucosalized surfaces of the nasal cavity and paranasal sinuses—through nasal endoscopy provides the examiner with information that is essential to the diagnosis and management of CRS.

HISTORY OF NASAL ENDOSCOPY

Historically, the anatomy of the nasal cavity and paranasal sinuses has intrigued mankind, and a rudimentary knowledge of the anatomy dates back to Egyptian tomb inscriptions (prior to 1500 B.C.) (1). Improved access to the nasal cavity and other orifices of the body was obtained with the development of the speculum by the Romans, dating to the 1st Century A.D. Since this time of speculae and mirror illumination, no meaningful advances occurred in the visualization of the body's cavities until the time of Philipp Bozzini (1773–1809) who developed the first rigid endoscope (2). Although he practiced as an urologist, he developed a system for rigid endoscopy that was suitable for use in many areas of the body, including the nasal cavity (3).

From this point, the candle illumination provided by Bozzini's system was enhanced as another urologist, Maximillian Nitze (with engineer Joseph Leiter), developed an endoscope in 1887 using a glowing platinum wire for illumination. Nitze also developed an optical system into the body of his endoscope that involved a series of glass lenses separated by air spacers. The next major advance was the development of the Hopkins rod lens system, developed by Harold Hopkins in 1960, which modified Baird's design of sending light and images down a flexible glass cable. His rod incorporated glass fibers for the transmission of light as well as a series of air lenses separated by glass spacers, and, by doing so, improved optical efficiency nine fold (4). This novel technology was fostered and manufactured by Karl Storz, who coupled Hopkins' endoscope with cold light illumination. Today, Hopkins rods are the standard for rigid nasal endoscopy, and their coupling with a distal xenon light source provide excellent illumination without the morbidity of "hot light" from the scope's tip.

Pioneering work in the realm of nasal endoscopy began in the mid- to late 1970s via the work of Brister, Messerklinger, Draf, and Terrier. The tenets of increased accessibility, less discomfort, and simplified documentation resounded as rigid and flexible nasal endoscopy became more widespread in the 1980s (5). However, it was the introduction of endoscopic diagnosis and surgery of the paranasal sinuses by otorhinolaryngologists in Europe in the mid-1980s that made this phenomenon pervasive and allowed the anatomy and physiology of the sinonasal cavity to be better understood (6,7). Stammberger's introduction of this technique sparked interest in the anatomy and physiology of the sinonasal cavity that had been somewhat quiescent since the time of Emil Zuckerkandl in the late 19th century, whose scientific approach to sinus anatomy and function is still deemed "state of the art" and "enabled the foundation of modern sinus surgery with his first book in 1882," according to Stammberger (8).

MODERN NASAL ENDOSCOPY

Modern endoscopy entails the use of a light source with cable, a camera, and, most importantly, an endoscope. Storz revolutionized the endoscope by combining Hopkins's optical system with a means to deliver "cold" light. This was done by using flexible glass cables inside the scope that transmitted light with minimal loss via a phenomenon known as total internal reflection. Until this time, illumination for endoscopy had been unchanged since Nitze incorporated a distal light bulb decades earlier. This method was fraught with complications due to the excessive heat created by the bulb, as over 90% of all electrical energy put into the light source was dissipated as heat at the distal end of the scope. Hopkins and Storz increased illumination and decreased morbidity with "cold" light, taking advantage of a scope transmitting only light with a high efficiency that is emitted from a distal light source.

The light carried in the fiberoptic glass cables of the endoscope is generated by a light source and is carried to the scope via a cable. Today, xenon light sources are state of the art as they provide a wide spectrum of light wavelengths that approximates that of the sun. This was an improvement over halogen, whose narrower spectral characteristics provided less illumination and more distortion of color. The color temperature of xenon light is approximately 6000 K, which is similar to the temperature on the surface of the sun and helps explain why its color is so true. The marriage of a strong and bright external light source to the cold and efficiently transmitting glass fibers inside the modern endoscope allows unparalleled illumination.

The modern rigid endoscope is very similar to that developed by Hopkins and Storz. Although they are available in diameters as small as 0.5 mm, the majority of sinonasal endoscopes are either 4.0 or 2.7 mm ("pediatric") endoscopes. The standard 4.0 mm scope is most useful in clinical practice, as each 10% increase in diameter results in a 46% increase in illumination. A variety of different angled telescopes are available that allow illumination and visualization of a field at a fixed angle from the axis of the endoscope. Although the endoscope itself is straight, an angle-of-view prism is incorporated into the distal tip of the scope allowing visualization and illumination at a defined angle from the working axis of the endoscope. In a clinical setting, nasal endoscopy is generally carried out with 0°, 30°, 45°, and 70° endoscopes and allows visualization of structures that may not be in the line of site of the scope.

Flexible scopes have become the workhorse of otolaryngic endoscopy primarily due to their versatility. In a clinical setting, these endoscopes can be used in the pharynx and larynx as well as in the nasal cavity. However, they do have shortcomings. Due to their flaccid nature, single-handed maneuvering can be challenging and may pose a problem when a hand is needed for instrumentation. In addition, the optical quality of flexible endoscopy is inferior to that provided by a Hopkins rod, as the flexible scopes rely on transmission of the image back to the observer via fiberoptics (Fig. 1). Technological advances are improving flexible endoscopy as "chip tip" scopes are now available that incorporate a charge-coupled device chip at the distal end of the scope. This captures the image at the

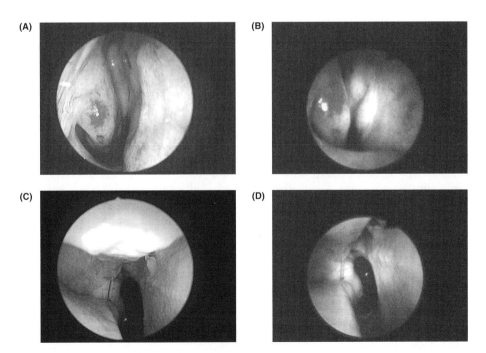

FIGURE 1 (*See color insert.*) The anterior and posterior right nasal cavity is examined in the same patient with the same sized rigid (**A, C**) and flexible (**B, D**) endoscopes. Rigid scopes carry more light to the object and have superior optics resulting in a better image quality. Flexible scopes rely on bundles of optical fibers to transmit the image back to the examiner, thereby decreasing the optical quality and giving a more pixilated or grainy image.

distal end of the scope and relays the information digitally to the observer rather than depending upon transmission of the image via bundles of fiberoptic cables.

NASAL ENDOSCOPY IN THE DIAGNOSIS OF CRS

The ability to survey the sinonasal cavity using nasal endoscopy and interpret the findings is a precious tool that gives objective findings to the diagnostician. The ability to do this is a skill or a learned craft that has classically belonged to those in the field of Otorhinolaryngology. However, it has been documented that primary care physician visits account for 87% of all patient visits for rhinosinusitis (9); in general, these physicians diagnose and treat CRS without the use of this valuable tool. In 1997, the Task Force on Rhinosinusitis (sponsored by the American Academy of Otolaryngology-Head and Neck Surgery) took this and other factors into account as they established a definition for rhinosinusitis that made it possible for all physicians to make an appropriate diagnosis. To this end, the Task Force on Rhinosinusitis defined CRS using a set of patient-reported symptoms—enabling the diagnosis to be made from a patient's subjective history alone (Table 1). Although head and neck physical examination elements (as well as nasal endoscopy) could further support the diagnosis, the presence or absence of these did not affect the final diagnosis.

The 1997 definition of CRS also allowed standardized reporting and served as a basis upon which to further define the disease. The omission of objective parameters, such as nasal endoscopy and imaging, was addressed as the Task Force stated they were not required for diagnosis but did provide helpful information, especially in recalcitrant cases. The natural progression of academic medicine sought to identify and analyze objective disease in this patient population that met the diagnosis of CRS. This was done through the investigation of nasal endoscopy and imaging in patients with documented CRS.

Casiano studied preoperative patients with the purpose of evaluating the ability of nasal endoscopy to predict computed tomography (CT) evidence of disease. These patients, for the most part, had been maximally treated medically and had preoperative CT performed as well as nasal endoscopy. He concluded that endoscopic examination could be correlated with predictable radiographic findings as endoscopy had a sensitivity of 74% and a specificity of 84%. When the sensitivity of endoscopy was further analyzed, it was seen that this was somewhat lower than expected due to a high number of "false negatives"—that is, patients

TABLE 1 Symptomatic Diagnosis of CRS (1997 Task Force on Rhinosinusitis)

Major criteria	Minor criteria
Facial pain of pressure	Headache
Purulent anterior or posterior nasal drip	Fever
Hyposmia or anosmia	Halitosis
Nasal obstruction	Fatigue
Facial congestion or fullness	Dental pain
	Ear pain, pressure, or fullness
	Cough

In 1997, the Task Force on Rhinosinusitis defined chronic sinusitis as the presence of two or more major criteria or one major and two minor criteria for at least 12 weeks.
Source: Adapted from Ref. 9.

with normal endoscopy for a certain area but radiographic evidence of disease. Of these "false negatives," 98% had only minimal mucosal thickening on CT (10).

Stankiewicz and Chow also investigated the role of nasal endoscopy in patients meeting the Rhinosinusitis Task Force definition of CRS (11). In contrast to Casiano's study, this population consisted of patients on their initial referral to an otolaryngologist who met the symptomatic criteria outlined in 1997. These patients were objectively evaluated by sinonasal endoscopy and CT on the same day as diagnosis in an attempt to compare endoscopy to CT findings and symptomologic diagnosis. Of the 78 people who met the subjective criteria, only 43 (55%) of them had objective (endoscopic or CT) evidence of disease. Of these 43 patients, 17 (22%) had both endoscopic evidence and CT evidence, six (8%) had endoscopic evidence alone, and 20 (26%) had CT evidence alone.

Stankiewicz and Chow also correlated endoscopic findings and CT findings. They concluded that the sensitivity of nasal endoscopy in the diagnosis of CRS was low at 46%, which was felt to be due in part to the fact that the "true positives" used in their calculations may not have had the disease at all. Although the sensitivity found in this study may not be currently applicable (due to different diagnostic criteria for CRS), the data from their positive and negative predictive values are relevant. They found that if nasal endoscopy was normal, 78% of these patients had no or very minimal CT abnormalities. Conversely, if there was pathology seen on endoscopy, 74% had positive CT scans.

These two studies provided important data on nasal endoscopy as they correlated endoscopic information with other objective data (CT) and analyzed them in well-defined populations with CRS. Not only did this add to the validity of nasal endoscopy, but it also added to a growing body of support that exposed weaknesses in the subjective diagnosis of CRS. Other information supporting these shortcomings of symptomatic diagnosis came from investigations of radiographic imaging and microbiology in patients who met the 1997 subjective criteria for CRS. All these led to a definition revision in 2003 that required objective findings for the diagnosis.

In 2003, the CRS Task Force supported by the Sinus and Allergy Health Partnership (SAHP) amended the 1997 criteria, and these definitions were endorsed by the American Academy of Otolaryngology-Head and Neck Surgery, the American Rhinologic Society, and the American Academy of Otolaryngic Allergy. In addition to the prerequisite of 12 weeks of symptoms of CRS (Table 1), physical examination findings consistent with sinonasal inflammation are required to make a clinical diagnosis. Again, taking into account that 87% of rhinosinusitis visits are to primary care physicians, this had to be carefully defined and delineated as to enable any physician to potentially make a diagnosis. Therefore, many of the objective criteria needed to establish the presence of rhinosinusitis can be established using anterior rhinoscopy (Fig. 2), which is recommended to be performed in the decongested state. These objective criteria are detailed in Table 2.

Nasal endoscopy by a trained professional allows a detailed evaluation of the sinonasal cavity in a patient with CRS, with special attention to the middle meatus and sphenoethmoidal recess. By allowing the anterior rhinoscopic examination to suffice for the clinical diagnosis of CRS, the SAHP empowered patient-care providers to obtain objective evidence without necessarily precisely visualizing the drainage tracts of the paranasal sinuses. In their report, the SAHP detail both "clinical" and "research" criteria required for diagnosis, with research criteria

(A)   (B)

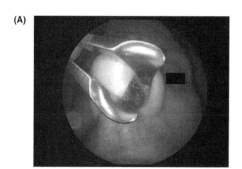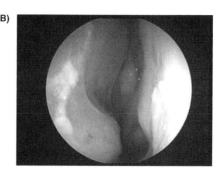

FIGURE 2 (*See color insert.*) Anterior rhinoscopy should be performed in the native and decongested state. Excellent illumination is provided directly by a headlight or indirectly by a head mirror. A nasal speculum (**A**) increases visualization and allows for visualization of the anterior nasal cavity (**B**). Although polyps and purulence of the middle meatus may be visualized, anterior rhinoscopy is more adept in evaluating the nasal septum and inferior turbinate pathology, as is the case in this patient with a large septal spur running near the floor of the left nasal cavity.

requiring nasal endoscopy and/or CT evidence of disease. Two separate groups of criteria were delineated in order to reduce the number of false positives that may be incurred with the use of anterior rhinoscopy alone; this infers the notion that nasal endoscopy is superior to anterior rhinoscopy in the accurate diagnosis of CRS (Fig. 3).

By creating "research criteria" for CRS that require endoscopy and/or CT evidence of sinonasal inflammation, the SAHP Task Force allowed more specific data to be collected and compared regarding many aspects of CRS. This allowed a more uniform reporting of disease and a more specific definition that would ultimately facilitate comparisons of findings from different investigators in a more precise and reproducible manner. Although this may seem basic, it is pervasive as it strictly delineates populations that meet even stricter criteria for CRS and allows similar populations to be studied and compared among observers. By establishing a firmer diagnosis in the clinical realm, patient care will be impacted as well.

TABLE 2   Objective Requirements for the Diagnosis of CRS (SAHP, 2003)

Physical examination evidence
  Anterior rhinoscopy findings
    Discolored nasal drainage
    Nasal polyps
  Polypoid edema
  Nasal endoscopy findings
    Any of the above
    Edema, erythema, or granulation tissue involving the middle meatus or ethmoid bulla
Radiographic evidence
  Computed tomography
    Mucosal thickening, air-fluid level, or bone changes
Plain sinus radiograph
  Water's view with > 5 mm mucosal thickening or air-fluid level

The Sinus and Health Allergy Partnership (SAHP) revised the diagnostic criteria for CRS by stating that objective evidence for disease must be present in addition to 12 or more weeks of symptoms.

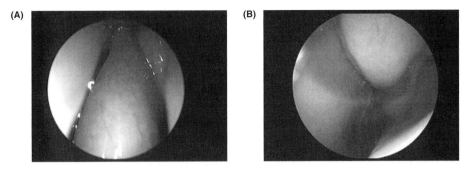

FIGURE 3 Nasal endoscopy improves visualization of those structures seen by anterior rhino-scopy. The polyp present in the anterior-lateral left middle meatus in (**A**) was not visible on anterior rhinoscopy. Unlike rhinoscopy, endoscopy is also able to assess the posterior nasal cavity and detect pathology in that area. (**B**) The figure reveals purulent drainage in the posterior middle meatus in this same patient whose osteomeatal complex was obstructed by a small polyp.

Ironically, setting rigid diagnostic criteria will also serve to analyze these means by which the disease is defined. The understanding of the role of nasal endoscopy diagnosis will benefit from this standardization as like groups are more reliably compared. For instance, there are several studies that objectively evaluate the use of nasal endoscopy in the diagnosis of CRS besides those of Casiano and Stankiewicz and Chow that are referenced here; however, their methods and inclusion criteria vary thereby making it difficult to compare the studies to each other (12). This is by no means a reflection on the work of these investigators, but more so a consequence of the prior Rhinosinusitis Task Force diagnostic criteria that led to the selection of a patient population that was very difficult to study objectively and compare between investigators.

NASAL ENDOSCOPY AND THE MANAGEMENT OF PATIENTS WITH CRS

Once the diagnostic dilemmas are elucidated, there are many uses of nasal endo-scopy in the management of those diagnosed with CRS. Evaluation of therapeutic interventions, access for therapy, and evaluation of the postoperative patient are all areas where nasal endoscopy is of benefit.

Evaluation of Treatment Effects

In the clinic, the endoscope can serve as a tool to the surgeon to help identify anatomic entities that predispose to CRS. Pinpointing anatomic anomalies in the clinic is crucial to success in the operating room. Endoscopy allows visualization of these structures in a three-dimensional manner and helps one understand the natural physiology of the patient. As discussed by Stammberger, proficient nasal endoscopy requires a thorough knowledge of the anatomy and physiology of the sinuses; we feel a corollary of this also holds true, namely that proficient nasal endoscopy also leads to a deeper understanding of the anatomy and physiology of the paranasal sinuses. Through these means, endoscopy can help identify structures that may be amenable to surgical repair, especially if medical manage-ment fails. Two-dimensional images from radiographic studies are brought to life with a full understanding of the true structure of the paranasal sinuses by relating these findings to endoscopy.

When a patient is being treated medically, it is important to follow the progression of disease or response to therapy. In the clinical setting, nasal endoscopy is unparalleled in its ability to follow the mucosal response to therapy in CRS. Nasal endoscopy offers a quick and cost-effective evaluation of the sinonasal cavity, and careful documentation or photo–documentation allows the observer to compare a patient's response over a prolonged period of time. Due to the high correlation of endoscopic and CT findings (10) objective evaluation involving nasal endoscopy during the medical management of CRS is recommended and does not incur the expense, morbidity, and inconvenience of serial CT scans.

Access to the Sinonasal Cavity for Diagnostic Purposes

Endoscopy allows access to the sinonasal cavity that facilitates both medical and surgical treatment for CRS. First and foremost, endoscopy allows access to the site of infection and inflammation and allows directed cultures to be performed. Collection of purulent sinonasal secretions with a suction trap or a culture swab under endoscopic visualization allows culture and identification of the offending microorganism. Sensitivities of the pathogen to antibiotics are generally performed as well and allow for the administration of culture-directed antibiotics. This allows for much more precise antimicrobial therapy and protects against the development of antimicrobial resistance systemically as well as in the sinonasal cavity. It also quantifies microbial levels and allows these results from bacterial plating to help guide management.

The historic gold standard for maxillary sinus culture is the maxillary sinus puncture via the inferior meatus or canine fossa approach. This invasive method allows the transmucosal collection of sinus contents through direct aspiration or irrigation. It is relatively morbid compared to endoscopic swab, painful for the patient, and difficult to perform in the outpatient setting. The use of endoscopically obtained middle meatus cultures as a noninvasive method to determine the bacteriology of maxillary sinusitis has been recently reviewed by our group. A meta-analysis of the modern data reveals the concordance rate between endoscopically obtained middle meatal swab and maxillary puncture to be 82%. In maxillary sinusitis, it is felt that this high concordance rate makes the use of endoscopic swab the procedure of choice. In addition, since other paranasal sinuses are generally not amenable to transmucosal puncture, this study suggests that endoscopically obtained cultures from purulent nasal secretions near sinus ostia are highly suggestive of the microbiology of that sinus (13).

Nasal endoscopy can also be used in the evaluation of bacterial rhinosinusitis in the intensive care unit (ICU) patient, but the concordance of culture results between these and maxillary antral puncture is somewhat lower in this patient population. Due to the instrumentation of the nasal and oral cavities in this patient population, radiographic findings consistent with rhinosinusitis are frequently found upon CT scanning. In this setting, it has been shown that endoscopic evidence of middle meatal purulence is actually a better predictor than CT (78% vs. 47%) for the diagnosis of antral tap-proven bacterial sinusitis (14). Therefore, this method is much more effective in the screening of ICU patients than CT, a very commonly used technique.

There are many studies documenting the microbiology of rhinosinusitis, but the question is how these culture results change patient management. Antibiotic resistance in CRS is a problem at the patient level as well as the population level. The first line of management by the primary care physician is generally an empiric, broad-spectrum antibiotic. Repeated administration of broad-spectrum empiric therapy, especially in the setting of resistant organisms, is both futile and irresponsible. In a review of the medical management of postoperative patients, we found that the use of endoscopic culture results changes the antibiotic therapy chosen in approximately one-third of patients.

In addition to detecting and analyzing microbial pathogens, direct access offered by nasal endoscopy allows documentation and quantification of inflammatory mediators. The presence of Charcot-Leyden crystals, fungal hyphae, or allergic mucin provides the endoscopist with the ability to diagnose allergic fungal rhinosinusitis in a patient with CRS (15). Without the access provided by endoscopy, identification and treatment of this and other comorbid factors would be very difficult. Similarly, the delineation of nasal polyposis via endoscopy allows the examiner to assess its impact on the natural drainage pathways of the paranasal sinuses. For instance, polyposis on the medial aspect of the middle turbinate has a functional impact distinct from those present in the middle meatus. Endoscopy can differentiate this as well as assess the response of these polyps to topical and systemic therapy.

Endoscopy can also be used to evaluate mucociliary flow and the dynamic changes of the sinonasal cavity. This is of particular importance in patients with accessory maxillary sinus ostia as well as those who have undergone a prior maxillary antrostomy that did not communicate with the natural ostium. These posterior fontanel ostia are known for their ability to recirculate mucus in and out of the maxillary sinus and cause dysfunction leading to chronic infection. Endoscopically, this is best visualized with a 30° or 45° endoscope with particular attention to the lateral nasal wall. In doing so, the transport of mucopus can be seen to emanate out of the posterior fontanel antrostomy and travel anteriorly along the lateral nasal wall only to re-enter the maxillary sinus through its natural ostium. This dynamic phenomenon is typically not appreciated by even the highest quality CT.

Nasal endoscopy can be used to sample other tissue in addition to purulent secretions. For instance, biopsy of the nasal respiratory mucosa is required for the evaluation of ciliary dysmotility, the presence of which can predispose patients to recurrent infections. Sinonasal tumors may also be misdiagnosed as CRS or may present alongside CRS. Evaluation and biopsy of suspicious soft tissue within the sinonasal cavity may lead to the diagnosis of malignancy or benign entities such as inverting papilloma.

Evaluation of the Operative and Postoperative Patient

Although the correlation between radiographic and endoscopic findings is always important for a full comprehension of anatomy and pathophysiology, it is even more important in operative patients. This allows the surgeon to formulate an operative plan and to survey the intranasal landscape for pathology as well as patient-specific factors. Correlation between endoscopy and radiographs also may help identify sources of potential pitfalls, and the recognition of entities such as a low skull base, an uncinate process with abnormal insertion, paradoxically shaped turbinates, septal deviation, the presence of Haller and Onodi cells, and other structures may help avoid intraoperative complications and maximize disease management.

Nasal endoscopy is crucial in the management of the postoperative patient. First, postoperative debridements facilitate the return of a normally mucosalized sinonasal cavity. They facilitate healing and allow the surgeon to make slight modifications in the operative field, such as lysis of webs or removal of clots. The use of angled scopes and surgical instrumentation in the clinic setting is challenging to the budding rhinologist yet is a key to successful outcomes. Postoperative care in this manner should continue until the cavity is re–epithelialized (16).

Functional endoscopic sinus surgery (FESS) generally enlarges the paranasal sinus ostia and therefore allows the endoscopist better visualization and access. In many instances, the mucosa inside the sinus cavities is amenable to visualization, especially using the techniques outlined above. Larger communications between the nasal cavity and paranasal sinuses also allow more precise introduction of instrumentation for diagnostic and therapeutic purposes. Intrasinus disease is generally easier to characterize, monitor, and access in the postoperative state.

In the realm of modern surgery, FESS is relatively unique insofar as the operative site can be routinely seen and accessed with the quick and relatively simple technique of nasal endoscopy. Kennedy analyzed his outcomes in 120 patients following FESS and noted only 45% of these patients had "normal" endoscopy at their final follow-up. These findings did not always correlate with disease state and subjective symptoms, as had been previously described; symptom improvement did not correlate well with resolution of disease. This reinforced the tenet that the use of the endoscopic examination allows persistent disease to be identified, diagnosed, and treated before it becomes symptomatic. This also highlights the need for appropriate medical therapy in postoperative patients and the need for careful rhinoscopy in the evaluation and follow-up of operative disease. Kennedy's study also noted that the objective (endoscopic) outcome was highly dependent upon preoperative CT staging of disease (16).

One of the longest and most detailed analyses of functional endoscopic sinus surgery sought to analyze endoscopic postoperative results and compare them to recurrence of disease as one of its primary objectives. Here, it was found that those with endoscopic evidence of an inflamed sinonasal cavity at 1.5 years were more likely to have recurrence of disease and need revision surgery. Subjective data were not predictive of recurrence. Therefore, nasal endoscopy in postoperative patients can help differentiate a population more likely to fail surgical intervention (17).

PHYSICAL EXAMINATION IN PATIENTS WITH CRS

First, however, a discussion of physical examination findings in CRS patients is warranted. A thorough head and neck examination as well as a pulmonary examination is warranted; however, with the exception of anterior rhinoscopy, these are generally nonspecific. Classically, pain and/or pressure from each sinus cavity may be referred to an area of the head: maxillary, ethmoid, frontal, and sphenoid inflammation have been correlated with infraorbital, lacrimal, forehead, and vertex/occiput discomfort, respectively (18). Despite these subjective descriptors, there are no data to support that percussion of these areas provides any meaningful diagnostic information. Similarly, external transillumination has been classically described yet has failed to show any accurate diagnostic correlation with rhinosinusitis (19).

Anterior rhinoscopy should be performed and carefully documented on each patient visit. Although this examination may seem rudimentary and basic to the practicing otorhinolaryngologist, it may be daunting to the primary care physician. It provides fast and reliable visualization of the anterior nasal cavity and does not require expensive fiberoptic equipment. The necessary tools for this important examination include a nasal speculum, a head mirror, and a light source. No matter how basic it may seem, the source of illumination is of utmost importance in this examination. The use of indirect illumination with a head mirror allows the transmission of reflected light into the nasal cavity and, by means of being hands-free, avoids line-of-sight issues incurred by handheld light sources. By changing the focal length between the mirror and the subject, indirect illumination also allows the examiner an improved depth of field. It is also cheaper and easier to maintain than a fiberoptic headlight.

With the nasal speculum placed in the vestibule, examination of the nasal cavity using anterior rhinoscopy ensues. This should be performed in the native and decongested state. First, the septum is examined for perforation, mucosal changes, spurs, and deviation. The character and degree of deviation is noted, especially any contact with the middle turbinate or compromise of the nasal airway. The turbinates are also assessed for their degree of congestion as well as their mucosal state. In patients without obstructed views, the middle turbinate and middle meatus are generally visible. Close inspection should evaluate for the presence of polyps, erythema, edema, or purulent secretions in the middle meatus. A view of the posterior nasal cavity (including the sphenoethmoidal recess) is generally not possible with anterior rhinoscopy. Again, the valuable information from anterior rhinoscopy cannot be underscored; according to the Task Force on Rhinosinusitis, the most significant finding on clinical examination in patients with rhinosinusitis is purulent secretions in the nasal cavity (9).

After initial anterior rhinoscopy is performed, the nose is decongested with an alpha-agonist, and the examination should be repeated in the decongested state allowing improved visualization of the middle meatus. If nasal endoscopy is planned, a topical anesthetic is also applied at this time. Although different administration systems exist, the multi-use Venturi nasal atomizer has proved to be a cost-effective and safe method to apply these agents (20). Although the data are somewhat conflicting, investigations into the ideal preparation for endoscopy have recommended a variety of preparations (21–23). We find 1% lidocaine and 0.1% tetrahydrozoline administered by a Venturi atomizer the most effective for decongestive and anesthetic purposes. The use of cocaine for diagnostic endoscopy is discouraged although it is an effective anesthetic and decongestive agent to use for postoperative debridements.

Nasal endoscopy should then be performed in a systematic fashion in order to fully evaluate all areas in question. First, the endoscope is passed along the floor of the nose, lateral to the inferior turbinate, and back into the nasopharynx. This allows visualization of the inferior meatus, the opening of the nasolacrimal duct, the inferiolateral nasal wall, and the nasopharynx, including the adenoid pad, Eustachian tube orifice, and fossa of Rosenmuller. The second pass is made medial to the middle turbinate at an angle of 30°. This allows access to the sphenoethmoidal recess, the posterior septum, and superior turbinate. The third pass is into the middle meatus and allows visualization of the osteomeatal complex, lateral nasal wall, and frontal recess. Access lateral to the middle turbinate may be difficult; if so, this can be achieved by "rolling" the endoscope into the middle meatus from the anterio-inferior aspect of the middle turbinate or by medially displacing the middle turbinate with an instrument such as a rigid suction catheter or a cerumen curette.

The choice of endoscope is variable, and the types of endoscopes commonly used are discussed above. Although some may argue that flexible endoscopy is more cost-effective in the office setting (10), we feel that the improved illumination and visualization provided by the 4 mm rigid endoscope makes it the best choice. In addition, its rigid character allows the examiner a free hand to suction, manipulate, collect specimens, and debride. Although the 0° endoscope is the easiest to maneuver in the nasal cavity, angled rigid endoscopes can be used to visualize structures that are not in the direct line of sight and offer superior visualization of the lateral nasal wall, skull base, and frontal recess. Specifically, we feel the lateral nasal wall is best visualized with the 30° endoscope, the skull base with the 30° or 45°, and the frontal recess with the 45° or 70°. In post-surgical patients, angled rigid endoscopes can offer a view of the paranasal sinus contents. In a postoperative patient, the floor of the sphenoid can be easily visualized with a 30° endoscope turned upside-down, and the anterior and lateral walls of the maxillary sinus can be inspected with an upside-down 70°. Depending on the preferences of the examiner and specific patient factors, it is common to use multiple rigid endoscopes during one examination. We commonly use the 30° and the 45° or 70° to complete our three passes.

There are limitations of endoscopy, as nasal access and visualization does not always lead to an accurate representation of what is occurring in a paranasal sinus. This is especially the case in patients who have never undergone sinus surgery, as the sinus ostia are in their native state and do not allow visualization into the sinus cavity. Moreover, even in patients who have had FESS, there may be areas that cannot be visualized with endoscopy, the degree of which depends somewhat on the extent of surgery. In these instances, evaluation of the nasal mucosa in the area of the sphenoethmoidal recess and the osteomeatal complex provides information that must be extrapolated to infer what is going on inside the nearby sinuses. The accuracy of this inference depends on many factors, including the specific finding seen on endoscopic examination.

Staging systems have been proposed to document the status of the mucosa upon nasal endoscopy. Endoscopic findings are used to stage allergic fungal rhinosinusitis as established by Kuhn in 1997, and each stage reflects an incremental increase in visible disease upon endoscopy (Table 3). This staging system is straightforward and easy to understand; it allows the mucosal changes to be documented in a straightforward manner and is reproducible. This study also asserted that nasal endoscopy is the most efficacious modality to follow the medical management of patients with allergic fungal rhinosinusitis, and it is especially useful in this population to help guide the use of systemic steroids (24).

There have been numerous staging systems for the documentation of CRS, the myriad of which reflects the difficulty in objectively quantifying the disease. This has led to discrepancies in disease reporting, which makes comparisons

TABLE 3   Endoscopic Staging System for Allergic Fungal Sinusitis

Stage	Criteria
0	No evidence of disease
1	Edematous mucosa
2	Polypoid mucosa
3	Polyps and fungal debris (allergic fungal mucin)

Source: From Ref. 23.

TABLE 4 Scores of Endoscopic Appearance (as defined by the 1997 Task Force on Rhinosinusitis)

Characteristic	0	1	2
Polyps	None	Confined to MM	Beyond MM
Discharge	None	Clear and thin	Thick and purulent
Edema	None	Mild	Severe
Scarring	None	Mild	Severe
Crusting	None	Mild	Severe

A score is formulated for each side (maximum score possible per side = 20). *Abbreviation*: MM, middle meatus.
Source: From Refs. 9, 25.

between studies difficult, and confounds associations between observers. The 1997 Task Force on Rhinosinusitis addressed these shortcomings and recommended the modified Lund-Mackay scoring system for radiographic patient assessment, especially for research purposes (25). This system has been shown to have the highest intraobserver and interobserver agreement (26). Radiographic staging of disease was chosen as it was shown by Kennedy that radiographic findings were the major determinant for prognosis when all preoperative patient factors were taken into account (16).

In addition to recommending a radiographic system for the staging of CRS, the Task Force on Rhinosinusitis supported the use of scoring other patient variables including symptoms, operative history, and endoscopic appearance. These scores were fashioned in a reproducible manner but were not included in the staging system. The endoscopic findings scored included the presence of polyps, discharge, edema, scarring, and crusting (26). These are further detailed in Table 4.

CONCLUSION

Although the nasal endoscope is seen by many as a useful tool allowing visualization and access to the sinonasal cavity in the operating room, its most important and powerful use takes place in the clinic. Nasal endoscopy has evolved along with the definition of CRS itself and allows the facile surveillance of the pathologic anatomic site. It allows access for diagnosis, characterization, and therapy and offers visualization that promotes comprehension of the disease process. It has a high sensitivity and specificity, correlates well with CT, and contributes greatly to medical decision-making. Although the nasal endoscope may help win the proverbial "battle" in the operating room, the understanding and application of nasal endoscopy in the diagnosis and clinical management is vital in winning the war against CRS.

REFERENCES

1. Stammberger H. History of rhinology: anatomy of the paranasal sinuses. Rhinology 1989; 27:197–210.
2. Enrico De Divitiis, Paolo Cappabianca. Endoscopic endonasal transsphenoidal surgery. In: Leonhard M, Cappabianca P, de Divitiis E, eds. The Endoscope, Endoscopic Equipment and Instrumentation. New York: Springer-Verlag, 2003, 9–19.
3. Sircus W, Flisk E. Milestones in the evolution of endoscopy: a short history. J R Coll Physicians Edinb 2003; 33:124–34.
4. Jennings CR. Harold Hopkins. Arch Otolaryngol Head Neck Surg 1998; 124:1042.

5. Yamashita K. Endonasal flexible fiberoptic endoscopy. Rhinology 1983; 21:233–7.
6. Stammberger H. Endoscopic endonasal surgery concepts in treatment of recurring rhinosinusitis. Otolaryngology Head Neck Surg 1986 94:143–55.
7. Kennedy DW. Functional endoscopic sinus surgery: technique. Arch Otolaryngol 1985; 111:643–9.
8. Stammberger H. History of rhinology: anatomy of the paranasal sinuses. Rhinology 1989; 27:197–210.
9. Lanza D, Kennedy D. Adult rhinosinusitis defined. Otolaryngol Head Neck Surg 1997; 117(3 Pt 2):S1–7.
10. Casiano RR. Correlation of clinical examination with computer tomography in paranasal sinus disease. Am J Rhinol 1997; 11(3):193–6.
11. Stankiewicz JA, Chow JM. Nasal endoscopy and the definition and diagnosis of chronic rhinosinusitis. Otolaryngol Head Neck Surg 2002; 126:623–7.
12. Hughes R, Jones N. The role of nasal endoscopy in outpatient management. Clin Otolaryngol 1998; 23:224–6.
13. Dubin MG, Ebert CS, Coffey CS, Melroy CT, Sonnenburg RE, Senior BA. Concordance of middle meatal swab and maxillary sinus aspirate in acute and chronic sinusitis: a meta analysis. Am J Rhinol 2006; 20(1):77–83.
14. Skoulas I, Helidonis E, Kountakis S. Evaluation of sinusitis in the intensive care unit patient. Otolaryngol Head Neck Surg 2003; 128:503–9.
15. Bent JP, Kuhn FA. Diagnosis of allergic fungal sinusitis. Otolaryngol Head Neck Surg 1994; 111:580–8.
16. Kennedy D. Prognostic factors, outcomes and staging in ethmoid sinus surgery. Laryngoscope 1992; 102:1–18.
17. Senior B, Kennedy D, Tanabodee J, Kroger H, Hassab M, Lanza D. Long-term results of functional endoscopic sinus surgery. Laryngoscope 1998; 108:151–7.
18. Hadley JA, Schaeffer SD. Clinical evaluation of rhinosinusitis: history and physical examination. Otolaryngol Head Neck Surg 1997; 117(3 Pt 2):S7–11.
19. Spector SL, Lotan A, English G, Philpot I. Comparison between transillumination and the roentgenogram in diagnosing paranasal sinus disease. J Allergy Clin Immunol 1981; 67: 22–6.
20. Dubin MG, White DR, Melroy CT, Gergan MT, Rutala WA, Senior BA. Multi-use Venturi nasal atomizer contamination in a clinical rhinologic practice. Am J Rhinol 2004; 18:151–6.
21. Sadek S, Scott A, White A, Wilson P, Carlin W. The efficacy of topical anesthesia in flexible nasendoscopy: a double blind randomized controlled trial. Clin Otolaryngol 2001; 26:25–8.
22. Cain A, Murray D, McClymont L. The use of topical nasal anesthesia before flexible nasendoscopy. Clin Otolaryngol 2002; 27:485–8.
23. Smith J, Rockley T. A comparison of cocaine and 'co-phenylcaine' local anesthesia in flexible nasendoscopy. Clin Otolaryngol 2002; 27:192–6.
24. Kupferberg FB, Bent JP, Kuhn FA. Prognosis for allergic fungal sinusitis. Otolaryngol Head Neck Surg 1997; 117:35–41.
25. Lund VJ, Kenney DW. Staging for rhinosinusitis. Otolaryngol Head Neck Surg 1997; 117(3 Pt 2):S35–40.
26. Oluwole M, Russell N, Tan L, et al. A comparison of computerized tomographic staging systems in chronic sinusitis. Clin Otolaryngol 1996; 21:91–5.

14 Role of Steroids in the Treatment of Rhinosinusitis with and Without Polyposis

Wytske Fokkens

Department of Otorhinolaryngology, Academic Medical Centre, Amsterdam, The Netherlands

INTRODUCTION

The introduction of topically administered glucocorticoids has improved the treatment of upper [rhinitis, nasal polyps (NP)] and lower (asthma) airway inflammatory disease. The clinical efficacy of glucocorticoids may depend in part on their ability to reduce airway eosinophil infiltration by preventing their increased viability and activation. Both topical and systemic glucocorticoids may affect eosinophil function by both directly reducing eosinophil viability and activation (1–4) or by indirectly reducing the secretion of chemotactic cytokines by nasal mucosa and polyp epithelial cells (5–8). The potency of these effects is lower in nasal polyps than in nasal mucosa suggesting an induced inflammatory resistance to steroid treatment in chronic rhinosinusitis (CRS)/nasal polyposis (4,6).

The new generation of nasal corticosteroid preparations have strong local anti-inflammatory effects and negligible systemic side effects. They come as sprays, powders, and/or drops. The best effect of intranasal steroids is obtained with optimal mucosal contact. This can be achieved by rinsing the nose some time before spraying and, if obstruction is prominent, opening the nasal cavity with a local decongestant in the first 1–2 weeks of treatment.

The biological action of glucocorticoids is mediated through activation of intracellular glucocorticoid receptors (GR) (9), expressed in many tissues and cells (10). Two human isoforms of GR have been identified, GRα and GRβ, which originate from the same gene by alternative splicing of the GR primary transcript (11). Upon hormone binding, GRα enhances anti-inflammatory or represses proinflammatory gene transcription, and exerts most of the anti-inflammatory effects of glucocorticoids through protein–protein interactions between GR and transcription factors, such as AP-1 and NF-κB. The GRβ isoform does not bind steroids but may interfere with the GR function. There may be several mechanisms accounting for the resistance to the anti-inflammatory effects of glucocorticoids, including an overexpression of GRβ or a downexpression of GRα. Increased expression of GRβ has been reported in patients with NP (12,13) while downregulation of GRα levels after treatment with glucocorticoids (14,15) has also been postulated to be one of the possible explanations for the secondary glucocorticoid resistance phenomenon.

Most of the mechanistic studies of corticosteroid action in patients with chronic RS come from studies of nasal polyposis. Treatment of NP with topical glucocorticoids reduced the local tissue infiltration with eosinophils and T lymphocytes and suppressed the local production of Th-2 cytokines, particularly interleukin-4 (IL-4) and IL-13 (16). Endothelial P-selectin expression was also strongly suppressed, and this may in part account for the ability of topical corticosteroids to suppress tissue eosinophil infiltration. In this study, local production of IL-5 was also reduced, but this effect was not statistically significant after four weeks of intranasal fluticasone treatment (16).

POTENTIAL INDICATIONS FOR CORTICOSTEROIDS IN RHINOSINUSITIS
Acute/Intermittent Rhinosinusitis Without Nasal Polyps

In acute RS, nasal corticosteroids have usually been studied as adjunctive therapy to oral antibiotic treatment. Most of these studies have shown a significant adjunctive effect on symptoms, but not on computed tomography (CT) scan findings (17–22). No side effects of local corticosteroids were seen on this presumably bacterially infected mucosa. One study showed a faster resolution when intranasal steroids were used in addition to an antibiotic (20), probably the most important study parameter in this self-limiting disease.

Studies are underway which compare nasal steroids to antibiotics as a single treatment in patients with acute RS. The first data (only published as abstract) showed significant reduction of symptomatology in acute RS over placebo and an antibiotic alone. The evidence for adjunctive therapy to systemic antibiotics is level I, but as a single therapy no (published) data are available (Table 1).

Persistent (Chronic) Rhinosinusitis Without Nasal Polyps

The evidence for an effect of local intranasal steroids in persistent RS is limited but positive (23–27). In the groups that looked at differences in the responses between allergic and nonallergic patients, there was either no difference or the effect was better in the patients who did not show allergy (Table 2) (25).

Persistent (Chronic) Rhinosinusitis with Nasal Polyps

In studies on the treatment of NP, it is of value to look separately at the effect on rhinitis symptoms associated with polyposis and the effect on the size of NP per se. Only placebo-controlled studies will be considered.

Local (topical) corticosteroids have a documented effect on bilateral NP and also on symptoms associated with NP such as nasal blockage, secretion, and sneezing but the effect on the sense of smell is not high (28–38). There is a high evidence level (I) for effect on polyp size and nasal symptoms associated with nasal polyposis. For individual symptoms, blockage responds best to corticosteroids but improvement in the sense of smell is not so obvious. Some studies show a dose–response (36) up to 800 µg. The magnitude of effect of local corticosteroids may also differ depending on the method of administration; however, comparative trials related to this issue are not available (Table 3).

Postoperative Treatment with Topical Corticosteroids for CRS with NP to Prevent Recurrence of Nasal Polyps

The effect of postoperative intranasal steroids on the recurrence rate of NP after polypectomy is well documented and the evidence level is Ib (38–43). Two studies describe the effect after FESS in a group of patients who underwent FESS after inadequate response to at least three months of local corticosteroid treatment. The studies show conflicting results for reasons that are not clear (Table 4) (44,45).

TABLE 1 Treatment with Intranasal Corticosteroids in Acute/Intermittent Rhinosinusitis Without Nasal Polyposis

Study	Drug	Antibiotic	Number of patients	Effect	X-ray
Qvarnberg et al. (17)	Budesonide	Erythromycin	20	Significant effect on nasal symptoms, facial pain, and sensitivity; final clinical outcome did not differ	Mucosal thickening = no effect
Meltzer et al. (18)	Mometasone furoate	Amoxicillin/ clavulanate	407	Significant effect in congestion, facial pain, headache, and rhinorrhea. No significant effect in postnasal drip	No statistical difference in CT outcome
Nayak et al. (19)	Mometasone furoate	Amoxicillin/ clavulanate	967	Total symptom score was improved (nasal congestion, facial pain, rhinorrhea, and postnasal drip)	No statistical difference in CT outcome
Dolor et al. (20)	Fluticasone propionate	Cefuroxime axetil	95	Significant effect.Effect measured as time to clinical success depending on patients, self-judgment of symptomatic improvement	Not done
Barlan et al. (21)	Budesonide	Amoxicillin/ clavulanate	89 (children)	Improvement in cough and nasal secretion seen at the end of the second week of treatment in the budesonide group	Not done
Meltzer et al. (22)	Flunisolide	Amoxicillin/ clavulanate	180	Significant effect: overall score for global assessment of efficacy was greater in the group with flunisolide	No effect on X ray

Prophylactic Treatment of Intermittent Rhinosinusitis

There is very low evidence for a prophylactic effect of nasal corticosteroids in preventing intermittent (acute) RS (Table 5).

In a study by Puhakka et al. (46) fluticasone propionate (FP) (200 μg four times daily) or placebo were used for six days in 199 subjects with an acute common cold, 24–48 hours after the onset of symptoms to study the preventive effects of FP on risk for the development of acute RS. The frequency of RS at day seven in subjects positive for rhinovirus, based on X-ray, was not significantly different between the groups.

Cook et al. randomised 227 subjects with recurrent episodes of RS to continue on fluticasone or placebo after an acute episode of RS. Although the total

TABLE 2 Treatment with Nasal Corticosteroids in Persistent (Chronic) Rhinosinusitis Without Nasal Polyposis

Study	Drug	Number	Time	Symptoms	Other effects
Parikh et al. (23)	Fluticasone propionate	22	16 wk	Not significant	Acoustic rhinometry not significant
Lavigne et al. (24)	Intrasinus budesonide	26	3 wk	Total symptom score significantly improved	T-cells, eosinophils, mRNA for IL-4, and IL-5 significantly improved
Cuenant et al. (25)	Tixocortol irrigation	60	11 days	Nasal obstruction significantly improved	Maxillary ostial patency significantly improved
Sykes et al. (26)	Dexamethasone + tramazoline	50	4 wk	Discharge, obstruction, and facial pain significantly improved	Plain X ray and nasal airway resistance and mucociliary clearance significantly improved
Lund et al. (27)	Budesonide	134	20 wk	Significant symptom improvement	Significant improvement in airway using PNIF

number of recurrences was not statistically different, the mean number of days to first recurrence was 97.5 and 116.6 respectively (P = 0.011) (47).

Systemic Steroids in Acute/Intermittent Rhinosinusitis
Gehanno et al. (48) performed a placebo-controlled trial to evaluate the effect of adding 8 mg of methylprednisolone three times daily for five days as adjunctive therapy to 10 days treatment with amoxicillin-clavulanate potassium in patients with acute RS. Criteria for enrollment were: symptoms <10 days, craniofacial pain, purulent nasal discharge with purulent drainage from the middle meatus, and opacities of the sinuses on X-ray or CT scan. No difference was seen in therapeutic outcome at day 14 between the groups (N = 417) but at day four there was a significant reduction of headache and facial pain in the steroid group (evidence level: I b). Recently, Klossek et al. showed the efficacy of a short course of oral prednisone (3 days), versus placebo, in the treatment of the functional signs of acute maxillary RS with severe pain in adults in addition to an appropriate antibiotic (49).

Systemic Steroids in Persistent (Chronic) Rhinosinusitis with Nasal Polyps
There are no double-blind studies performed on single treatment with systemic steroids in patients with NP without concomitant treatment with topical steroids (49–53). Open studies performed with the combination of systemic and topical steroids indicate that they are effective in polyp reduction and in improving nasal symptoms associated with NP, even the sense of smell. The effect is reversible (50) (evidence level: III) (Table 6).

There is also no study available on depot injection of corticosteroids or local injection into polyps or the inferior turbinate. These types of treatment are actually obsolete because of the risk of fat necrosis at the site of the injection or blindness following endonasal injection.

TABLE 3 Treatment with Nasal Corticosteroids in Persistent Rhinosinusitis with Nasal Polyposis

Study	Drug	Number	Treatment time (wk)	Effect on nasal symptoms	Objective measures	Effect on polyps
Mygind et al. (28)	BDP	35	3	Total symptom score[a]	None	N.S.
Deuschl and Drettner (30)	BDP	20	4	Blockage[a]	Rhinomanometry[a]	N.S.
Holopainen et al. (31)	Bud	19	16	Total symptom score[a]	Nasal peak flow[a] Eosinophilia[a]	Yes
Tos et al. (32)	Bud	138	6	Total symptom score[a] Sense of smell[a]	Polyp size	Yes
Vendelo Johansen et al. (29)	Bud	91	12	Blockage[a] Sneezing[a] Secretion[a] Sense of smell N.S.	Nasal peak Inspiratory flow[a]	Yes
Lildholdt et al. (33)	Bud	116	4	Blockage[a] Sneezing[a] Secretion[a] Sense of smell N.S.	Nasal peak Expiratory flow[a]	Yes
Holmberg et al. (34)	FP/BDP	55	26	Over all assessment[a]	Nasal peak Inspiratory flow[a]	Yes in BDP
Keith et al. (35)	FPND	104	12	Blockage[a] Rhinitis[a] Sense of smell N.S.	Nasal peak Inspiratory flow[a] Olfactory test N.S.	N.S.
Penttila et al. (36)	FP	142	12	Blockage[a] Rhinitis[a] Sense of smell N.S.	Nasal peak Inspiratory flow[a] Olfactory test[a]	Yes
Lund et al. (37)	FP/BDP	29	12	Blockage[a] Rhinitis N.S.	Nasal peak Inspiratory flow[a] Acoustic Rhinometry[a]	Yes FP
Hadfield et al. (38)	BM	46 CF children	6	N.S.	Polyp size	Yes

Abbreviations: BM, betamethasone; FP, fluticasone propionate; BDP, beclomethasone dipropionate; Bud, budesonide; N.S., not significant.
[a]Stag sig.

TABLE 4 Nasal Corticosteroids in the Postoperative Treatment of Persistent Rhinosinusitis with Nasal Polyps to Prevent Recurrences of Nasal Polyps

Study	Drug	Number	Treatment time (wk)	Effect on nasal symptoms	Effect on polyp recurrence (method of test)
Drettner et al. (39)	Flunisolide	22	12	Total nasal score (blockage, secretion sneezing)[a]	N.S. (anterior rhinoscopy)
Virolainen and Puhakka (no statistics) (40)	BDP	40	52	Blockage	Yes (anterior rhinoscopy)
Karlsson and Rundcrantz (41)	BDP	40	120	Not described	Yes (anterior rhinoscopy)–
Dingsor et al. (42)	Flunisolide	41	52	Blockage[a] Sneezing[a]	Yes (anterior rhinoscopy)–
Hartwig et al. (43)	BUD	73	26	Blockage N.S.	Yes (anterior rhinoscopy)
Dijkstra et al. (44)	FP	162	52	N.S.	N.S. (nasal endoscopy)
Rowe-Jones et al. (45)	FP	109	260	Overall visual analog score	Yes (endoscopic polyp score and total nasal volume)

Abbreviations: BM, betamethasone; FP, fluticasone propionate; BDP, beclomethasone dipropionate; Bud, budesonide; N.S., not significant.
[a]Stag sig.

Surgical Treatment Versus Steroids in Nasal Polyps

In two open studies Lildholdt et al. (50,51) compared single injections of 14 mg betametasone to intranasal polypectomy without any difference in outcome 12 months after treatment with subsequent local steroids in both groups, as measured by mean nasal score or mean score of sense of smell. In a study by Blomqvist et al. (54) 32 patients were pretreated with systemic steroids (prednisolone for 14 days) and budesonide for four weeks, after which unilateral FESS was performed and intranasal steroids given for an additional 12 months to both sides. The sense of smell improved after treatment with systemic and local steroids. Surgery had an additional beneficial effect on nasal obstruction and secretion that persisted over the study period but no additional effect was observed on sense of smell. The authors concluded that surgical treatment is indicated after steroid treatment if nasal obstruction persists but not if hyposmia is the primary symptom (level III).

To date, too little data are available to determine whether there is any difference between surgery and steroid therapy in the long-term outcome of patients with nasal polyposis.

TABLE 5 Treatment with Nasal Corticosteroids in Prophylaxis of Intermittent (Acute) Rhinosinusitis

Study	Drug	Number	Time (wk)	Effect	Comments
Puhakka et al. (46)	FP	199	1	N.S.	Common cold
Cook et al. (47)	FP	227	11	Increased time to first recurrence, decreased frequency of acute rhinosinusitis	

Abbreviations: FP, fluticasone propionate; N.S., not significant.

TABLE 6 Treatment with Systemic Corticosteroids in Persistent (Chronic) Rhinosinusitis with Nasal Polyps

Study	Drug	Number	Dose/time	Effect symptoms	Effect polyps	Evidence
Lildholdt et al. (50)	Betametamethasone/ budesonide	16	14 mg/52 wk	Yes	Yes	III
Lildholdt et al. (51)	Betametamethasone/ BDP	53	?/52 wk	Yes	Yes	III
van Camp and Clement (52)	Prednisolone 60 mg	25	2 wk	72%	Yes 10/22	III
Damm et al. (53)	Budesonide + fluocortolone	20	?	Yes	?	III

Abbreviation: BDP, beclomethasone dipropionate.

Surgical Treatment Versus Steroids in CRS

To our knowledge no studies have been published to date comparing surgery and topical corticosteroids in the treatment of chronic RS.

Topical Corticosteroids in the Treatment of Pediatric Rhinosinusitis

Only one study suggests that topical corticosteroids may be a useful ancillary treatment to antibiotics in childhood acute RS, effective in reducing the cough and nasal discharge earlier in the course of disease (21). There are a large number of studies showing that local corticosteroids are effective and safe in children with rhinitis (55–59). However there are no studies showing significant efficacy in children with chronic RS either with or without NP.

CONCLUSION

Chronic RS is a multifactorial disease and comprises a vicious cycle of pathophysiologic, anatomic, and constitutive factors. Treatment is aimed to break the vicious cycle: reducing mucosal inflammation and swelling, controlling infection, and restoring aeration of the nasal and sinus mucosa. Pharmacologic treatment, including treatment with local or systemic corticosteroids, is the cornerstone of dealing with the disease. If symptoms persist after aggressive pharmacologic treatment, surgical treatment should be considered.

REFERENCES

1. Xaubet A, Mullol J, Lopez E, et al. Comparison of the role of nasal polyp and normal nasal mucosal epithelial cells on in vitro eosinophil survival. Mediation by GM-CSF and inhibition by dexamethasone. Clin Exp Allergy 1994; 24:307–17.
2. Mullol J, Xaubet A, Lopez E, Roca-Ferrer J, Picado C. Comparative study of the effects of different glucocorticosteroids on eosinophil survival primed by cultured epithelial cell supernatants obtained from nasal mucosa and nasal polyps. Thorax 1995; 50:270–4.
3. Mullol J, Xaubet A, Lopez E, et al. Eosinophil activation by epithelial cells of the respiratory mucosa. Comparative study of normal mucosa and inflammatory mucosa. Med Clin (Barc) 1997; 109:6–11.
4. Mullol J, Lopez E, Roca-Ferrer J, et al. Effects of topical anti-inflammatory drugs on eosinophil survival primed by epithelial cells. Additive effect of glucocorticoids and nedocromil sodium. Clin Exp Allergy 1997; 27:1432–41.

5. Mullol J, Xaubet A, Gaya A, et al. Cytokine gene expression and release from epithelial cells. A comparison study between healthy nasal mucosa and nasal polyps. Clin Exp Allergy 1995; 25:607–15.
6. Mullol J, Roca-Ferrer J, Xaubet A, Raserra J, Picado C. Inhibition of GM-CSF secretion by topical corticosteroids and nedocromil sodium. A comparison study using nasal polyp epithelial cells. Respir Med 2000; 94:428–31.
7. Roca-Ferrer J, Mullol J, Lopez E, et al. Effect of topical anti-inflammatory drugs on epithelial cell-induced eosinophil survival and GM-CSF secretion. Eur Respir J 1997; 10:1488–95.
8. Xaubet A, Mullol J, Roca-Ferrer J, et al. Effect of budesonide and nedocromil sodium on IL-6 and IL-8 release from human nasal mucosa and polyp epithelial cells. Respir Med 2001; 95:408–14.
9. Leung DY, Bloom JW. Update on glucocorticoid action and resistance. J Allergy Clin Immunol 2003; 111:3–22; quiz 23.
10. Pujols L, Mullol J, Roca-Ferrer J, et al. Expression of glucocorticoid receptor alpha- and beta-isoforms in human cells and tissues. Am J Physiol Cell Physiol 2002; 283: C1324–31.
11. Oakley RH, Sar M, Cidlowski JA. The human glucocorticoid receptor beta isoform. Expression, biochemical properties, and putative function. J Biol Chem 1996; 271: 9550–9.
12. Hamilos DL, Leung DY, Muro S, et al. GRbeta expression in nasal polyp inflammatory cells and its relationship to the anti-inflammatory effects of intranasal fluticasone. J Allergy Clin Immunol 2001; 108:58–68.
13. Pujols L, Mullol J, Benitez P, et al. Expression of the glucocorticoid receptor alpha and beta isoforms in human nasal mucosa and polyp epithelial cells. Respir Med 2003; 97:90–6.
14. Knutsson PU, Bronnegard M, Marcus C, Stierna P. Regulation of glucocorticoid receptor mRNA in nasal mucosa by local administration of fluticasone and budesonide. J Allergy Clin Immunol 1996; 97:655–61.
15. Pujols L, Mullol J, Perez M, et al. Expression of the human glucocorticoid receptor alpha and beta isoforms in human respiratory epithelial cells and their regulation by dexamethasone. Am J Respir Cell Mol Biol 2001; 24:48–57.
16. Hamilos DL, Thawley SE, Kramper MA, Kamil A, Hamid QA. Effect of intranasal fluticasone on cellular infiltration, endothelial adhesion molecule expression, and proinflammatory cytokine mRNA in nasal polyp disease. J Allergy Clin Immunol. 1999; 103:78–87.
17. Qvarnberg Y, Kantola O, Salo J, Toivanen M, Valtonen H, Vuori E. Influence of topical steroid treatment on maxillary sinusitis. Rhinology 1992; 30:103–12.
18. Meltzer EO, Charous BL, Busse WW, Zinreich SJ, Lorber RR, Danzig MR. Added relief in the treatment of acute recurrent sinusitis with adjunctive mometasone furoate nasal spray. The Nasonex Sinusitis Group. J Allergy Clin Immunol 2000; 106:630–7.
19. Nayak AS, Settipane GA, Pedinoff A, et al. Effective dose range of mometasone furoate nasal spray in the treatment of acute rhinosinusitis. Ann Allergy Asthma Immunol 2002; 89:271–8.
20. Dolor RJ, Witsell DL, Hellkamp AS, Williams JW Jr, Califf RM, Simel DL. Comparison of cefuroxime with or without intranasal fluticasone for the treatment of rhinosinusitis. The CAFFS Trial: a randomized controlled trial. JAMA 2001; 286:3097–105.
21. Barlan IB, Erkan E, Bakir M, Berrak S, Basaran MM. Intranasal budesonide spray as an adjunct to oral antibiotic therapy for acute sinusitis in children. Ann Allergy Asthma Immunol 1997; 78:598–601.
22. Meltzer EO, Orgel HA, Backhaus JW, et al. Intranasal flunisolide spray as an adjunct to oral antibiotic therapy for sinusitis. J Allergy Clin Immunol 1993; 92:812–23.
23. Parikh A, Scadding GK, Darby Y, Baker RC. Topical corticosteroids in chronic rhinosinusitis: a randomized, double-blind, placebo-controlled trial using fluticasone propionate aqueous nasal spray. Rhinology 2001; 39:75–9.
24. Lavigne F, Cameron L, Renzi PM, et al. Intrasinus administration of topical budesonide to allergic patients with chronic rhinosinusitis following surgery. Laryngoscope 2002; 112:858–64.

25. Cuenant G, Stipon JP, Plante-Longchamp G, Baudoin C, Guerrier Y. Efficacy of endonasal neomycin-tixocortol pivalate irrigation in the treatment of chronic allergic and bacterial sinusitis. ORL J Otorhinolaryngol Relat Spec 1986; 48:226–32.
26. Sykes DA, Wilson R, Chan KL, Mackay IS, Cole PJ. Relative importance of antibiotic and improved clearance in topical treatment of chronic mucopurulent rhinosinusitis. A controlled study. Lancet 1986; 2:358–60.
27. Lund VJ, Black JH, Szabo LZ, Schrewelius C, Akerlund A. Efficacy and tolerability of budesonide aqueous nasal spray in chronic rhinosinusitis patients. Rhinology 2004; 42:57–62.
28. Mygind N, Pedersen CB, Prytz S, Sorensen H. Treatment of nasal polyps with intranasal beclomethasone dipropionate aerosol. Clin Allergy 1975; 5:158–64.
29. Vendelo Johansen L, Illum P, Kristensen S, Winther L, Vang Petersen S, Synnerstad B. The effect of budesonide (Rhinocort) in the treatment of small and medium-sized nasal polyps. Clin Otolaryngol 1993; 18:524–7.
30. Deuschl H, Drettner B. Nasal polyps treated by beclomethasone nasal aerosol. Rhinology 1977; 15:17–23.
31. Holopainen E, Grahne B, Malmberg H, Makinien J, Lindqvist N. Budesonide in the treatment of nasal polyposis. Eur J Respir Dis Suppl 1982; 122:221–8.
32. Tos M, Svendstrup F, Arndal H, et al. Efficacy of an aqueous and a powder formulation of nasal budesonide compared in patients with nasal polyps. Am J Rhinol 1998; 12:183–9.
33. Lildholdt T, Rundcrantz H, Lindqvist N. Efficacy of topical corticosteroid powder for nasal polyps: a double-blind, placebo-controlled study of budesonide. Clin Otolaryngol 1995; 20:26–30.
34. Holmberg K, Juliusson S, Balder B, Smith DL, Richards DH, Karlsson G. Fluticasone propionate aqueous nasal spray in the treatment of nasal polyposis. Ann Allergy Asthma Immunol 1997; 78:270–6.
35. Keith P, Nieminen J, Hollingworth K, Dolovich J. Efficacy and tolerability of fluticasone propionate nasal drops 400 microgram once daily compared with placebo for the treatment of bilateral polyposis in adults. Clin Exp Allergy 2000; 30:1460–8.
36. Penttila M, Poulsen P, Hollingworth K, Holmstrom M. Dose-related efficacy and tolerability of fluticasone propionate nasal drops 400 microg once daily and twice daily in the treatment of bilateral nasal polyposis: a placebo-controlled randomized study in adult patients. Clin Exp Allergy 2000; 30:94–102.
37. Lund VJ, Flood J, Sykes AP, Richards DH. Effect of fluticasone in severe polyposis. Arch Otolaryngol Head Neck Surg 1998; 124:513–8.
38. Hadfield PJ, Rowe-Jones JM, Mackay IS. A prospective treatment trial of nasal polyps in adults with cystic fibrosis. Rhinology 2000; 38(2):63–5.
39. Drettner B, Ebbesen A, Nilsson M. Prophylactive treatment with flunisolide after polypectomy. Rhinology 1982; 20:148–58.
40. Virolainen E, Puhakka H. The effect of intranasal beclomethasone dipropionate on the recurrence of nasal polyps after ethmoidectomy. Rhinology 1980; 18:8–18.
41. Karlsson G, Rundcrantz H. A randomized trial of intranasal beclomethasone dipropionate after polypectomy. Rhinology 1982; 20:144–8.
42. Dingsor G, Kramer J, Olsholt R, Soderstrom T. Flunisolide nasal spray 0.025% in the prophylactic treatment of nasal polyposis after polypectomy. A randomized, double blind, parallel, placebo controlled study. Rhinology 1985; 23:48–58.
43. Hartwig S, Linden M, Laurent C, Vargo AK, Lindqvist N. Budesonide nasal spray as prophylactic treatment after polypectomy (a double blind clinical trial). J Laryngol Otol 1988; 102:148–51.
44. Dijkstra MD, Ebbens FA, Poublon RM, Fokkens WJ. Fluticasone propionate aqueous nasal spray does not influence the recurrence rate of chronic rhinosinusitis and nasal polyps 1 year after functional endoscopic sinus surgery. Clin Exp Allergy 2004; 34:1395–400.
45. Rowe-Jones JM, Medcalf M, Durham SR, Richards DH, Mackay IS. Functional endoscopic sinus surgery: 5 year follow up and results of a prospective, randomised,

stratified, double-blind, placebo controlled study of postoperative fluticasone propionate aqueous nasal spray. Rhinology 2005; 43(1):2–10.

46. Puhakka T, Makela MJ, Malmstrom K, EO, et al. The common cold: effects of intranasal fluticasone propionate treatment. J Allergy Clin Immunol 1998; 101(6 Pt 1): 726–31.

47. Cook C, Meltzer EO, Goode-Sellers S, Prillaman B, Witham L, Philpot E. Fluticasone propionate aqueous nasal spray decreases frequency of recurrence and increases time to recurrence of acute sinusitis. J Allergy Clin Immunol 2002; 109:S86 (abstract).

48. Gehanno P, Beauvillain C, Bobin S, et al. Short therapy with amoxicillin-clavulanate and corticosteroids in acute sinusitis: results of a multicentre study in adults. Scand J Infect Dis 2000; 32:678–84.

49. Klossek JM, Desmonts-Gohler C, Deslandes B, et al. Treatment of functional signs of acute maxillary rhinosinusitis in adults. Efficacy and tolerance of administration of oral prednisone for 3 days. Presse Med 2004; 33:303–9.

50. Lildholdt T, Rundcrantz H, Bende M, Larsen K. Glucocorticoid treatment for nasal polyps. The use of topical budesonide powder, intramuscular betamethasone, and surgical treatment. Arch Otolaryngol Head Neck Surg 1997; 123:595–600.

51. Lildholdt T, Fogstrup J, Gammelgaard N, Kortholm B, Ulsoe C. Surgical versus medical treatment of nasal polyps. Acta Otolaryngol 1988; 105:140–3.

52. van Camp C, Clement PA. Results of oral steroid treatment in nasal polyposis. Rhinology 1994; 32:5–9.

53. Damm M, Jungehulsing M, Eckel HE, Schmidt M, Theissen P. Effects of systemic steroid treatment in chronic polypoid rhinosinusitis evaluated with magnetic resonance imaging. Otolaryngol Head Neck Surg 1999; 120:517–23.

54. Blomqvist EH, Lundblad L, Anggard A, Haraldsson PO, Stjarne Pl. A randomized controlled study evaluating medical treatment versus surgical treatment in addition to medical treatment of nasal polyposis. J Allergy Clin Immunol 2001; 107:224–8.

55. Passalacqua G, Albano M, Canonica GW, et al. Inhaled and nasal corticosteroids: safety aspects. Allergy 2000; 55:16–33.

56. Scadding GK. Corticosteroids in the treatment of pediatric allergic rhinitis. J Allergy Clin Immunol 2001; 108(1 Suppl.):S58–64.

57. Fokkens WJ, Cserhati E, dos Santos JM, et al. Budesonide aqueous nasal spray is an effective treatment in children with perennial allergic rhinitis, with an onset of action within 12 hours. Ann Allergy Asthma Immunol 2002; 89:278–84.

58. Fokkens WJ, Scadding GK. Perennial rhinitis in the under 4s: a difficult problem to treat safely and effectively? A comparison of intranasal fluticasone propionate and ketotifen in the treatment of 2–4-year-old children with perennial rhinitis. Pediatr Allergy Immunol 2004; 15:261–6.

59. Baena-Cagnani CE. Safety and tolerability of treatments for allergic rhinitis in children. Drug Saf 2004; 27:883–98.

Adjuvant Therapies in the Treatment of Acute and Chronic Rhinosinusitis

Mark D. Scarupa
Institute for Asthma and Allergy, Johns Hopkins Asthma and Allergy Center, Chevy Chase, Maryland, U.S.A.

Michael A. Kaliner
George Washington University Hospital, Chevy Chase, Maryland, U.S.A.

INTRODUCTION

Acute and chronic rhinosinusitis (CRS) are conditions frequently encountered by primary care physicians and sub-specialists alike. While the selection of appropriate antibiotic therapy is clearly important in bringing about resolution of symptoms, a great number of secondary or adjuvant therapies are available and often prescribed to patients. With the exception of nasal corticosteroids, there are relatively few controlled trials in the literature confirming the benefits of these adjunctive therapies for the treatment of rhinosinusitis.

Adjuvant therapies are typically considered to hasten the resolution of infection, improve symptoms, or to prevent recurrence in patients prone to repeated infection. Though the presence of infectious organisms is a cardinal feature of sinus infections, ostial obstruction, impaired mucociliary clearance, increased mucus viscosity and volume, and the presence of inflammatory mediators, all contribute to creating an environment conducive to infection. It is these alterations in the nasal-sinus environment and the attributed symptoms that adjunctive therapies attempt to influence.

ADJUNCTIVE THERAPIES CONSIDERED IN ALL PATIENTS WITH SINUS DISEASE
Nasal Saline Lavage

Nasal/sinus irrigation with saline has long been used as an adjunctive therapy for the management of acute and CRS as well as a part of postoperative management. There are numerous studies examining the efficacy of different devices for delivering saline to the nasal and sinus cavities. Furthermore, there has been interest in whether isotonic or hypertonic saline is of greater benefit. With the exception of nasal corticosteroids, saline nasal washings are perhaps the only adjuvant therapy where a relative wealth of clinical trials exists supporting their use.

Saline can be introduced into the nasal sinus cavity as a fine mist using relatively small volume (a few milliliters) or larger volumes (4–12 ounces) can be used in a douching fashion. A dental waterpik used with a Grossan adaptor tip as well as a nasal nebulizer can also be used for this purpose. A study comparing three techniques has been published: saline douches, sprays delivered by a metered spray bottle, or nebulization via a RinoFlow (Respironics) device (1). In this study, radiolabeled saline was used to monitor nasal/sinus saline distribution in postoperative patients with chronic sinus disease and in healthy controls. All three devices irrigated the anterior and posterior nasal cavity adequately. Douching, however, achieved a better distribution into the maxillary sinus and frontal recess than the other methods. In fact, the spray technique did not penetrate either the maxillary sinus or anterior recess in any patients including those who were postoperative. Nebulized saline only reached the maxillary sinuses in one third of patients. None of the techniques adequately penetrated the frontal or sphenoid sinuses. Other studies using higher volume spray bottles have shown considerable penetration into the maxillary sinuses (2).

Saline lavages can be either isotonic or hypertonic. A study of pediatric patients with CRS examined the effect of hypertonic saline (3.5%) washing versus normal saline (0.9%) (3). After four weeks of treatment, both groups had significantly decreased post-nasal drip scores. However, only the hypertonic saline group had a significant improvement in cough score and an improvement in radiographic scores. Other studies have shown similar benefits from hypertonic saline washes. In a long-term study, adult patients with CRS were randomized to receive either hypertonic saline (2.0% saline buffered with baking soda) washing for six months or continuation of their usual sinus care (4). Subjects receiving hypertonic saline washes had improved sinus symptom scores by two different measures, required less frequent antibiotics and had more two-week periods free of rhinosinusitis symptoms than did controls.

There have been numerous other controlled studies using nasal irrigation in patients with chronic sinus disease. The majority have shown benefit (5–8). An exception is a study by Adam et al. where adults who had the diagnosis of the common cold or acute bacterial sinusitis were examined. The study reported no improvement with hypertonic saline introduced by a spray. However, it is unclear what volume of nasal spray was used (9).

Mechanistically, hypertonic saline seems to improve mucociliary function in vivo. In a study of healthy volunteers without significant sinus disease, 3% hypertonic saline, but not normal saline, both buffered to pH of 7.6, acutely improved mucociliary clearance as measured by saccharine testing (10). Keojampa et al. reported that both buffered normal and 3% hypertonic saline improved ciliary function although hypertonic saline led to a significantly greater improvement (11). In vitro, a study using cryopreserved mucosa from patients who had undergone transnasal surgery of the pituitary demonstrated that both normal and hypertonic saline (both 7% and 14.4% NaCl) had a detrimental effect on ciliary beat frequency (12). At both 7% and 14.4% NaCl, ciliostasis occurred within five minutes of saline application. However, this study was conducted entirely on cryopreserved tissue in vitro, and intermediate concentrations of hypertonic saline were not examined.

Experience in our clinic with 3% hypertonic saline lavage has been overwhelmingly positive. The majority of our patients tolerate a relatively large volume lavage and feel that it improves them symptomatically and results in less frequent sinus infections. Essentially all patients with rhinosinusitis are maintained on once or twice daily saline lavages. Patients are instructed to use the washings prophylactically and to increase the washing frequency if symptoms worsen.

Decongestants

Decongestants cause constriction of the capacitance vessels in the nasal mucosa leading to decreased blood volume and reduction in turbinate thickness. In theory, this should minimize ostial obstruction due to turbinate swelling and thus provide relief of symptoms and improved drainage. Both oral and topical decongestants act on alpha and, to a lesser extent, beta adrenergic receptors leading to vasoconstriction. Radiographically, application of 1% phenylephrine hydrochloride leads to markedly reduced turbinate size and reduced mucosal thickening in the ethmoid infundibulum (13). Anecdotally, patients report relief of symptoms when using topical decongestants such as oxymetazoline or oral decongestants such as pseudoephedrine.

In a study of 118 patients with allergic rhinitis but not sinusitis, Shaikh reported that patients using 1% ephedrine-saline nasal wash every 48 hours for four weeks had improved nasal symptoms and inspiratory peak flow (14). In another prospective study, patients with acute bacterial sinusitis were treated with three weeks of amoxicillin/clavulanic acid and were randomized to receive 3% saline, fluticasone propionate, once daily 0.05% oxymetazoline, or no additional treatment (15). Though there was no significant difference in clinical outcome between the groups, the groups receiving saline and oxymetazoline had statistically significant increased mucociliary clearance as measured by the saccharin method.

An in vitro study using nasal respiratory tissue from healthy volunteers incubated with varying concentrations of phenylephrine found the opposite result, with the topical decongestant impairing ciliary function (16). Results of experiments with animal models have suggested that oxymetazoline might actually cause an increase in inflammation during acute bacterial sinusitis, though this suggestion has not been confirmed in humans (17).

A potential side effect of topical decongestants is the development of rebound nasal congestion or rhinitis medicamentosa. The rule of thumb is to advise patients to use a nasal decongestant for no more than 3–5 days consecutively. In 10 healthy volunteers who used 0.05% oxymetazoline nightly for four weeks, 80% developed nasal congestion in the evening before medication administration (18). The nasal obstruction appeared in some patients after as little as one week. However, even at week four, the obstruction was relieved by the nightly dose of oxymetazoline and within 48 hours of discontinuation, evening nasal congestion ended. This study suggests that using topical decongestants for up to four weeks may not lead to significant rebound and that this treatment rarely leads to more permanent tissue changes.

Oral decongestants are one of the most common active ingredients found in over-the-counter cough and cold medications and therefore are extensively used in patients with rhinosinusitis. Despite their frequent use, studies are lacking as to their efficacy in the treatment of sinus disease. There are numerous studies documenting the benefit of pseudoephedrine alone or in combination with antihistamines for the treatment of rhinitis. These studies have shown that congestion is consistently improved. Similar to topical decongestants, most patients report significant relief of symptoms when taking oral decongestants. Both topical and systemic decongestants can raise blood pressure making them relatively contraindicated in patients with hypertension.

In our clinic, topical nasal decongestants are used in an attempt to prevent upper respiratory tract infections or acute allergic inflammation from progressing into acute bacterial rhinosinusitis. We instruct patients with a history of recurrent rhinosinusitis to use nasal decongestants for 3–7 days at the first sign of a cold or congestion, along with nasal saline lavages, in an attempt to prevent acute bacterial rhinosinusitis from developing.

Topical Antiseptics and Antibiotics

Topical antibiotics and antiseptics have been used as adjunctive therapy, prophylaxis, and as primary therapies in the treatment of rhinosinusitis. Antiseptics may be mixed with saline and used for nasal washing in an attempt to sterilize or at least decrease the number of potential pathogens in the nasal-sinus cavity. Dilute solutions of povidone-iodine (e.g. Betadine®) and hydrogen peroxide have been used although there are no published studies which support their use. Anecdotally, at high concentrations, both agents can be very irritating to the nasal mucosa.

N-chlorotaurine (NCT) is an antiseptic that has been studied in the treatment of otitis externa and refractory rhinosinusitis (19). NCT is an endogenous antimicrobial that generates oxidants. It has activity against gram-positive bacteria, gram-negative bacteria, and fungal organisms. One case report was published using NCT for the treatment of refractory sinusitis in an immunosuppressed heart transplant patient (20). The compound was reportedly well tolerated and effective.

Tobramycin is probably the most commonly used topical antibiotic in the treatment of sinus disease. The drug has especially good activity against *Pseudomonas*, a species difficult to eradicate in some CRS patients. In a randomized trial assessing tobramycin delivered through a large particle nebulizer versus nebulized saline, Desrosiers and Salas-Prato found equal improvement of symptoms, quality of life scores, and mucosal appearance (21). In the population of CRS patients refractory to conventional medical and surgical interventions, tobramycin seemed to hasten improvement in pain scores. However, this treatment led to the development of nasal congestion. The authors concluded that tobramycin provided little additional benefit. Tobramycin is frequently used via nebulization into the lungs in patients with cystic fibrosis (CF). Patients with CF are also prone to sinus disease and anecdotally seem to benefit from using nebulized tobramycin intranasally.

Gentamycin (40 mg) and dexamethasone (2 mg) were instilled into the sinus antrum of 18 asthmatics with CRS. In this noncontrolled study, patients reported subjective improvement after the seven consecutive days of washings (22). Forced expiratory volume in one second (FEV_1) also significantly improved. Furthermore, there was a reduction in eosinophil cationic protein and tryptase levels in the patients' sinus fluid. However, without a control group, it is difficult to assess whether the effect was caused by gentamycin, dexamethasone, or the combination of the two.

There is currently great interest in the role of *Staphylococcus aureus* superantigens in nasal polyposis and hyperplastic sinus disease. Studies have shown increased *S. aureus* nasal colonization in patients with polyps and the presence of immunoglobulin E (IgE) antibodies directed against *S. aureus* enterotoxins (23). Both mupirocin and bacitracin are topical antibiotics with good activity against sensitive *Staphylococcus* species. No studies have specifically used either of these medications in hyperplastic sinus disease although both are commonly used to decrease *Staphylococcus* nasal carriage. An article published over 30 years ago described the use of nebulized bacitracin in patients with sinus disease (24). The author reported 100 of 100 patients cured, with an average of 3.17 treatments required to cure. There are also many reports of aerosolized penicillin being used to treat sinus disease in the 1940s (25,26).

In an in vitro study, Gosepath et al. observed the effect of topical antibiotics, antifungals, and antiseptics on the mucociliary activity of nasal respiratory cells (27).

Nasal respiratory cells were harvested from healthy individuals and exposed to solutions containing different concentrations of ofloxacin, betadine, hydrogen peroxide, amphotericin B, itraconazole, and clortrimazole. Ciliary beat frequency decreased after exposure to all agents at all concentrations. The authors concluded that although topical agents may be able to decrease intranasal pathogens, they also inhibit mucociliary clearance which is potentially detrimental. Furthermore, the degree of mucociliary inhibition was dose dependent, thus lower, rather than higher, concentrations of topical agents may be more beneficial.

There seems to be no role for intranasal antibiotics or antiseptics in the treatment of uncomplicated acute rhinosinusitis. In resistant CRS with or without polyposis, topical antimicrobials may be useful, particularly in patients with excessive mucus production and colonization with either *S. aureus* or a gram-negative rod, such as *Pseudomonas*. The presence of these bacteria should first be confirmed by culture and the antimicrobial susceptibility of the organism determined. Intranasal mupiricin is useful for patients colonized with *S. aureus* or in those with impetiginous crusting or secretions. Topical aminoglycoside treatment with either gentamycin or tobramycin (100 mg/l in saline solution) is useful for patients colonized with gram-negative bacteria.

Guaifenesin

Guaifenesin has long been a staple ingredient of over-the-counter cough and cold preparations. It has been best studied for cough, bronchitis, and other lower respiratory symptoms. In the bronchioles, it seems to increase respiratory tract fluid secretion, decreasing mucus viscosity, and helping to loosen phlegm. Its exact mechanism of action is poorly understood.

The potential benefit of guaifenesin as add-on therapy in rhinosinusitis is twofold. The drug has been shown to thin lower respiratory secretions (mucolytic action), and it can be surmised that it may be able to do the same in the upper airway. Potentially, decreasing the viscosity of mucus in the nose and paranasal sinuses would allow for improved mucociliary clearance of infectious mucus, thereby allowing the sinuses to more adequately drain. Secondly, a common feature of both acute and CRS is cough caused by post-nasal drip. Guaifenesin potentially has some antitussive effects.

As an antitussive agent, guaifenesin has been studied in controlled trials in adults with upper respiratory tract infections and cough. In a study comparing guaifenesin alone versus the combination of guaifenesin with either codeine or dextromethorphan, no difference was found between the groups when examining cough frequency, cough quality, sleep disturbance, or absenteeism (28). The authors concluded that guaifenesin was equally efficacious alone as in combination, although there was no placebo arm. Other studies have demonstrated the antitussive effects of both dextromethorphan and codeine (29). Kuhn et al. used both objective (cough count by recording) and subjective questionnaires to assess cough in young people with the common cold (30). No difference in cough frequency was found between patients receiving guaifenesin versus those receiving vehicle. Patients in the treatment group did report a subjective thinning in mucus quality.

Only one limited study has examined the role of guaifenesin in CRS. Using subjective scoring measures, 23 male patients with HIV, chronic nasal congestion, and mucoid postnasal drainage were randomized to receive either 1200 mg of guaifenesin or placebo taken twice daily for three weeks (31). Patients with evidence of an acute infection by radiograph were excluded. Patients treated with guaifenesin reported a significant decrease in nasal congestion at week three and a thinner quality of postnasal drainage at weeks two and three when compared with placebo. The quantity of postnasal drainage was not altered.

Guaifenesin is extremely safe and well tolerated with few potential drug interactions. There are very limited data supporting its use in patients with sinus disease, although patients do report some anecdotal benefit. Studies consistently report that mucus is perceived as less viscous after guaifenesin use, although multiple other subjective and objective measures have failed to demonstrate superiority to placebo. Guaifenesin should be considered as a symptom-relieving add-on therapy in patients complaining of thick tenacious mucous, especially in hypertensive patients for whom decongestants are contraindicated.

ADJUNCTIVE THERAPIES CONSIDERED IN SPECIFIC POPULATIONS
Antihistamines
In both adults and children, underlying allergic rhinitis predisposes patients to develop sinusitis. In adult and pediatric patients with rhinosinusitis, 55% were found to have allergic rhinitis (32). Similarly, in a population of Chinese children, Chen et al. found a link between allergic rhinitis, asthma, and atopic dermatitis with increased risk of sinopulmonary infection (33). Mechanistically, underlying allergic rhinitis can lead to nasal mucosa inflammation and ostial obstruction. Inflammatory mediators released during allergen exposure may also interfere with mucociliary function (34).

Antihistamines, either oral or intranasal, are frequently used by patients with allergic rhinitis as symptom relievers. Oral antihistamines typically decrease nasal itch, rhinorrhea, and sneezing. There is some evidence for a mild decongestive activity with the newer nonsedating antihistamines as well. In a multi-center, randomized, double-blind, placebo-controlled, parallel-group study, 139 patients with a history of allergic rhinitis and acute sinusitis diagnosed by symptoms, rhinoscopy, and radiograph were given loratadine or placebo along with conventional therapies (antibiotics and oral corticosteroids) (35). In the loratadine group, sneezing and nasal obstruction symptom scores were significantly improved when compared with the placebo group as was improvement as assessed by a blinded physician. Studies using a similar compound, desloratadine, have shown that the drug leads to both improved inspiratory nasal peak-flow and decreased subjective nasal congestion symptom scores when compared with placebo (36).

In an ovalbumin-sensitized mouse model, Kirtsreesakul et al. examined the effect of desloratadine during acute sinus infection (37). Sensitized mice were intranasally inoculated with *Streptococcus pneumoniae* and then observed for symptoms during allergen challenges. Additionally, nasal lavage was cultured and analyzed. In the desloratadine-treated group, symptoms were decreased, and lavage fluid demonstrated less infectious organisms and phagocytes.

In the UnitedStates, there is currently only one available topical antihistamine nasal spray, azelastine, although others are undergoing clinical trials. Azelastine is approved for the treatment of both allergic and nonallergic rhinitis. Azelastine functions as an H_1 receptor antagonist and also inhibits the formation of leukotrienes, cytokines, kinins, and the generation of superoxide free radicals (38). It also interferes with the expression of intercellular adhesion molecules.

To date there are no clinical trails using azelastine for rhinosinusitis. However, as the drug has decongestant effects without the potential for causing rhinitis medicamentosa, it may relieve some rhinosinusitis symptoms and perhaps aid in sinus drainage. It may also be used as a chronic maintenance medication in patients with CRS who have either allergic or nonallergic rhinitis as the underlying cause of chronic nasal inflammation.

It is unclear whether antihistamines are effective add-on therapies for rhinosinusitis. It is also unclear whether the potential decongesting properties are unique to loratadine and desloratadine or are present in other antihistamines. As a class, antihistamines certainly are safe and well tolerated thus making them worthwhile in allergic individuals who have rhinitis with or without sinusitis.

Antileukotrienes

Cysteinyl leukotrienes (LTC4, LTD4, and LTE4) increase vascular permeability, promote mucus secretion, and cause chemotaxis of inflammatory cells. Each of these actions may be relevant to the pathophysiology of sinus disease. Leukotrienes are clearly present in the inflamed nasal/sinus tissue of patients with chronic sinusitis, particularly those with aspirin sensitivity and/or polyposis (39–41). In a study of 34 patients with CRS, 22 with aspirin sensitivity, Sousa et al. found elevated numbers of inflammatory leukocytes expressing the $CysLT_1$ receptor (42). These cells were in a significantly greater abundance in aspirin-sensitive patients. However, in non-aspirin sensitive patients, $CysLT_1$ receptor expressing cells were also elevated.

To date there are no placebo-controlled trials using leukotriene receptor antagonists (LTRAs) or 5-LO inhibitors in the treatment of rhinosinusitis. Parnes and Chuma treated 40 patients with polyposis and rhinosinusitis with either zafirlukast or zileuton (43). The majority (72%) experienced subjective improvement with a significant decrease in headache, facial pain and pressure, ear discomfort, dentalgia, purulent nasal discharge, postnasal drip, congestion, fever, and anosmia. Half of the patients were reported to have stabilization of polyposis on endoscopic examination. A similar study found 50% subjective improvement and endoscopic stabilization in aspirin-sensitive patients with chronic sinus disease (44). Although studies employing zileuton have consistently shown symptom improvement, objective measures such as inspiratory nasal peak flow have not been altered by antileukotrienes (45). Case reports also suggest that antileukotrienes may play a role in the treatment of allergic fungal rhinosinusitis (46). Zileuton was also shown to reduce rhinorrhea and improve sense of smell in aspirin-sensitive asthmatic patients in a double-blind, placebo-controlled trial (47).

Immunotherapy

Whereas conventional immunotherapy (IT) has been shown to be of benefit in the treatment of allergic rhinitis, conjunctivitis, allergic fungal rhinosinusitis (AFRS), and asthma, there are only a few studies examining the role of IT in rhinosinusitis or allergic fungal rhinosinusitis. As there is an increased incidence of rhinosinusitis in atopic individuals, many patients with rhinosinusitis are placed on IT to treat the underlying allergic rhinitis with the hope that such treatment might reduce rhinosinusitis as well. In a study of 114 patients with a history of rhinitis and radiographic evidence of rhinosinusitis, Nathan et al. examined multiple subjective measures in patients receiving conventional aeroallergen IT (48). Patients who received IT for at least one year, with a mean duration of 3.3 years, reported a 61% improvement in sinus pain, 50% improvement in nasal purulent mucus, and a 49% improvement in nasal congestion. Furthermore, there was a 54% reduction in nasal/sinus surgical procedures and 74% fewer days lost from work or school. In an earlier study involving 72 allergic patients undergoing functional endoscopic sinus surgery, IT given before or after surgery did not influence middle meatal patency, synechiae formation, or polyp recurrence (49).

Although AFRS is relatively rare, there are more publications on the use of IT in this disorder than for treatment of conventional rhinosinusitis. The exact mechanism of AFRS is not entirely understood, but it likely involves Gell and Coombs type I and III hypersensitivity directed at colonizing fungi in the paranasal sinuses. The most frequently implicated fungal species include *Bipolaris, Aspergillus, Curvularia, Alternaria,* and *Helminthosporium* (50). In a group of 22 AFRS patients, Folker et al. placed 11 on IT directed at relevant fungal organisms following sinus surgery (50). The other 11 patients received routine care without IT. The mean duration of IT was 33 months. Patients receiving IT had significantly improved sinus-specific quality of life scores, improved CRS symptom scores, improved endoscopic mucosal staging scores, and required less topical and oral corticosteroids. Follow-up studies by the same group have shown equally impressive results (51). Furthermore, IT-treated patients were shown to require significantly fewer postoperative office visits and fewer repeat surgeries (52).

Other Adjuvants

Other therapies exist to treat the symptoms associated with rhinosinusitis and to hasten resolution of symptoms, although even less data exist supporting their efficacy. Patients are frequently encouraged to increase intake of fluids. In theory, this treatment may thin secretions aiding in their removal. Steam and hot compresses anecdotally help relieve some sensations of facial pain and pressure. Steam additionally may loosen nasal and chest secretions making mucus more easily expectorated.

Analgesics such as aspirin, nonsteroidal anti-inflammatory drugs (NSAIDs), cyclooxygenase-2 inhibitors, and acetaminophen can minimize sinus pain. Of course, aspirin and NSAIDs need to be avoided in patients with aspirin-sensitive sinus disease. Narcotic pain medications are rarely required for acute rhinosinusitis.

Therapies directed at shrinking and/or stabilizing nasal polyps certainly play a role in the chronic management of sinus disease. There is now a good deal of data supporting the role of aspirin desensitization in patients with aspirin-sensitive nasal and lower respiratory disease (see Chapter 17) (53). Intranasal furosemide has been demonstrated in one study to have an inhibitory effect on nasal polyp tissue (54).

SUMMARY AND RECOMMENDATIONS FOR TREATMENT

There is good evidence supporting the use of antibiotics, nasal corticosteroids, and probably saline lavage in the treatment of both acute and CRS. There is minimal evidence for the use of other adjuvants, although many add-on therapies have such anecdotal benefit that they have become common additions to the regimens of most patients undergoing treatment for sinus disease. Although there are few studies examining the use of oral decongestants, and the studies using topical decongestants are conflicting, patients almost universally report relief of facial pressure and pain after using such medications. Whether decongestants hasten the resolution of infection remains debatable. Guaifenesin may help reduce the symptom of postnasal drainage, but there are no controlled trials demonstrating this effect.

Adjuvants intended to alter disease outcome have even less supporting evidence. Case series using topical antibiotics and antiseptics have been conflicting, and further studies are needed. The same can be said for the use of allergen immunotherapy. While immunotherapy certainly provides relief of allergic nasal, ocular, and lower respiratory symptoms, the question remains as to whether IT also improves CRS. Antihistamines and antileukotrienes provide symptom relief in allergic patients but as yet have no proven benefit for CRS. Zileuton may be useful for rhinosinusitis in association with aspirin-sensitive asthma.

Our approach in the management of rhinosinusitis typically depends on the chronicity and relative complexity of the sinus disease. In patients with uncomplicated rhinosinusitis, use of an appropriate antibiotic coupled with 4–7 days of a topical decongestant along with nasal saline douching is usually adequate to both cure and provide symptom relief.

In patients with more complicated disease, prophylactic strategies are implemented in an attempt to decrease the frequency of infection and thus minimize the number of antibiotic courses required. Frequently, patients use daily lavage with hypertonic saline, nasal corticosteroids, and intermittent decongestants. In patients with underlying allergies contributing to nasal inflammation, antihistamines, antileukotrienes, and IT may be added.

When CRS patients develop acute infection, our usual recommendations are to increase the frequency of performing hypertonic saline lavage, use oral and topical decongestants, and prescribe a prolonged course of appropriate antibiotics. A short course of oral steroids may also be helpful to reduce inflammation and promote clearance of infection. A retrospective analysis of patients with CRS seems to indicate that an aggressive approach is of benefit. Twenty-six out of forty patients with CRS disease given prolonged antibiotics, oral steroids, nasal saline lavages, and nasal corticosteroids had symptom benefit at eight weeks (55). Similarly, an approach using four weeks of antibiotics, nasal saline lavage, nasal corticosteroids, and topical decongestants also had overwhelmingly positive outcomes (32). In patients who have persistent symptoms despite such treatment, it is critical to ascertain whether there is a persistent sinus infection. It is extremely useful to obtain sinus mucus samples for bacterial culture and sensitivity and fungal stains and cultures and to base therapy on the results of these tests. As previously mentioned, topical antibiotics or antiseptics may be useful both in acute treatment and at times for chronic maintenance/prophylaxis. Finally, guaifenesin, warm compresses, oral analgesics, and steam are worth considering in any patient with rhinosinusitis as safe and potentially beneficial symptom relievers.

REFERENCES

1. Wormald PJ, Cain T, Oates L, et al. A comparative study of three methods of nasal irrigation. Laryngoscope 2004; 114:2224–7.
2. Olson DE, Rasgon BM, Hilsinger RL. Radiographic comparison of three methods for nasal saline irrigation. Laryngoscope 2002; 112:1394–8.

3. Shoseyov D, Bibi H, Shai P, et al. Treatment with hypertonic saline versus normal saline was of pediatric chronic sinusitis. J Allergy Clin Immunol 1998; 101:602–5.
4. Rabago D, Zgierska A, Mundt M, Barrett B, Bobula J, Maberry R. Efficacy of daily hypertonic saline nasal irrigation among patients with sinusitis: a randomized controlled trial. J Fam Pract 2002; 51:1049–55.
5. Tomooka LT, Murphy C, Davidson TM. Clinical study and literature review of nasal irrigation. Laryngoscope 2000; 220:1189–93.
6. Heatley DG, McConnell KE, Kille TL, et al. Nasal irrigation for the alleviation of sinonasal symptoms. Otolaryngol Head Neck Surg 2001; 125:44–8.
7. Bachmann G, Hommel G, Michel O. Effect of irrigation of the nose with isotonic salt solution on adult patients with chronic paranasal sinus disease. Eur Arch Otorhinolaryngol 2000; 257:537–41.
8. Seaton TL. Hypertonic saline for chronic sinusitis. J Fam Prac 1998; 47:94.
9. Adam P, Stiffman M, Blake R. A clinical trial of hypertonic saline nasal spray in subjects with the common cold or rhinosinusitis. Arch Fam Med 1998; 7:39–43.
10. Talbot AR, Herr TM, Parsons DS. Mucociliary clearance and buffered hypertonic saline solution. Laryngoscope 1997; 107:500–3.
11. Keojampa BK, Nguyen MH, Ryan MW. Effects of buffered saline solution on nasal mucociliary clearance and nasal airway patency. Otolaryngol Head Neck Surg 2004; 131:679–82.
12. Boek WM, Keles N, Graamans K, et al. Physiologic and hypertonic saline solutions impair ciliary activity in vitro. Laryngoscope 1999; 109:396–9.
13. Stringer SP, Mancuso AA, Avino AJ. Effect of a topical vasoconstrictor on computed tomography of paranasal sinus disease. Laryngoscope 1993; 103:6–12.
14. Shaikh WA. Ephedrine-saline nasal wash in allergic rhinitis. J Allergy Clin Immunol 1995; 96:597–600.
15. Inanh S, Oxturk O, Korkmaz M, et al. The effects of topical agents of fluticasone propionate, oxymetazoline, and 3% and 0.9% sodium chloride solutions on mucociliary clearance in the therapy of acute bacterial rhinosinusitis in vivo. Laryngoscope 2002; 112:320–5.
16. Min YG, Yun YS, Rhee CS, et al. Effects of phenylephrine on ciliary beat in human respiratory epithelium: quantitative measurement by video-computerized analysis. Laryngoscope 1998; 108:418–21.
17. Bende M, Fukami M, Arfors KE, et al. Effect of oxymetazoline nose drops on acute sinusitis in the rabbit. Ann Otol Rhinol Laryngol 1996; 105:222–5.
18. Yoo JK, Seikaly H, Calhoun KH. Extended use of topical nasal decongestants. Laryngoscope 1997; 107:40–3.
19. Neher A, Nagl M, Appenroth E, et al. Acute otitis externa: efficacy and tolerability of N-chlorotaurine, a novel endogenous antiseptic agent. Laryngoscope 2004; 114:850–4.
20. Gstottner M, Nagl M, Pototschnig C, et al. Refractory rhinosinusitis complicating immunosuppression: application of N-chlorotaurine, a novel endogenous antiseptic agent. ORL J Otorhinolaryngol Relat Spec 2003; 65:303–5.
21. Desrosiers MY, Salas-Prato M. Treatment of chronic rhinosinusitis refractory to other treatments with topical antibiotic therapy delivered by means of a large-particle nebulizer: results of a controlled trial. Otolaryngol Head Neck Surg 2001; 125:265–9.
22. Kalogjera L, Vagic D, Baudion T. Effect of endosinusal treatment on cellular markers in mild and moderate asthmatics. Acta Otolaryngol 2003; 123:310–3.
23. Gevaert P, Holtappels G, Johansson SG, et al. Organization of secondary lymphoid tissue and local IgE formation to Staphylococcus aureus enterotoxins in nasal polyp tissue. Allergy 2005; 60:71–9.
24. Hopp ES, McGarvey WK. The treatment of paranasal sinusitis with aerosol bacitracin. Laryngoscope 1972; 82:1419–24.
25. Mutch N, Rewell RD. Penicillin by inhalation. Lancet 1945; 1:650–2.
26. Bryson V, Samsone E, Laskin S. Aerosolization of penicillin solutions. Science 1944; 100:33–5.

27. Gosepath J, Grebneva N, Mossikhin S, et al. Topical antibiotic, antifungal, and antiseptic solutions decrease ciliary activity in nasal respiratory cells. Am J Rhinol 2002; 16:25–31.
28. Croughan-Minibane MS, Petitti DB, Rodnick JE, Eliaser G. Clinical trial examining effectiveness of three cough syrups. J Am Board Fam Prac 1993; 6:109–15.
29. Empey DW, Laitinen GA, Bye CE, et al. Comparison of the antitussive effects of codeine phosphate 20 mg, dextromethorphan 30 mg and noscapione 30 mg using citric acid-induced cough in normal subjects. Eur J Clin Pharmacol 1979; 16:393–7.
30. Kuhn JJ, Hendley JO, Adams KF, et al. Antitussive effect of guaifenesin in young adults with natural colds. Chest 1982; 82:713–8.
31. Wawrose SF, Tami TA, Amoils CP. The role of guaifenesin in the treatment of sinonasal disease in patients infected with the human immunodeficiency virus (HIV). Laryngoscope 1992; 102:1225–8.
32. McNally PA, White MV, Kaliner MA. Sinusitis in an allergist's office: analysis of 200 consecutive cases. Allergy Asthma Proc 1997; 18:169–75.
33. Chen CF, Wu KG, Hsu MC, Tang RB. Prevalence and relationship between allergic disease and infectious diseases. J Microbiol Immunol Infect 2001; 34:57–62.
34. Kirtsreesakul V, Naclerio RM. Role of allergy in rhinosinusitis. Curr Opin Allergy Clin Immunology 2004; 4:17–23.
35. Braun JJ, Albert JP, Michel FB, et al. Adjunct effect of loratadine in the treatment of acute sinusitis in patients with allergic rhinitis. Allergy 1997; 52:650–5.
36. Bhatia S, Baroody FM, de Tineo M, et al. Increased nasal airflow with budesonide compared with desloratadine during the allergy season. Arch Otolaryngol Head Neck Surg 2005; 131:223–8.
37. Kirtsreesakul V, Blair C, Yu X, et al. Desloratadine partially inhibits the augmented bacterial responses in the sinuses of allergic and infected mice. Clin Exp Allergy 2004; 34:1649–54.
38. Lal D, Corey JP. Vasomotor rhinitis update. Curr Opin Otolaryngol Head Neck Surg 2004; 12:243–7.
39. Georgitis JW, et al. Increase in cysteinyl LTs in nasal lavage from patients with chronic sinusitis. Int Arch Allergy Immunol 1995; 106:416.
40. Steinke JW, Bradley D, Arango P, et al. Cysteinyl leukotriene expression in chronic hyperplastic sinusitis-nasal polyposis: importance to eosinophilia and asthma. J Allergy Clin Immunol 2003; 111:342–9.
41. Pérez-Novo CA, Watelet JB, Claeys C, Van Cauwenberge P, Bachert C. Prostaglandin, leukotriene, and lipoxin balance in chronic rhinosinusitis with and without nasal polyposis. J Allergy Clin Immunol 2005; 115:1189–96.
42. Sousa AR, Parikh A, Scadding G, et al. Leukotriene-receptor expression on nasal mucosal inflammatory cells in aspirin-sensitive rhinosinusitis. NEJM 2002; 347:1493–9.
43. Parnes SM, Chuma AV. Acute effects of antileukotrienes on sinonasal polyposis and sinusitis. Ear Nose Throat J 2000; 79:18–20.
44. Ulualp SO, Sterman BM, Toohill RJ. Antileukotriene therapy for the relief of sinus symptoms in aspirin triad disease. Ear Nose Throat J 1999; 78:604–6, 608, 613.
45. Wilson AM, White PS, Gardiner Q, et al. Effects of leukotriene receptor antagonist therapy in patients with chronic rhinosinusitis in a real life rhinology clinic setting. Rhinology 2001; 39:142–6.
46. Schubert MS. Antileukotriene therapy for allergic fungal sinusitis. J Allergy Clin Immunol 2001; 108:466–7.
47. Dahlen B, Nizankowska E, Szczeklik A, et al. Benefits from adding the 5-lipoxygenase inhibitor zileuton to conventional therapy in aspirin-intolerant asthmatics. Am J Respir Crit Care Med 1998; 157:1187–94.
48. Nathan RA, Santilli J, Rockwell W, et al. Effectiveness of immunotherapy for recurring sinusitis associated with allergic rhinitis as assessed by the Sinusitis Outcomes Questionnaire. Ann Allergy Asthma Immunol 2004; 92:668–72.
49. Nishioka GJ, Cook PR, Davis WE, et al. Immunotherapy in patients undergoing functional endoscopic sinus surgery. Otolaryngol Head Neck Surg 1994; 110:406–12.

50. Folker RJ, Marple BF, Mabry RL, Mabry CS. Treatment of allergic fungal sinusitis: a comparison trial of postoperative immunotherapy with specific fungal antigens. Laryngocope 1998; 108(11, Part 1):1623–7.
51. Mabry RL, Mabry CS. Allergic fungal sinusitis: the role of immunotherapy. Otolaryngol Clin North Am 2000; 33:433–40.
52. Bassichis BA, Marple BE, Mabry RL, Newcomer MT, Schwade ND. Use of immunotherapy in previously treated patients with allergic fungal sinusitis. Otolaryngol Head Neck Surg 2001; 125:487–90.
53. Stevenson DD, Hankammer MA, Mathison DA, et al. Aspirin desensitization treatment of aspirin-sensitive patients with rhinosinusitis-asthma: long-term outcomes. J Allergy Clin Immunol 1996; 98:751–8.
54. Passali D, Bernstein JM, Passali FM, et al. Treatment of recurrent chronic hyperplastic sinusitis with nasal polyposis. Arch Otolaryngol Head Neck Surgery 2003; 129:656–9.
55. Subramanian HN, Schechtman KB, Hamilos DL. A retrospective analysis of the treatment and time to relapse after intensive medical treatment for chronic sinusitis. Am J Rhinol 2002; 16:303–12.

16 Allergic Fungal Sinusitis

Mark S. Schubert
*Department of Medicine, University of Arizona College of Medicine, and
Allergy Asthma Clinic, Ltd., Phoenix, Arizona, U.S.A.*

INTRODUCTION

Fungal rhinosinusitis occurs as either tissue-invasive or tissue-noninvasive disease. There are three types of invasive and two types of noninvasive disease (Table 1). The various types of fungal rhinosinusitis are distinguishable histopathologically and clinically. Allergic fungal rhinosinusitis (AFRS), also known as allergic fungal sinusitis, is a distinct type of noninvasive fungal rhinosinusitis that represents more of an allergic/hypersensitivity response to the presence of small numbers of extramucosal fungi living within the sinus cavity(s) rather than a fungal infection per se. The fungi are found growing within a characteristic extramucosal peanut-buttery mucus inspissate of many compressed pyknotic eosinophils along with their degranulation products, known as allergic mucin (1–4). AFRS is analogous in many ways to allergic bronchopulmonary aspergillosis (ABPA), a hypersensitivity disease of the lung (2,4–5,8).

Allergic fungal rhinosinusitis is also a form of chronic hypertrophic sinus disease, or chronic rhinosinusitis (CRS) (4,9). Chronic rhinosinusitis also called by other names including CRS, chronic rhinosinusitis with nasal polyps, and hyperplastic sinusitis, is a common chronic sinonasal eosinophilic-lymphocytic inflammatory respiratory condition characterized clinically by chronically recurring sinonasal mucosal hypertrophy, hyperplasia, and edematous polyp formation, and immunologically by its similarity to asthma (9,10). Indeed, the clinical and immunologic similarities between AFRS, CRS, asthma, and other chronic eosinophilic-lymphocytic respiratory disorders suggest that they all have related or shared pathophysiology(s) (9). This chapter compares and contrasts AFRS as both a type of fungal rhinosinusitis and as a type of CRS. The differential diagnosis, diagnostic criteria, and current approach to treatment are reviewed.

AFRS CLINICAL PRESENTATION

Allergic fungal rhinosinusitis has an incidence of between 5–10% of all CRS going to surgery (1,11–13). The southern and southwestern United States appear to have the highest incidence of disease, presumably because the fungi that cause AFRS are indigenous to these areas. Most cases of AFRS are due to the dematiaceous fungi ("phaeohyphomycosis") that include *Bipolaris, Curvularia, Exserohilum*, and *Alternaria* spp.; *Aspergillus* spp. ("hyalohyphomycosis") are also found in some cases (4,5).

Patients with AFRS have chronic unilateral or bilateral CRS with nasal polyps (4,5,8,14). They tend to be young, immunocompetent, and have inhalant allergy (atopy) (5). They may give a history for previous sinus surgery because AFRS is highly recurrent (5,14). They commonly describe nasal cast production,

TABLE 1   Types of Fungal Rhinosinusitis

Invasive fungal rhinosinusitis
Acute necrotizing fungal rhinosinusitis
Chronic invasive fungal rhinosinusitis
Granulomatous invasive fungal rhinosinusitis
Noninvasive fungal rhinosinusitis
Fungal ball (sinus mycetoma)
Allergic fungal rhinosinusitis

Source: From Ref. 6.

green to black rubbery formed elements made of allergic mucin, expelled from the nose (5). The sinus computed tomography (CT) is always abnormal (Fig. 1), often showing areas of increased contrast ("hyperattenuation") within the paranasal sinuses that represent inspissated allergic mucin (4,5,14). Extrasinus extension of AFRS from the paranasal sinuses into the orbit or into the cranium has been reported (5,15), although this does not represent tissue or bone invasion with fungi. Rather, the bone appears to be resorbed due to juxtaposition and pressure from the expanding fungal-containing allergic mucin mass. This may cause proptosis and facial asymmetry (Fig. 1).

Patients with AFRS are immunocompetent both by clinical history and laboratory evaluations (5,14). Allergy skin testing shows multiple positives to common aeroallergens, including the etiologic AFRS organism (5). Total serum immunoglobulizn (IgE) is usually elevated, although typically not as high as with ABPA (4,5). However, a normal total serum IgE in AFRS can also occasionally be seen (5). The total serum IgE appears to act as an "allergic acute phase reactant" in AFRS, similar to that seen in ABPA, rising with disease exacerbations and falling with remissions (7). Other laboratory parameters should be normal. For example,

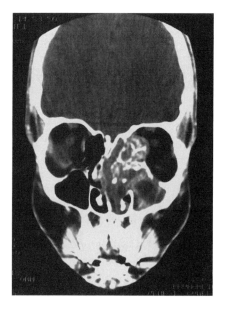

FIGURE 1   Sinus CT scan (tissue window) of an AFRS patient.

significant peripheral eosinophilia or an elevated erythrocyte sedimentation rate is generally not seen (5).

AFRS PATHOPHYSIOLOGY

It is likely that AFRS can develop in a patient with pre-established CRS, but can also occur de novo as the cause of the CRS (14). The host's inflammatory response to the presence of the etiologic fungi within the sinuses allows the formation and accumulation of extramucosal allergic mucin, which serves as the substrate for continued fungal growth and persistence. Inflammation-induced injury to the mucosal epithelium causes impairment in sinonasal mucociliary transport with resultant functional sinus obstruction. Functional sinus obstruction further promotes the accumulation and inspissation of allergic mucin. Allergic mucin itself likely contributes to mucosal inflammation and injury because it is an eosinophil-rich proinflammatory material that includes eosinophil degranulation products that are mucosal and epithelial cell-toxic (16). Subsequent mucosal hypertrophy, hyperplasia, and polyp formation eventually lead to anatomic sinus obstruction with trapping of an expanding fungal-containing allergic mucin mass. This ongoing "AFRS sinusitis cycle" allows the perpetuation of an inflammatory milieu conducive to the continued development and persistence of AFRS (14).

The striking association of dematiaceous fungi and *Aspergillus*, but paucity of other fungi reported from AFRS surgical sinus cultures, together with the findings of fungal-specific IgE and IgG, and an elevated total serum IgE that fluctuates with disease activity (5,14), suggests that the involved fungi have important physicochemical properties that make them "sinonasophilic," and immunogenic properties that result in CRS.

Recent research has shown that AFRS and other forms of CRS are associated with the human leukocyte antigen (HLA) class II major histocompatibility (MHC) genes of the HLA-DQ3 family (17). Many other chronic inflammatory diseases are also associated with MHC class II genes, suggesting that CRS rhinosinusitis disorders share mechanisms of immunopathogenesis at a fundamental level with other common chronic inflammatory disorders.

The MHC class II genes code for cell surface molecules on professional antigen-presenting cells (such as dendritic cells) that bind foreign antigenic protein fragments (peptides) and present them to T cell receptors on T cells, allowing the T cells to "see" and be activated by the foreign antigen. This manifests ultimately in humoral and cell-mediated antigen-specific immune responses. When analyzed and compared to other CRS patients without AFRS, with and without the presence of atopy, it was concluded that the HLA-DQ3 association with AFRS and other forms of CRS included factors in addition to antigen presentation specificities (17). For example, it has recently been speculated that microbial superantigens serve as an important immunostimulatory factor that lead to the intensity and chronicity of inflammation seen in AFRS and other common forms of CRS (9). A number of microbial superantigens are currently known, including those that cause staphylococcal food poisoning and toxic shock syndrome; as such they represent one mechanism of microbial virulence. Superantigens act by binding to the sides of the MHC class II molecule and T cell receptor on the antigen-presenting cell and the T cell, respectively, forming a molecular bridge that bypasses antigen specificity and causes activation of subsets of T cells expressing particular V-region gene elements. Involvement of microbial superantigens has already been shown or

TABLE 2 AFRS Diagnostic Criteria

Characteristic allergic mucin seen on surgical sinus histopathology or grossly at surgery
Fungal stain-positive for hyphae within the allergic mucin or surgical sinus fungal culture-positive
Sinus mucosal inflammatory infiltrate—small lymphocytes, plasma cells, eosinophils without
  necrosis, granulomas or fungal invasion
Other fungal diseases are excluded; no histologic evidence of invasive fungal disease
Evidence of AFRS etiologic fungal-specific IgE by skin testing or in vitro testing[a]

[a]Technical limitations, such as a negative surgical sinus fungal culture, may preclude this as a diagnostic criteria
  in selected cases; see Figures 2, 3, and 4.
Source: Adapted from Refs. 5, 29.

implicated in a number of other chronic inflammatory diseases, including atopic dermatitis, psoriasis, chronic severe asthma, Kawasaki's disease, rheumatoid arthritis, multiple sclerosis, type I diabetes, and inflammatory bowel diseases (9).

DIAGNOSIS OF AFRS

Histopathologic criteria must be met when diagnosing any form of fungal rhinosinusitis. Diagnostic criteria for AFRS are listed in Table 2. Characteristic allergic mucin must be seen, a fungal stain (e.g., Gomori's methenamine silver stain) and/or surgical sinus fungal cultures must be positive, and the sinus mucosal histopathology should show an "allergic" or "asthmatic" inflammatory infiltrate of lymphocytes and eosinophils. In addition, other fungal diseases must be excluded.

The diagnosis of AFRS is most easily facilitated when the allergic mucin is found histopathologically to stain positively for fungal elements (Fig. 2). However, it is important to distinguish AFRS from the other noninvasive fungal rhinosinusitis disorder, fungal ball (sinus mycetoma) (Table 1). In fungal ball, multitudes of fungal hyphae are compressed into a mass, usually without the presence of allergic mucin, whereas in AFRS only sparse numbers of fungal hyphae are present within allergic mucin (4,11,14).

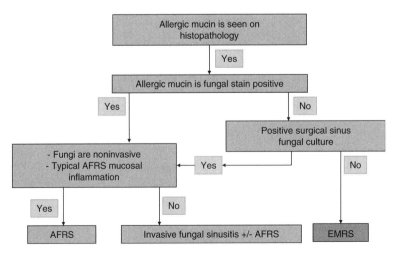

FIGURE 2 For diagnosis of AFRS. Presence of allergic mucin by histopathology or grossly; allergic mucin either stains positive for fungal hyphae or the surgical sinus fungal culture is positive; no histological evidence for fungal tissue-invasion.

Unfortunately, surgical sampling limitations may occasionally provide specimens from AFRS surgery in which no fungal hyphae can be found within the allergic mucin. To diagnose AFRS in these cases, the surgical fungal culture must be positive (Fig. 2). If allergic mucin is present but is fungal stain-negative, and if the surgical fungal culture is negative, the diagnosis of exclusion is eosinophilic mucin rhinosinusitis (EMRS) (Figs. 2 and 3) (4,18), although a better name for this type of CRS would have been allergic mucin rhinosinusitis because the "eosinophilic mucin" is actually allergic mucin. Inspissated allergic mucin in EMRS also hyperattenuates on sinus CT and is radiographically similar to the fungal-containing allergic mucin present in AFRS, demonstrating that the allergic mucin itself is involved in the radiographic hyperattenuation seen in AFRS (19). Although some patients with EMRS may actually have AFRS that is not diagnosed due to surgical sampling error, patients with "true" EMRS do not have AFRS despite the presence of characteristic allergic mucin, and the involvement of fungi will not be found on any previous or subsequent surgeries for recurrent CRS.

If an EMRS patient is atopic to common aeroallergens on allergy testing, they can also be considered an "AFRS candidate" (Fig. 3) but cannot be diagnosed with AFRS in the absence of a positive fungal stain or fungal culture. However, if the EMRS patient is nonatopic, it is unlikely they have AFRS because common inhalant atopy is nearly always present in AFRS (4,8,14). Interestingly, many EMRS patients have the triad of CRS, asthma, and aspirin/nonsteroidal antiinflammatory drug hypersensitivity (acetyl salicylic asid (ASA) triad) (4).

Surgical sampling error may also occasionally deprive the pathologist of histopathologic allergic mucin for fungal staining despite its characteristic presence grossly at surgery and its description in the operative report. To diagnose AFRS in such cases, the surgical sinus fungal culture must be positive, along with the other diagnostic criteria (Fig. 4).

The presence of a sinus CT showing CRS with areas of hyperattenuation, description of characteristic allergic mucin grossly or histopathologically, inhalant

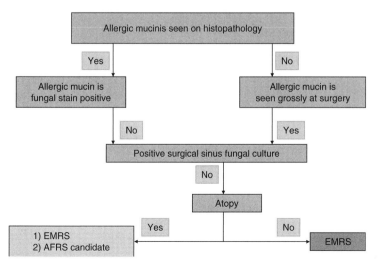

FIGURE 3 For diagnosis of AFRS candidate. Allergic mucin is present histopathologically or grossly; fungal stain and surgical sinus fungal culture are negative; presence of inhalant atopy (particularly for dematiaceous fungi).

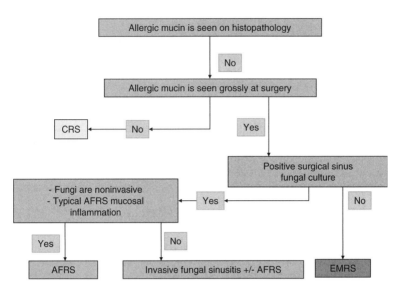

FIGURE 4 For diagnosis of AFRS. Allergic mucin is seen grossly (but not histopathologically); surgical sinus fungal culture is positive; no histological evidence for fungal tissue-invasion.

atopy, and immunocompetence are all found in AFRS but are not in themselves diagnostic for AFRS since similar findings can be present in non-AFRS CRS including EMRS. However, these clinical findings will always be present in an AFRS patient and will support the diagnosis of AFRS. Allergy skin test positivity to the etiologic AFRS mold is present in all patients with AFRS, but is insufficient to diagnose AFRS because these molds also cause common inhalant atopy, such as allergic rhinitis. The diagnosis of AFRS would have to be questioned, however, when a patient with suspected AFRS is allergy skin test-negative to the mold cultured from sinus surgery. It would be very unlikely that this mold was the causative AFRS organism since fungal-specific IgE to the etiologic mold is always present in AFRS (4,5). This might occur when allergic mucin is seen at surgery but histopathologic fungal stain is negative in the setting of a positive surgical fungal culture. This underscores the need for careful surgical sampling for culture, because accidental nasal contamination can easily lead to false-positive fungal and bacterial cultures, representing a pitfall to be avoided in the diagnosis of AFRS (4,8,14).

TREATMENT OF AFRS

Surgical treatment alone, without postoperative medical management, leads to AFRS recurrence rates of up to 100% depending on the expert referenced (4,8). Adequate surgical removal of diseased mucosa and allergic mucin is an important first step in the treatment of any AFRS patient. Unfortunately, there are no fully controlled studies published for the medical treatment of AFRS. The closest we have to such a study is the large eight year retrospective study of 67 AFRS patients from Phoenix, AZ, where half were given postoperative oral corticosteroids (OCS) utilizing a specific protocol for up to one year, and the other half were otherwise treated similarly with allergy medications and allergen immunotherapy, but were not given OCS (7). Results showed the OCS-treated group to have substantially less rhinosinusitis activity and surgical recurrence rates compared to those not treated with OCS. The rationale behind using OCS for AFRS was based on previous failures with systemic antifungals for AFRS and the success with OCS treatment for the analogous lung disease, ABPA. The OCS protocol for AFRS was 0.5 mg prednisone/kg every AM for two weeks postoperatively, followed by 0.5 mg/kg every other AM for two weeks, then gradually tapering to 5–7.5 mg every other AM by three months postoperatively, then maintaining 5 mg every other AM for the duration of treatment. Patients were typically treated with OCS for one year. AFRS recurrence was further reduced by using a short "burst" of OCS during intercurrent episodes of acute rhinosinusitis, with antibiotics if indicated, with rapid taper to the baseline OCS dose. Because of the clinical success and lack of significant side effects reported with the careful use of this OCS protocol, together with many additional published cases using OCS for AFRS, the consensus is that postoperative OCS treatment for AFRS should strongly be considered. However, it is recommended that patients undergo an initial evaluation to rule out significant contraindications to the use of OCS, such as a positive purified protein derivative (PPD) skin test or evidence for high-risk infectious disease, cataracts, glaucoma, osteoporosis, history for avascular osteonecrosis, diabetes, hematologic disease, or immunocompromised state (4,8).

Other medical treatments commonly used for AFRS include antihistamines, nasal corticosteroids, and allergen immunotherapy to the relevant aeroallergens involved in the patient's inhalant atopy (4,8,14). A case report of the successful use of the oral antileukotriene montelukast in AFRS has also been reported (20). The rationale behind using allergy medications and allergen immunotherapy is that these patients have underlying atopy as an AFRS risk factor, and any treatment that can realistically reduce the conditions conducive to AFRS relapse and need for continuation of OCS should be considered.

Topical antifungals via nose spray or nebulizer have not been adequately studied for AFRS. Such treatment might eventually be shown to be helpful in AFRS but would potentially be problematic due to difficulty in getting medicine to the deep sinus cavities. There are, however, several published placebo-controlled studies using either tobramycin or amphotericin B nasal spray or lavage for patients with non-AFRS CRS. One study reported clinical worsening with tobramycin (21). One study using an intranasal spray of amphotericin B found no difference from placebo (22); however, a study using a larger volume amphotericin B nasal irrigation reported borderline improvement in mucosal thickening with active treatment (23). However, a recent large, double-blind, placebo-controlled, multicenter study confirmed the lack of efficacy of sinonasal amphotericin B for patients with recurrent CRS both with and without nasal polyps (30). In yet another study, using high-dose oral terbinifine failed to show improvement in mucosal thickening or CRS symptoms compared to placebo (24).

The amphotericin B studies were prompted because Ponikau et al. hypothesized that most patients with any form of CRS actually have AFRS or undefined fungal-related immunopathogenesis at some level (25). The authors had reached this conclusion because virtually all CRS patients in their study had had a multitude of different fungi cultured from transnasal acquisition of mucus, but this study has been criticized because their control patients without sinus disease also showed the same result, likely reflecting nasal contamination by this culturing protocol (26–28). Such nasal contamination leads to false-positive sinus culture results and is a pitfall to be avoided in the diagnosis of AFRS (4,8,14). It still remains to be proved whether fungi really play any role in the pathogenesis of the common forms of non-AFRS CRS.

The total serum IgE should be followed postoperatively in AFRS patients at intervals as it can help guide medical-surgical decision-making (7). A rising total serum IgE is associated with AFRS recurrence, and a falling IgE is associated with remission, analogous to that seen in ABPA.

CONCLUSION

The most common form of fungal rhinosinusitis is AFRS. Like other forms of CRS, it is often associated with high surgical recurrence rates and a difficult clinical course. Treatment is challenging, requiring close medical-surgical cooperation for the best long-term outcomes. Recent recognition that AFRS and other common forms of CRS are chronic inflammatory diseases has led to a further understanding of their immunopathogenesis, and possible relationships to other common inflammatory diseases. Additional studies of the immunopathogenesis, genetics, role of microbes, and optimal surgical and medical treatment approaches for AFRS and other forms of CRS are needed to ultimately improve the clinical outcome for all of these patients.

REFERENCES

1. Katzenstein AA, Sale SR, Greenburger PA. Allergic *Aspergillus* sinusitis: a newly recognized form of sinusitis. J Allergy Clin Immunol 1983;72:89–93.
2. Gourley DS, Whisman BA, Jorgensen NL, et al. Allergic Bipolaris sinusitis: clinical and immunopathologic characteristics. J Allergy Clin Immunol 1990; 85:583–91.
3. Bent JP III, Kuhn FA. Diagnosis of allergic fungal sinusitis. Otolaryngol Head Neck Surg 1994; 111:580–8.
4. Schubert MS. Allergic fungal sinusitis. Otolaryngol Clin North Am 2004; 37:301–326.
5. Schubert MS, Goetz DW. Evaluation and treatment of allergic fungal sinusitis. I. Demographics and diagnosis. J Allergy Clin Immunol 1998; 102:387–94.
6. deShazo RD, Chapin K., Swain RE. N Engl J Med 1997; 337:254–59.
7. Schubert MS, Goetz DW. Evaluation and treatment of allergic fungal sinusitis. II. Treatment and follow-up. J Allergy Clin Immunol 1998; 102:395–402.
8. Schubert MS. Allergic fungal sinusitis: Pathogenesis and management strategies. Drugs 2004; 64:363–374.
9. Schubert MS. A superantigen hypothesis for the pathogenesis of chronic hypertrophic rhinosinusitis, allergic fungal sinusitis, and related disorders. Ann Allergy Asthma Immunol 2001; 87:181–8.
10. Hamilos DL. Chronic sinusitis. J Allergy Clin Immunol 2000; 106:213–27.
11. Ferreiro JA, Carlson BA, Cody DT. Paranasal sinus fungus balls. Head Neck 1997; 19:481–6.
12. Ence BK, Gourley DS, Jorgensen NL, et al. Allergic fungal sinusitis. Am J Rhinol 1990; 4:169–78.
13. Collins MM, Nair SB, Wormald PJ. Prevalence of noninvasive fungal sinusitis in South Australia. Am J Rhinol 2003; 17:127–32.
14. Schubert MS. Medical treatment of allergic fungal sinusitis. Ann Allergy Asthma Immunol 2000; 85:90–101.
15. McClay JE, Marple B, Kapadia L, et al. Clinical presentation of allergic fungal sinusitis in children. Laryngoscope 2002; 112:565–9.
16. Khan DA, Cody TC III, George TJ, et al. Allergic fungal sinusitis: an immunohistologic analysis. J Allergy Clin Immunol 2000; 106:1096–1101.
17. Schubert MS, Hutcheson PS, Graff RJ, Santiago L, Slavin RG. HLA-DQB1*03 in allergic fungal sinusitis and other chronic hypertrophic rhinosinusitis disorders. J Allergy Clin Immunol 2004; 114:1376–83.

18. Ferguson BJ. Eosinophilic mucin rhinosinusitis: a distinct clinicopathological entity. Laryngoscope 2000; 110:799–813.
19. Schubert MS. Fungal rhinosinusitis: diagnosis and therapy. Curr Allergy Asthma Rep 2001; 1:268–76.
20. Schubert MS. Antileukotriene therapy for allergic fungal sinusitis. J Allergy Clin Immunol 2001; 108:466–7.
21. Desrosiers MY, Salas-Prato M. Treatment of chronic rhinosinusitis refractory to other treatments with topical antibiotic therapy delivered by means of a large-particle nebulizer: results of a controlled trial. Otolaryngol Head Neck Surg 2001; 125:265–9.
22. Weschta M, Rimek D, Formanek M, et al. Topical antifungal treatment of chronic rhinosinusitis with nasal polyps: A randomized, double-blind clinical trial. J Allergy Clin Immunol 2004; 113:1122–8.
23. Ponikau JU, Sherris DA, Weaver A, Kita H. Treatment of chronic rhinosinusitis with intranasal amphotericin B: A randomized, placebo-controlled, double-blind pilot trial. J Allergy Clin Immunol 2005; 115:125–31.
24. Kennedy DW, Kuhn FA, Hamilos DL, et al. Treatment of chronic rhinosinusitis with high-dose oral terbinafine: a double blind, placebo-controlled study. Laryngoscope. 2005; 115:1793–9.
25. Ponikau JU, Sherris DA, Kern EB, et al. The diagnosis and incidence of allergic fungal sinusitis. Mayo Clin Proc 1999; 74:877–84.
26. Kuhn FA, Javer AR. Allergic fungal sinusitis: a four year follow-up. Am J Rhinol 2000; 14:149–56.
27. Dibbern DA, Dreskin SC. Allergic fungal sinusitis. Mayo Clin Proc 2000; 75:122. [Letter to the Editor].
28. Page EH. Allergic fungal sinusitis. Mayo Clin Proc 2000; 75:122. [Letter to the Editor].
29. Meltzer EO, Hamilos DL, Hadley JA, et al. Rhinosinusitis: establishing definitions for clinical research and patient care. Published simultaneously in J Allergy Clin Immunol 2004; 114(6 Suppl.):155–212 and Otolaryngol Head Neck Surg 2004; 131(6 Suppl.): S1–62.
30. Ebbens FA, Scadding GK, Badia L, et al. Amphotericin B nasal lavages: not a solution for patients with chronic rhinosinusitis. J Allergy Clin Immunol 2006; 118:1149–56.

17 Medical Management of Rhinosinusitis Comorbidities—Asthma, Aspirin Sensitivity, Gastroesophageal Reflux, Immune Deficiencies

Raymond G. Slavin

Division of Allergy and Immunology, Department of Internal Medicine, St. Louis University School of Medicine, St. Louis, Missouri, U.S.A.

INTRODUCTION

This monograph is largely concerned with patterns of illness, pathophysiology, and management of chronic rhinosinusitis (CRS). It is important to realize that CRS does not occur alone but may, in many instances, exist in association with other medical conditions or comorbidities. Some of these associated conditions may predispose to the development of CRS. Some may be worsened by the presence of CRS. Finally, some may simply be seen as co-existent. It is the intent of this chapter to discuss four co-morbid conditions commonly seen in CRS, to delve into the pathophysiologic mechanisms, and finally deal with their management.

ASTHMA
Association of Rhinosinusitis and Asthma

The association between bronchial asthma and paranasal sinusitis has been noted for many years. A number of clinical studies performed as early as the 1920s and 1930s emphasized rhinosinusitis as a trigger for worsening of asthma (1,2). This relationship was eventually disputed because of the then prevailing notions that sinus changes simply reflected a disease of the entire respiratory membrane and that management of rhinosinusitis would have little effect on the course of lower respiratory tract disease. In the past two decades, however, the relationship between the upper and lower airways has been re-examined.

One piece of evidence that demonstrates a strong relationship between rhinosinusitis and asthma is a study conducted in the Los Angeles Children's Hospital that showed that 75% of pediatric patients admitted with status asthmaticus had abnormal sinus radiographs (3). Another study from Finland that was performed in adults reported abnormal sinus films in 87% of adults with asthma exacerbations (4). In a report from the Netherlands, 84% of adults with severe asthma showed sinus computed tomography (CT) abnormalities (5). A more recent study (6) looked at 35 patients with severe asthma taking corticosteroids every day and 34 patients with mild to moderate asthma. The authors found that all the subjects with severe asthma had abnormalities as revealed in the CT scans of the sinuses compared with 88% of the individuals with mild to moderate asthma.

There has been a suggestion that the association between CRS and asthma is strong only in those with extensive sinus disease. It appears that peripheral blood eosinophil level is a good marker for extensive rhinosinusitis. In a study by

Newman et al. (7), 104 patients undergoing sinus surgery had their CT scans reviewed for extent of disease and total serum IgE as well as specific IgE antibodies to common inhalant antigens measured, and a peripheral blood sample analyzed for total eosinophil count. The authors found that among the patients with peripheral eosinophilia, 87% had extensive sinus disease as found by CT scan.

The previously cited study from the Netherlands (5) showed that the vast majority of patients with severe asthma not only had sinus CT abnormalities but that the extent of sinus disease was also positively related to airway inflammation. This was reflected by the increased eosinophil count in induced sputum and peripheral blood, as well as the level of nitric oxide (NO) in exhaled air. This is indicative of an association between sinonasal and lower airway inflammation in patients with severe asthma.

The overriding question is whether the association between rhinosinusitis and asthma represents an epiphenomenon—that is, are rhinosinusitis and asthma manifestations of the same underlying disease process in different parts of the respiratory tract, or are they causally related? Can rhinosinusitis trigger bronchial asthma? (8).

Although more clinical evidence is needed, some data suggest that difficult-to-treat asthma can be better controlled if the coexisting rhinosinusitis is addressed, either with medications or surgery. This indicates evidence for an etiologic role of rhinosinusitis in lower airway disease.

Results of Medical Therapy of Rhinosinusitis on Asthma

Currently, no controlled study has been performed in adults that demonstrates improvement in asthma symptoms by medically treating patients with rhinosinusitis. There are, however, a number of studies of children that show a significant improvement in the asthmatic state with appropriate antibiotic treatment for coexistent rhinosinusitis. In a study by Rachelefsky et al. (9), 79% of the children were able to discontinue bronchodilator medication after the rhinosinusitis was medically treated. Pulmonary function test results were normal in 67% of patients who had demonstrated pretreatment abnormalities. Similar results were reported in another group of children from the University of Pittsburgh (10).

Another similar study carried out by Oliveira and Sole (11) looked at improvement of bronchial hyperresponsiveness (BHR) in children treated for sinusitis. The authors studied 46 atopic and 20 normal children. Methacholine challenges were done both before and 30 days after the sinusitis was treated with nasal saline, antibiotics, antihistamine, or decongestant, along with 5 days of prednisone. The authors found that the only patients who showed a decrease in their sensitivity to methacholine after treatment were those with rhinitis and asthma with opacified maxillary sinuses at entry and those who had normal sinus radiographs at 30 days into the study. Therefore, the authors concluded that children with allergic rhinitis and sinusitis with asthma had improvements in their BHR to methacholine and their symptoms decreased, with their sinuses responding appropriately to medical therapy.

Effects of Surgical Therapy of Rhinosinusitis on Asthma

There is evidence in the literature that patients with medically resistant rhinosinusitis demonstrate improvement in their asthma after definitive nasosinus surgery. One study looked at 205 adult patients with the aspirin triad, all of whom were steroid-dependent (12). The aspirin triad, sometimes called Samters triad or, more recently, aspirin exacerbated airway disease (AERD), includes nasal polyps, asthma, and aspirin sensitivity. These patients underwent functional endoscopic sinus surgery (FESS). After the procedure, 40% of the patients were able to discontinue their daily steroids for asthma control, and another 44% were able to decrease the dose of steroids to either every other day or only bursts. This study is particularly notable because patients with AERD have notoriously difficult-to-treat asthma. Another study looked at 20 patients between 16 and 72 years of age with asthma and CRS. These patients also underwent FESS. After the procedure, 70% reported the frequency of asthma to be less, and 65% reported less severe asthma. Notably, there was a 75% reduction in hospitalizations and an 81% reduction in emergency room and urgent care clinic visits in the year after they underwent FESS (13).

In children too, the effect of FESS on CRS and asthma is promising. Parsons and Phillips (14) reported a reduction of 89% in chronic cough and a 96% decrease in asthma after FESS in 52 children 7 months to 17 years of age. Additionally, the number of asthma exacerbations per month decreased from 6.7 to 2.5 and emergency room visits declined by 79%. Manning et al. (15) studied 14 steroid-dependent childhood asthmatic patients, six of whom were immune-deficient. After FESS, 11 of the children showed improvement in their asthma, there was a decrease in school days lost from 22.23 to 14.5, and a decrease in days in hospital from 21.4 to 6.

A study by Dunlop et al. (16) looked at 50 patients with asthma who had undergone endoscopic surgery. A total of 20% had reduction in the amount of inhaled corticosteroids required, and there were significant decreases in the use of oral corticosteroids and hospitalizations in the year after the surgery. Similarly, Dhong et al. (17) observed 19 patients who underwent endoscopic sinus surgery for rhinosinusitis. These patients demonstrated significant improvements in diurnal and nocturnal asthma symptoms and had improvements in asthma medication scores. No changes were noted in pulmonary function tests. In an adult outcome study by Gliklich and Metson (18), it was noted that patients with pre-existing asthma had the greatest improvement in overall health measures after sinus surgery. However, Goldstein et al. (19) performed a retrospective medical record analysis on 13 patients with asthma who underwent FESS for medically refractory CRS and found no significant change in group mean asthma symptoms, asthma medication usage, pulmonary function test results, and number of emergency room visits or hospitalizations.

Ikayama et al. (20) studied 42 patients with CRS, 50 patients with stable asthma, 50 patients with chronic bronchitis, and 40 patients with allergic rhinitis and compared their methacholine BHR. They found that BHR of subjects with CRS was less than that of the subjects with asthma but was similar to those with chronic bronchitis or allergic rhinitis in both its prevalence and degree. The authors further examined patients with CRS and bronchial asthma who had undergone endoscopic surgery. They noted that after the surgical treatment, the patients had a significant decrease in their BHR with improvements in both nasal symptoms and sinus lesions. Therefore, adequate therapy of CRS appears to reduce BHR.

Mechanisms Relating Rhinosinusitis with Asthma

Although the exact mechanism that links rhinosinusitis with asthma is unknown, a number of possibilities have been suggested. Four such theories involve the eosinophil, inflammatory mediators, neural reflexes, and circulating factors (Table 1).

TABLE 1   Mechanisms Relating Chronic Rhinosinusitis to Asthma

Eosinophils
Inflammatory mediators
Neural reflexes
Circulating factors

Eosinophils
It is well known that the eosinophil has a role in mediating bronchial epithelial injury in patients with chronic asthma. The role of the eosinophil in chronic inflammatory disease of the paranasal sinuses has been evaluated by examining tissues of patients undergoing surgery for CRS. In one such study, it was shown that whereas sinus tissues of patients with sinusitis and concomitant asthma, allergic rhinitis, or both had a large number of infiltrated eosinophils, patients with a history of chronic sinusitis alone did not have them (21). More recent studies, however, have argued that the major site of eosinophil accumulation in CRS is the mucus, and that the majority of CRS patients, regardless of whether they have asthma, show striking eosinophil accumulation extramucosally (22).

Immunofluorescent studies have demonstrated a remarkable association between the presence of extracellular deposition of major basic protein and damage to sinus mucosa. The large amount of tissue eosinophils seen in patients with chronic hyperplastic sinusitis has been shown to correlate with local cytokine production, particularly granulocyte–macrophage colony-stimulating factor (GM-CSF) and interleukin-3 (IL-3) (23). The histopathologic examination of the paranasal sinus epithelium has revealed it to be similar to that described in bronchial asthma (24). The eosinophil may act as an effector cell in chronic inflammatory disease in the paranasal respiratory epithelium, which points to the possibility that sinus disease in patients with bronchial asthma may have the same underlying mechanism of damage to the epithelial tissue.

Inflammatory Mediators
Another theory proposes that rhinosinusitis may act as an aggravator of bronchial asthma by local stimulation of irritant receptors by inflammatory mediators and resulting bronchospasm. Georgitis et al. compared mediator levels in maxillary sinus lavages of patients undergoing surgery for chronic sinusitis to levels in nasal lavages of patients with allergic rhinitis (25). The levels of inflammatory mediators such as leukotrienes, prostaglandin D_2 (PGD_2), and histamine were significantly elevated in patients with CRS and were in the range associated with local inflammation and irritant receptor stimulation.

Another study, which used a radionucleotide technique, failed to demonstrate pulmonary aspiration of purulent nasal secretions. This indicates that the seeding of the lower airways with mucopurulent secretions is an unlikely cause of concomitant pulmonary disease. Therefore, it also seems unlikely that the local mediators of inflammation would be aspirated into the lungs (26). There is the possibility that the sinus secretions could set off reflexes in other parts of the respiratory tract that could worsen bronchial asthma.

Neural Reflexes
The postulated neuroanatomic pathways that may reflexly connect the paranasal sinuses to the lungs are: receptors in the nose, pharynx, and presumably those in

the paranasal sinuses that give rise to afferent fibers that, in turn, form part of the trigeminal nerve. The trigeminal nerve passes to the brain stem, where it can connect via the reticular formation with the dorsal vagal nucleus. From the vagal nucleus, parasympathetic efferent fibers travel in the vagus nerve to the bronchi. The cholinergic parasympathetic nervous system plays a role in maintaining resting bronchial muscle tone as well as in mediating acute bronchospastic responses. The vagus nerve provides the cholinergic motor supply to the airway smooth muscle.

Further insights into the mechanism of sinusitis-induced asthma have recently emerged. In a study of 106 patients with chronic sinusitis, histamine challenge to the lower airways before and after medical treatment was performed (27). Forced expiratory volume in 1 second (FEV1) was measured as an index of bronchial narrowing and mid-inspiratory flow (MIF50) was measured as an index of extrabronchial airway narrowing. Both intrabronchial and extrabronchial hyperreactivity decreased after treatment, with the reduction in extrabronchial hyperreactivity being more pronounced and preceding the intrabronchial hyperreactivity decline. The changes in intrabronchial and extrabronchial reactivity were strongly associated with pharyngitis, as determined by medical history, physical examination, and nasal lavage. The authors propose that airway hyperresponsiveness in rhinosinusitis might depend on pharyngobronchial reflexes triggered by seeding of the inflammatory process into the pharynx through postnasal drip of mediators and infected material from affected sinuses.

In a later study, these same authors demonstrated actual damage of the pharyngeal mucosa in patients with CRS marked by epithelial thinning and a striking increase in pharyngeal nerve fiber density. This favors increased access of irritants to submucosal nerve endings, inducing the release of sensory neuropeptides via axon reflexes with activation of a neural arch, resulting in reflex airway constriction (28).

Circulating Factors

As previously noted, the extent of sinus disease seen on CT has been correlated with peripheral blood and sputum eosinophilia. This suggests not simply a local phenomenon, but rather a systemic process. Patients with chronic hyperplastic rhinosinusitis have an intense inflammatory process of the upper airway. It could be hypothesized that the inflamed sinus tissue releases not only mediators and cytokines into the circulation, which would directly affect the lower airways, but also chemotactic factors that recruit eosinophils from the bone marrow and direct them to the upper and lower airways (29). Recent evidence supports the hypothesis of "cross-talk" in allergic inflammation, although the mechanism(s) of this effect remain unknown. Specifically, it was demonstrated that isolated allergen challenge of the lower airways provoked allergic inflammation not only in the lungs but also in the nasal mucosa (30). Similarly, it was shown that isolated nasal allergen challenge provokes inflammation not only in the nose but also in the lung (31). This implies not only a shared susceptibility but also the tendency of the disease in one airway compartment to provoke allergic inflammation in the other.

Conclusions

The concept of "one airway–one disease" initially proposed to emphasize the relationship between allergic rhinitis and asthma, should also be extended to the paranasal sinuses. There is no question that there is a high degree of coexistence of CRS and asthma. The probability that CRS plays an important pathogenetic role in asthma is supported by a number of studies, in both children and adults, indicating that appropriate medical or surgical therapy for CRS significantly improves asthma symptomatology.

The diagnostic index of suspicion for CRS must be high in any case of difficult-to-control asthma. By the same token, any patient with CRS should be questioned carefully for the existence of cough, dyspnea on exertion, or nocturnal awakenings with shortness of breath, all highly indicative of bronchial asthma.

ASPIRIN SENSITIVITY
Incidence
There is an increased association of nasal polyps with aspirin (ASA) sensitivity. About 40–80% of patients with ASA sensitivity have polyposis and about 15% of patients with polyposis have ASA sensitivity (32).

In 1968, Samter and Beers described a symptom complex of ASA sensitivity, steroid-dependent asthma, and nasal polyposis generally associated with CRS (33). Initially, symptoms of nasal congestion, rhinorrhea, post-nasal drip, and hyposmia develop in the third or fourth decade of life. Within a few years, nasal polyposis develops followed by asthma. Finally, ASA sensitivity is diagnosed. Some patients experience only lower respiratory tract reactions (34), others have reactions in the nose, sinuses, and eyes only (35), but the majority experience both upper and lower respiratory tract reactions (36). A commonly used term for this entity is "aspirin-exacerbated respiratory disease (AERD)". In a series of 300 patients with AERD, 99% had abnormal sinus radiographs or CT scans.

Mechanism
The mechanism of ASA-induced reactions includes inhibition of the cyclooxygenase enzyme, COX-1 (37). COX-1 inhibition by aspirin and other nonsteroidal anti-inflammatory drugs (NSAIDs), leads to a decrease in spontaneous synthesis of the anti-inflammatory PGE_2, decreased synthesis of PGD_2, and an enhanced activity of 5-lipoxygenase (38). Leukotriene C4 (LTC4) synthesis is overexpressed in eosinophils and mast cells. This leads to an overproduction of cysteinyl leukotrienes (cysLTs) that are released into the airways, resulting in signs and symptoms typical of nasal congestion, rhinorrhea, and bronchospasm after ASA exposure (39).

Diagnosis
The clinical picture most suggestive of AERD in an asthmatic is the continuous formation of nasal polyps and pansinusitis. However, the diagnosis of AERD cannot be made from clinical presentation alone. Approximately two-thirds of patients with an identical clinical picture never react to ASA or other NSAIDs (40). About 15% of patients with ASA-induced asthma and rhinitis are unaware of their ASA sensitivity, indicating that ASA challenge is necessary to diagnose the disease fully.

When oral challenges with ASA are used to detect sensitivity, the prevalence of AERD in adult asthmatic populations is between 9% and 20% (41,42). Among adult asthmatics with nasal polyps and pansinusitis, the prevalence of AERD increases to 34% (43). Adult asthmatics with a history of AERD had positive oral challenges to ASA between 66% and 97% of the time (36,42). It should be emphasized that oral challenges with ASA or NSAIDs can induce severe bronchospastic and nasal reactions. Therefore, physicians conducting these challenges should be experienced in the technique and prepared to treat bronchospastic reactions aggressively.

Treatment

To prevent exacerbations, the ingestion of ASA and COX-1-inhibiting NSAIDs must be avoided. Safe drugs for ASA-sensitive patients include acetaminophen and salsalate in ordinary doses and selective COX-2 inhibitors (celecoxib and rofecoxib) (37).

The clinical efficacy in patients with AERD of ASA desensitization followed by daily ASA treatment has been reported. An ASA desensitization protocol is shown in Table 2. During oral ASA challenges, desensitization is accomplished by reintroducing the dose of ASA that initiated the ASA reaction on the previous day. If there is no reaction to the same dose, the next highest dose is given and repeated until reactions cease. This process of escalating doses of ASA continues until the patient can tolerate 650 mg of ASA without any reactions. ASA challenges and desensitizations should be performed by physicians experienced in the procedure and prepared to treat severe asthmatic attacks. Patients must be monitored closely with hourly pulmonary function tests, close nursing observation, and facilities to treat severe bronchospastic complications.

The clinical efficacy of ASA desensitization followed by daily ASA treatment in patients with AERD has been reported. In a study, 65 patients with AERD underwent ASA desensitization followed by treatment with ASA 650 mg twice daily. While the patients were under treatment with ASA, objective clinical criteria demonstrated significant improvement in their clinical courses, particularly a reduction in sinusitis. Simultaneous requirements for systemic corticosteroids declined significantly (44).

In a more recent study (45), 172 patients with AERD were desensitized and treated with aspirin. By the first 6 months of aspirin treatment, there were significant reductions in the number of sinus infections, numbers of short courses of prednisone, and improvements in the sense of smell and general assessment of nasal, sinus, and asthma symptoms. Of the patients who completed a year or more of aspirin treatment, 87% experienced improvement. Results persisted for 1–5 years; 14% of patients discontinued ASA because of side effects, usually gastritis.

Since ASA desensitization treatment appears to be particularly effective in reducing upper airway mucosal congestion and inflammation, the ideal candidates for treatment are those patients with recurrent or CRS and nasal polyps who have recently had sinus surgery with removal of inflammatory tissue.

TABLE 2 Aspirin Desensitization Protocol

Time	Days			
	1	2	3	4
8:00 a.m.	12 mg	45 mg	150 mg	650 mg
12:00 p.m. (noon)	20 mg	60 mg	200 mg	
4:00 p.m.	30 mg	100 mg	325 mg	

GASTROESOPHAGEAL REFLUX DISEASE
Mechanism
Gastroesophageal reflux disease (GERD) has been suggested as a cause of sinusitis. The literature on this subject is confusing and controversial. Several terms have been used in the literature to describe the relationship between GERD and rhinosinusitis. These include: gastroesophageal, extraesophageal, supraesophageal, gastroesophagopharyngeal, laryngopharyngeal, nasopharyngeal, and duodenogastroesophagopharyngeal reflux. Although the meanings of these terms are somewhat different, for the sake of simplicity we shall refer to them collectively as GERD. The mechanism of GERD causing sinusitis is thought to be a direct reflux of gastric acid into the pharynx and subsequently to the nasopharynx, causing inflammation of the sinus ostium leading to sinusitis (46).

Results of GERD Therapy on Sinusitis
A study of 30 children with chronic sinusitis was performed using 24-hour monitoring with dual pH probes, one in the nasopharynx and the other in the distal esophagus. Nineteen (63%) showed GE reflux, well above the expected prevalence of 5% in the healthy general population. Of these 19, six (32%) demonstrated nasopharyngeal reflux. Seventy-nine percent had improvements in their sinusitis symptoms after treatment of GERD. The recommendation of the authors was that children with chronic sinusitis refractory to medical therapy be evaluated for GERD and treated before sinus surgery is considered (47).

A study of adults evaluated the prevalence of gastroesophagopharyngeal reflux (GEPR) in 11 CT-confirmed chronic sinusitis patients who had not responded to conventional therapy and 11 normal healthy controls. A three-site ambulatory esophagopharyngeal pH monitoring technique was used. Ambulatory pH monitoring documented GEPR in seven of 11 patients and two of 11 normal volunteers (48).

Another study involved 19 adult patients with chronic sinusitis, 18 of whom had sinus surgery. Sixty-eight percent had classic GERD symptoms and 78% had abnormal results on an esophageal pH probe. Twelve were treated with proton pump inhibitors, four were treated with proton pump inhibitors and prokinetics, and two had repeat surgery. Six months later, 12 (67%) had improvement in sinus symptoms, with four being dramatic. The authors suggest that medical therapy as a treatment for adults with chronic sinusitis be confined to patients with abnormal pH results (49).

In another study, 38 patients with refractory CRS symptoms following endoscopic sinus surgery (ESS) were compared to 10 CRS patients who had resolution of their symptoms following ESS (50). A control group of 20 asymptomatic, healthy controls without ESS was also included. The author used a special probe to monitor pH in the distal esophagus, 1 cm above the upper esophageal sphincter (UES), and in the nasopharynx. The special probe was designed to detect nasopharyngeal reflux (NPR). The author found that the refractory CRS patients had greater nasopharyngeal as well as upper and lower esophageal reflux. Of note, the nasopharyngeal pH was <4.0 in 39% versus 7% of control patients.

Diagnosis
Patients with symptomatic GERD may complain of heartburn, chest/epigastric/cervical pain, water brash, belching, indigestion, nausea, vomiting, dysphagia, and

halitosis. Hoarseness due to GERD is referred to as reflux laryngitis. Laryngopharyngeal reflux (LPR) is a recognized cause of chronic cough, and non-productive throat clearing (51). Many patients, however, have asymptomatic GERD and symptom frequency and severity correlate poorly with esophageal injury.

The diagnosis of GERD can be based on history and a favorable response to a trial of pharmacologic treatment. Ambulatory 24-hour esophageal pH monitoring is the most sensitive method for diagnosing GERD. The sensitivity of barium studies is not high but demonstration of barium reflux is of high positive predictive value.

With respect to establishing GERD as a contributive factor in refractory CRS cases, there is no consensus on which form of esophageal monitoring is the most informative. Most authors agree, however, that esophageal pH monitoring is helpful and should probably be done with a dual-probe monitor that can simultaneously record pH readings in the lower esophagus and 1–2 cm above the upper esophageal sphincter. The study of DelGaudio offered the innovative technique of simultaneously measuring pH in the nasopharynx (51).

While an association between GERD and sinusitis remains controversial and difficult to prove, it is important to consider this relationship. Certainly, patients with symptomatic GERD should be treated. Furthermore, in patients with sinusitis refractory to medical therapy, diagnostic testing and/or treatment for asymptomatic GERD should also be considered prior to surgical intervention.

Management

Lifestyle Changes

The goals of GERD treatment are relief of symptoms and healing of esophagitis (Table 3). First and foremost are dietary and lifestyle measures. This includes avoidance of large meals, maintaining ideal weight, wearing loose clothing, eating the evening meal at least three hours before retiring, avoiding recumbency for two hours after a meal, and elevating the head of the bed with six-inch blocks. Cessation of smoking is recommended, as well as avoidance of carbonated drinks, alcohol, peppermint, coffee, chocolate, and fatty acids. All these substances reduce the lower esophageal sphincter (LES) pressure. Citrus juices, alcohol, and tomato-based products are direct esophageal irritants. Medications that lower the LES pressure include calcium channel blockers, benzodiazepines, narcotics, nicotine, estrogen, and progesterone (52).

Pharmacotherapy

Proton pump inhibitors have a much greater antisecretory effect and esophageal healing rate than H_2 receptor antagonists. However, the clinician may be forced, through managed care restrictions, to first prescribe H_2 receptor antagonists: The

TABLE 3 Management of Gastroesophageal Reflux Disease

Lifestyle changes
    Pharmacotherapy
    H_2 receptor antagonists
    Proton pump inhibitors
    Prokinetic agents
Surgery
    Laparoscopic fundoplication

usual initial doses are cimetidine 800 mg twice a day or ranitidine 20 mg twice a day. If there is no response, a proton pump inhibitor should be started promptly, such as omeprazole 20 mg once a day or lansoprazole 30 mg once a day. The dose can be doubled in non-responsive patients.

Prokinetic agents effective in GERD include metaclopramide. The combination of an H_2-receptor antagonist and a prokinetic agent is often successful because it addresses two separate but interdependent components of GERD: acid exposure (H_2 receptor antagonist) and gastric emptying (prokinetic agent).

Surgery

The success of medical treatment of GERD, particularly with proton pump inhibitors, makes the need for surgery much less than in the past. The advantage of surgery over medical treatment is that fundoplication not only removes the acid insult but also prevents fluids from refluxing into the esophagus. Laparoscopic Nissen fundoplication is being used increasingly in the management of medically resistant GERD. The procedure is less invasive and is associated with lower morbidity rates than the previous "open" approach that requires thoracotomy/laporotomy.

IMMUNE DEFICIENCIES
Relationship of CRS

Immunodeficiency should be considered in any patient with recurrent or CRS. Particular consideration should be given to patients with more than three episodes of rhinosinusitis per year and those who have failed aggressive prior medical and/or surgical management (53). When the patient also has a history of recurrent otitis media, bronchitis, or bronchiectasis, suspicion should be heightened.

Diagnosis

Physical examination of a patient suspected to have congenital immune deficiency includes looking for absence of tonsillar tissue and findings associated with specific diseases such as ocular telangiectasis, skin and mucous membrane infection, eczema, clubbing, rales, rhonchi, petechiae, and purpura. The most common congenital immunodeficiency disorders are common variable immunodeficiency, Wiskott-Aldrich syndrome, ataxia telangiectasia, X-linked immunodeficiency with normal or increased IgM, and X-linked agammagobulinemia (54).

The majority of immunodeficient patients with recurrent sinusitis have defects in humoral immunity. However, there are subgroups that have combined humoral and cellular impairment (55). Prominent among these patients are those with acquired immune deficiency syndrome (AIDS) (56).

The indications for pursuing an extensive immunodeficiency evaluation depend on the age, history, physical examination, and lifestyle of the patient. In a child of <2 years of age with recurrent and possible life-threatening infections, one should proceed quickly. Infections with organisms of low pathogenicity should prompt the physician to think of a congenital immune deficiency. AIDS in either children or adults should also be an indication for evaluation of immune function.

Laboratory studies appropriate for evaluating immune deficiency include quantitative serum IgG-, IgA-, and IgM-specific antibody responses, complement evaluation and measurement of T-cell function by delayed hypersensitivity skin tests, and in vitro lymphocyte response to mitogens.

It is now realized that simple quantitation of circulating immune globulins is not enough to accurately diagnose humoral immune deficiency. Rather than a static measurement of existing levels, it is much more important to determine the dynamic response to an antigen. While the post-immunization response (measuring antibodies of the IgG isotype) to any protein antigen can be measured, the determination of the response to tetanus immunization is particularly advantageous since most patients have been immunized and 90–100% of children should have protective antibody titers after completing primary immunization (57). The response to polysaccharide antigen can be determined by measuring pre- and post-immunization responses to unconjugated pneumococcal vaccine (58).

In addition to total IgG deficiency, IgG subclass deficiency may cause recurrent infectious rhinosinusitis. These patients typically have low or undetectable IgG_2, IgG_3, or IgG_4 and yet have normal total serum IgG levels (59). Since a significant fraction of the immune response to carbohydrate antigens involves antibodies of the IgG_2 isotype, a deficiency of IgG_2 correlates with a poor response to polysaccharide-encapsulated organisms such as *Streptococcus pneumoniae, Haemophilus influenzae,* and *Moraxella catarrhalis* (59,60). Because there is a wide range of IgG_2 levels particularly in children under 8 years of age, a functional assessment of the immune response is necessary and more valuable than IgG subclass values per se.

Particular attention should be paid to patients with HIV infection since as many as 68% have recurrent or CRS (61). The increased likelihood of sinus disease correlates with CD4 T-cell deficiency. AIDS patients afford another example of abnormal specific antibody responses in the face of normal or even elevated total serum immunoglobulins. While there are case reports of AIDS patients who have infections due to atypical organisms, most rhinosinusitis infections in these patients are caused by the same organisms found in immunocompetent patients (62). Successful medical treatment generally involves a much longer period of aggressive medical therapy.

THERAPY

In patients with recurrent infections and antibody deficiency, intravenous immunoglobulin (IVIG) is approved as the replacement therapy. These conditions include X-linked agammaglobulinemia, common variable hypogammaglobulinemia, Wiskott-Aldrich syndrome and hyper-IgM syndrome. In addition, patients with IgG subclass deficiency who also demonstrate abnormal specific antibody production in response to vaccination may benefit from IVIG replacement therapy. There is no question that the use of IVIG in patients with immunoglobulin deficiency can prevent complications of rhinosinusitis including subperiosteal abscess, intracranial abscess, meningitis, and sepsis (63).

Occasionally, a patient may have normal total immunoglobulins but a poor pneumococcal vaccine response, and CRS may be the major, if not the only infectious process. These patients may experience resistant CRS unresponsive to medical and surgery therapy. In such cases, a trial of IVIG is warranted. Monthly therapy is given through the fall and winter. If the patient remains stable, therapy is discontinued during the summer.

REFERENCES

1. Gottlieb MS. Relation of intranasal sinus disease in the production of asthma. JAMA 1925; 85:105–9.
2. Bullen SS. Incidence of asthma in 400 cases of chronic sinusitis. J Allergy 1932; 4:402–8.
3. Fuller C, Richards W, Gilsanz V, et al. Sinusitis in status asthmaticus. J Allergy Clin Immunol 1990; 85:222.
4. Rossi OVJ, Pirila T, Laitinen J, et al. Sinus aspirates and radiographic abnormalities in severe attacks of asthma. Int Arch Allergy Immunol 1994; 103:209–16.
5. ten Brinke A, Grootendorst D, Schmidt JT, et al. Chronic sinusitis in severe asthma is related to sputum eosinophilia. J Allergy Clin Immunol 2002; 109:621–6.
6. Bresciani M, Paradis L, Des Roches A, et al. Rhinosinusitis in severe asthma. J Allergy Clin Immunol 2001; 107:73–80.
7. Newman L, Platts-Mills T, Phillips CD, et al. Chronic sinusitis: relationship of computed tomography findings in allergy, asthma, and eosinophilia. JAMA 1994; 271:363–7.
8. Borish L. Sinusitis to asthma: entering the realm of evidence-based medicine. J. Allergy Clin Immunol 2002; 9:606–8.
9. Rachelefsky G, Katz R, Siegel SC. Chronic sinus disease with associated reactive airway disease in children. Pediatrics 1984; 73:526–9.
10. Friedman R, Ackerman M, Wald E. Asthma and bacterial sinusitis in children. J Allergy Clin Immunol 1984; 74:185–9.
11. Oliveira C, Sole D. Improvement of bronchial hyperresponsiveness in asthmatic children treated for concomitant sinusitis. Ann Allergy Asthma Immunol 1997; 79:70–4.
12. English GM. Nasal polypectomy and sinus surgery in patients with asthma and aspirin idiosyncrasy. Laryngoscope 1986; 96:374–80.
13. Nishioka GJ, Cook PR, Davies WE, et al. Functional endoscopic sinus surgery in patients with chronic sinusitis and asthma. Otolaryngol Head Neck Surg 1994; 110:494–500.
14. Parsons D, Phillips S. Functional endoscopic surgery in children. Laryngoscope 1993; 103:899–903.
15. Manning S, Wasserman R, Silver R, Phillips DL. Results of endoscopic sinus surgery in pediatric patients with chronic sinusitis and asthma. Arch Otolaryngol Head Neck Surg 1994; 120:1142–5.
16. Dunlop G, Scadding GK, Lund VJ. The effect of endoscopic sinus surgery on asthma: management of patients with chronic rhinosinusitis, nasal polyposis, and asthma. Am J Rhinol 1999; 13:261–5.
17. Dhong H, Jung YS, Chung SK, Choi DC. Effect of endoscopic sinus surgery on asthmatic patients with chronic rhinosinusitis. Otolaryngol Head Neck Surg 2001; 124:99–104.
18. Gliklich R, Metson R. Effect of sinus surgery on quality of life. Otolaryngol Head Neck Surg 1997; 117:12–17.
19. Goldstein M, Grundfast S, Dunsky EH, et al. Effect of functional endoscopic sinus surgery on bronchial asthma outcomes. Arch Otolaryngol Head Neck Surg 1999; 125:314–9.
20. Ikayama M, Iijima H, Shimura S, et al. Methacholine bronchial hyperresponsiveness in chronic sinusitis. Respiration 1998; 65:450–7.
21. Harlin BL, Ansel DG, Lane SR, et al. A clinical and pathologic study of chronic sinusitis: the role of the eosinophil. J Allergy Clin Immunol 1988; 81:867–75.
22. Ponikau JU, Sherris DA, Kephart GM, et al. Striking deposition of toxic eosinophil major basic protein in mucus: implications for chronic rhinosinusitis. J Allergy Clin Immunol 2005; 116:362–9.
23. Hamilos DL, Leung DYM, Wood R, et al. Association of tissue eosinophilia and cytokine mRNA expression of granulocyte-macrophage colony-stimulating factor and interleukin-3. J Allergy Clin Immunol 1993; 91:39–48.
24. Ponikau JU, Sherris DA, Kephert EM, et al. Features of airway remodeling and eosinophilic inflammation in chronic rhinosinusitis. Is the histopathology similar to asthma? J. Allergy Clin Immunol 2003; 112:877–82.
25. Georgitis JW, Matthews BL, Stone B. Chronic sinusitis: characterization of cellular influx and inflammatory mediators in sinus lavage fluid. Int Arch Allergy Immunol 1995; 106:416–21.

26. Bardin PG, Van Heerden BB, Joubert JR. Absence of pulmonary aspiration of sinus contents in patients with asthma and sinusitis. J Allergy Clin Immunol 1990; 86:82–8.

27. Bucca C, Rolla G, Scappaticci E, et al. Extrathoracic and intrathoracic airway responsiveness in sinusitis. J Allergy Clin Immunol 1995; 95:52–9.

28. Rolla G. Cologrand P, Scappaticci E, et al. Damage of the pharyngeal mucosa and hyperresponsiveness of the airway in sinusitis. J Allergy Clin Immunol 1997; 100:52–7.

29. Denburg J, Sehmi R, Saito H, et al. Systemic aspects of allergic disease: bone marrow responses. J Allergy Clin Immunol 2000; 196(Suppl.):242–6.

30. Braunstahl GJ, Kleinjan A, Overbeek SE, Prins JB, Hoogsteden HC, Fokkens WJ. Segmental bronchial provocation induces nasal inflammation in allergic rhinitis patients. Am J Respir Crit Care Med 2000; 161:2051–7.

31. Braunstahl GJ, Overbeek SE, Kleinjan A, Prins JB, Hoogsteden HC, Fokkens WJ. Nasal allergen provocation induces adhesion molecule expression and tissue eosinophilia in upper and lower airways. J Allergy Clin Immunol 2001; 107:469–76.

32. Settipane GA. Epidemiology of nasal polyps. Allergy Asthma Proc 1996; 17:231–40.

33. Samter M, Beero RF. Intolerance to aspirin. Ann Int Med 1968; 68:975–82.

34. Stevenson DD. Diagnosis, prevention, and treatment of adverse reactions to aspirin and nonsteroidal anti-inflammatory drugs. J Allergy Clin Immunol 1984; 74:617–22.

35. Lumry WR, Curd JG, Zerger RS, et al. Aspirin-sensitive rhinosinusitis: the clinical syndrome and effects of aspirin administration. J Allergy Clin Immunol 1983; 71:580–7.

36. Pleskow WW, Stevenson DD, Mathison DA, et al. Aspirin-sensitive rhinosinusitis/asthma: spectrum of adverse reactions to aspirin. J Allergy Clin Immunol 1983; 71:574–9.

37. Szczeklik A, Stevenson DD. Aspirin-induced asthma: advances in pathogenesis and management. J Allergy Clin Immunol 1999; 104:5–13.

38. Pavord ID, Tattersfield AE. Bronchoprotective role for endogenous prostaglandin D E2. Lancet 1995; 345:436–42.

39. Cowburn AS, Sladek K, Soja J, et al. Overexpression of leukotriene C4 synthesis in bronchial biopsies from patients with aspirin-intolerant asthma. J Clin Invest 1998; 101:1–8.

40. Stevenson DD, Simon RA. Sensitivity to aspirin and nonsteroidal anti-inflammatory drugs. In: Middleton ES, Reed CE, Ellis EF, et al., eds. Allergy: Principles and Practice. 4th edn, vol. 3. St. Louis, MO: Mosby, 1993:1747–67.

41. McDonald J, Mathison DA, Stevenson DD. Aspirin intolerance in asthma: detection by challenge. J Allergy Clin Immunol 1972; 50:198–207.

42. Delaney JC. The diagnosis of aspirin idiosyncrasy by analgesic challenge. Clin Allergy, 1976; 6:177–81.

43. Weber RW, Hoffman M, Raine DA, et al. Incidence of bronchoconstriction due to aspirin, ozo dyes, non-ozo dyes, and preservatives in a population of perennial asthmatics. J Allergy Clin Immunol 1979; 64:32–7.

44. Stevenson DD, Hankammer MA, Mathison DA, et al. Aspirin desensitization treatment of aspirin sensitive rhinosinusitic-asthmatic patients: long term outcomes. J Allergy Clin Immunol 1996; 98:751–8.

45. Berges-Gimeno MP, Simon RA, Stevenson DD. Long-term treatment with aspirin desensitization in asthmatic patients with aspirin exacerbated respiratory disease. J Allergy Clin Immunol 2003; 111:80–6.

46. Barbero GJ. Gastroesophageal reflux and upper airway disease. Otolaryngol Clin North Am 1996; 29:27–38.

47. Phipps CD, Wood WE, Bigson WS, Cochran WJ. Gastroesophageal reflux contributing to chronic sinus disease in children: a prospective analysis. Arch Otolaryngol Head Neck Surg 2000; 126:831–6.

48. Ulualp SO, Toohill RJ, Hoffmann R, Shaker R. Possible relationship of gastroesophagopharyngeal acid reflux with pathogenesis of chronic sinusitis. Am J Rhinol 1999; 13:197–202.

49. diBaise JK, Huerter JV, Quigley EM. Sinusitis and gastroesophageal reflux disease. Ann Intern Med 1998; 129:1078–83.

50. DelGaudio JM. Direct nasopharyngeal reflux of gastric acid is a contributing factor in refractory chronic rhinosinusitis. Laryngoscope 2005; 115:946–57.

51. Franco RA Jr. Laryngopharyngeal reflux. Allergy Asthma Proc 2006; 27:21–5.

52. Theodoropoulos DS. Gastroesophageal reflux disease and asthma, Chapter 14. In: Slavin RG, Reisman RE, eds. Asthma. Philadelphia, PA: ACP, 2002:209–226.
53. Chee L, Graham SM, Carothers DG, et al. Immune dysfunction in refractory sinusitis in a tertiary care setting. Laryngoscope 2001; 111:233–5.
54. Rosen FS, Cooper M, Wedgwood R. The primary immunodeficiencies. Part I. N Engl J Med 1984; 311:235–42.
55. Polmar S. The role of the immunologist in sinus disease. J Allergy Clin Immunol 1992; 90:511–4.
56. Zurlo JJ. Fuertstein IM, Lebovics R, et al. Sinusitis in HIV infection. Am J Med 1992; 121:516–22.
57. Gross S, Blaiss MS, Herrod HG. The role of immunoglobulin subclasses and specific antibody determinations in the evaluation of recurrent infection in children. J Pediatr 1992; 121:516–22.
58. Tahkokallio O, Seppala IJ, Sarvas H, et al. Concentrations of serum immunoglobulins and antibodies to pneumococcal capsular polysaccharides in patients with recurrent or chronic sinusitis. Ann Otol Rhinol Laryngol 2001; 110:675–81.
59. Umetsu DT, Ambrosino DM, Quinti I, et al. Recurrent sinopulmonary infections and impaired antibody response to bacterial capsular polysaccharide antigen in children with selective IgG-subclass deficiency. N Engl J Med 1985; 313:1247–51.
60. Siber GR, Schur PH, Isenberg AC, et al. Correlation between serum IgG2 concentration and the antibody response to bacterial polysaccharide antigens. N Engl J Med 1980; 303:178–82.
61. Sprecht TJ, Rahm SJ, Longworth DI, et al. Frequency of sinusitis in AIDS patients. Proceedings of the IV International AIDS Conference. Stockholm, Sweden: University Publisher Group, Frederick, Maryland, 1988:399.
62. Janoff EN, Douglas JM, Gabriel M, et al. Class-specific antibody response to pneumococcal capsular antibodies in men infected with human immunodeficiency virus type 1. J Infect Dis 1988; 158:983–90.
63. Buckley RH, Shiff RI. The use of intravenous immunoglobulin in immune deficient diseases. N Engl J Med 1991; 325:110–7.

18 | Chronic Rhinosinusitis: Contrasts Between Children and Adult Patients

Rodney Lusk

Boys Town ENT Institute, Boys Town National Research Hospital, Omaha, Nebraska, U.S.A.

OVERVIEW

There is increasing evidence that acute and chronic rhinosinusitis (CRS) in children and adults is of different etiology and therefore warrants different treatment strategies. It is becoming more apparent that adult CRS has a relatively greater inflammatory component whereas childhood CRS has a relatively greater infectious component (1). This is secondary to immaturity of the pediatric immune system, the increased incidence of viral upper respiratory tract infections, and the smaller ostia to the sinuses in children. Concentrations of eosinophils in adult mucosa are greater than those noted in children (2) with a correspondingly higher incidence of atopic adults (86%) than children (43%). There is also a greater degree of collagen deposition and expansion of submucosal mucous glands in the adult sinus indicating more tissue remodeling and potentially greater irreversible scarring (2,3). The workup and treatment options for acute and CRS in children are therefore different than in adults. Certain systemic diseases are also more likely to occur in children. Immune deficiencies, cystic fibrosis, and ciliary dyskinesia are good examples. It must be realized that the disease processes between adults and children may be entirely different.

Chronic rhinosinusitis is a significant cause of morbidity in children. Cunningham et al. (4) prospectively evaluated children and their parents' perspective of the severity of their rhinosinusitis with the Child Health Questionnaire-Parent Form 50 and Child Health Questionnaire-Child Form 87. Children with rhinosinusitis were perceived by their parents as having more bodily pain and more limited physical activities than parental assessment of children with asthma, juvenile rheumatoid arthritis, and other chronic disorders.

PATHOPHYSIOLOGY

Rhinosinusitis is a multifactorial disease and therefore is difficult to accurately diagnose and treat. Viral infections are more frequent in children and often precede asthma attacks and sinus infections (5). Viral infections destroy the ciliary blanket and cause an inflammatory response that markedly alters the makeup of the mucosal epithelium. The mucus layer is a primary defense mechanism, and clearing of the layer is dependent on normal ciliary function. Since viral infection destroys the cilia, the secretions are not cleared from the sinuses, and their static accumulation provides an environment conducive for bacterial overgrowth and further mucosal damage. This secondary acute bacterial infection is associated with significant mucosal edema that is particularly problematic because of the small sinus ostia in children. The majority of acute infections clear when the cilia once again become functional. If the infection does not clear, and symptoms become persistent for a three month period or longer, the condition evolves into CRS.

There is increasing evidence that rhinosinusitis in children is more infectious in origin. Children have enlarged adenoid pads that harbor bacteria and can be associated with rhinosinusitis (6). There is a significant correlation between rhinosinusitis and infected adenoid core pathogens (6). The most common causes of infection of the sinuses in children include alpha-hemolytic *Streptococcus, Streptococcus pneumoniae, Haemophilus influenzae, Moraxella catarrhalis*, and *Staphylococcus aureus* (7). There is a higher incidence of *Staphylococcus aureus* in children when compared with adults. The exact correlation between anaerobes and rhinosinusitis is not yet known. Some investigators have noted a high incidence of anaerobes (8) while others have noted a much lower incidence (7). Ramadan et al. (9) used polymerase chain reaction (PCR) to help elucidate the true incidence of anaerobic infections in the sinuses (9). He found that PCR detected the presence of anaerobes four times more frequently than standard anaerobic culture techniques, which may account for some of the discrepancies in the literature.

OTHER CAUSES OR POTENTIAL RISK FACTORS FOR PEDIATRIC CHRONIC RHINOSINUSITIS
Age
Age is clearly a risk factor for rhinosinusitis; the younger the child the greater the incidence of recurrent acute and CRS. Some investigators have found age to be the most important factor and as the child matures the incidence of chronic respiratory tract infections markedly decreases (10). There appears to be a marked decrease in symptoms when children become 10 years of age or older (10). Age has also been found to be a more important factor than allergies (11).

Immature Immune Systems
Maternal immunoglobulins are detectable in the infant's circulation for approximately six months beyond which the infant must produce its own immunoglobulins. Children in day care settings are at greater risk of an infection because they are exposed to more viruses (12). Their symptoms are more frequent, and their respiratory symptoms more protracted. The average number of upper respiratory tract infections (URTIs) in infants can be as high as six per year with symptoms of each episode lasting as long as 2–3 weeks. As the immune system matures, the incidence of URTIs decreases.

Allergy
Although the exact relationship between allergies and rhinosinusitis is a subject of ongoing investigation, there appears to be an association. The incidence of complicated acute rhinosinusitis is higher in children with documented allergic rhinitis (10,13). Not all patients with CRS have allergies. Nguyen et al. reported that 59% of pediatric patients with chronic respiratory symptoms were skin test-positive and 58% had symptoms of CRS as documented with computed tomography (CT) scans (10). There is evidence that allergies are not as important as other factors such as age (11). Allergies evolve during childhood and testing is more problematic than in adults. Many allergists are hesitant to test children less than three years old. The decision to proceed with immunotherapy and medical

management prior to or subsequent to surgical treatment must be individualized for any given patient.

Adenoid Hypertrophy

An enlarged adenoid pad may completely obstruct the nasal airways and result in signs and symptoms consistent with rhinosinusitis. How large the adenoid pad must be to be associated with symptoms is debatable, and there is no consensus regarding the best way to assess the size of the adenoid pad. Flexible nasopharyngoscopy is well tolerated and can provide significant information regarding the size and status of the adenoid pad. There is evidence that adenoid hypertrophy is positively associated with skin test reactivity to mold spores (14). This same reactivity does not seem to be associated with animal dander or seasonal allergens. The adenoid pad may also be enlarged because of chronic adenoiditis secondary to bacteria growing in the crypts of the adenoid pad. The adenoiditis may also be the cause of CRS by infecting the region of the ostiomeatal complex.

Secondhand Smoke Inhalation

Intuitively, one would expect exposure to secondhand smoke to increase the risk of respiratory diseases including rhinosinusitis. There is suggestive evidence that both asthma and rhinosinusitis occur more frequently in children exposed to parents who smoke (15,16). Ramadan also found endoscopic sinus surgery to be less successful if the children were exposed to secondary smoke (17). There are also studies that children with recurrent otitis media are more likely to have exposure to environmental tobacco smoke than controls, but prospective follow up shows no significant difference in the clinical course of the children who were exposed to tobacco smoke compared to those who were not (18).

Anatomic Deformity

For many years it was felt that anatomic variations, such as septal deviation, concha bullosa, or infraorbital cells, were associated with an increased incidence of rhinosinusitis (19). These anatomic variations are less frequent in children, and significant septal deviation is infrequent in children. Septal deformity in the region of the osteomeatal complex (OMC) was thought to be associated with ostiomeatal narrowing and an increased risk of rhinosinusitis. There is now good evidence that septal deviation is not associated with an increased incidence of rhinosinusitis (20). There is a strong correlation between the presence of a concha bullosa and deviation of the septum to the contralateral side (21,22). However, an increased incidence of unilateral rhinosinusitis has not been associated with the septal deviation. The airway is usually maintained between a deviated septum and the lateral wall or the bullosa, suggesting that the deviation was not causing a mass effect. There was also no evidence of increased rhinosinusitis in these patients. The predominant conclusion in the literature indicates that there is no association between anatomic variants and CRS (20,23–25).

Gastroesophageal Reflux Disease

The incidence of gastroesophageal reflux disease (GERD) in the pediatric age group appears to be higher than in adults. Reflux has been known to be associated with other laryngeal pathology (26) and to negatively affect airway reconstruction

(27,28). Bothwell et al. (29) noted a higher incidence of GERD in children with CRS and also noted that if the GERD was medically managed the CRS improved enough to avert surgery in 89% of the children. Phipps et al. noted GERD in 63% of children with rhinosinusitis which is much greater than the 5% noted in normal children (30), and also noted that 32% of the children had reflux into the nasopharynx. They also noted a 79% improvement in symptoms when children were medically treated for their reflux. El-Serag et al. noted an increase in rhinosinusitis, 4.2% vs. 1.4%, in children (31) with GERD but this is not near the incidence cited by Barbero (32). Yellon et al. evaluated children who had positive esophageal biopsies of pathologic reflux and noted rhinosinusitis in only 10% of children (33). Suskind et al. noted a low incidence of rhinosinusitis in children with GERD significant enough to warrant antireflux surgery (34). In this study, the incidence of rhinosinusitis and otitis media was only 14% while 86% of the patients had some evidence of upper airway abnormalities, subglottic edema, reflex apnea, or recurrent croup. The lack of agreement regarding the role of GERD in CRS is probably due to the lack of good definitions and tools to study the disease process. GERD does appear to be a factor in some patients, however, our current state of knowledge does not allow us to predict how well their rhinosinusitis will respond to medical management.

Signs and Symptoms

The signs and symptoms of rhinosinusitis are nonspecific but similar in adults and children with some notable exceptions. Children rarely complain of headaches but manifest the pain as nonspecific irritability. Facial pain with pressure over the maxillary sinus is an unusual complaint in children. Facial tenderness is a rare finding in small children and is unreliable as an indicator of acute bacterial rhinosinusitis in older children and adolescents.

Younger children are more likely to have anterior purulent drainage. Nasal airway obstruction may be secondary to a variety of causes. Adenoid hypertrophy is rarely seen in adolescents and adults but frequently noted in younger children. The parameters which we have followed as most indicative of rhinosinusitis in children are (i) nasal airway obstruction, (ii) purulent rhinorrhea, (iii) headache, (iv) irritability, (v) day time cough, and (vi) night time cough. Night time cough is more frequent but day time cough appears to be more associated with CRS. All of these symptoms are nonspecific and cannot be used for clinical diagnosis on their own (10). One must use the context of all the symptoms to make the diagnosis, and this is unfortunately not an exact science. The physical examination of the nasal mucosa may show mild erythema and edema of then asal turbinates with mucopurulent discharge.

Imaging

It is generally agreed that imaging of the sinuses with plain films or CT scans is not necessary to make the diagnosis of rhinosinusitis in children (refer to Chapter 12) (35). This is somewhat different from the recommendations for adults where documentation of the disease with a CT scan is appropriate (36). This difference in recommendations is an attempt to reduce the potential longer term consequences of radiation exposure in children and to avoid sedation for CT scans. CT scans in children are appropriate under certain circumstances, such as evaluation of the anatomy in preparation for endoscopic sinus surgery (35). The CT scan should be obtained after the child has been treated with an appropriate long-term, 20–28-day, broad-spectrum antibiotic and topical nasal steroid sprays. The CT documents the extent of the rhinosinusitis and any anatomic abnormalities that might increase the risk of a complication. CT scans obtained when the patient is not on medical therapy could overestimate the severity of the disease and result in unnecessary surgery. Gwaltney et al. (37) demonstrated sinus disease with acute upper respiratory tract infections. One cannot assess chronicity of disease on a CT scan; therefore, the pediatric patient should be treated medically prior to the scan. A positive CT may be the focus of concern by anxious parents and result in significant pressure for the surgeon to intervene surgically. Proactive discussions with the parents regarding the significance of mild disease on CT scans can prevent this problem.

DIFFERENCES IN MEDICAL MANAGEMENT
Irrigation
Irrigating the nose has been noted to improve nasal physiology and help eradicate rhinosinusitis (38). This can be performed with hypertonic saline but requires fairly large amounts of fluid. Most children however will not allow irrigation of their nose with this volume of fluid. Most children will only spray their noses with saline and then blow the purulence from the nose. There is no evidence to support the effectiveness of this treatment in children.

Medical Management
There continues to be a debate regarding what constitutes adequate medical management. Some antibiotics, such as fluoroquinolones, which are effective for treatment of adult rhinosinusitis, are not available for children (39). Compliance can be a significant problem and most children require liquid medication which can be foul-tasting and difficult to administer. The following guidelines have been recommended for children with acute rhinosinusitis (35). For children less than 2 years of age with uncomplicated acute bacterial rhinosinusitis that is mild to moderate in degree of severity, who do not attend day care, and have not recently been treated with an antimicrobial, amoxicillin is recommended at either a usual dose of 45 mg/kg/day in two divided doses or a high dose of 90 mg/kg/day in two divided doses. If the child is allergic to amoxicillin, cefdinir (14 mg/kg/day in one or two doses), cefuroxime (30 mg/kg/day in two divided doses), or cefpodoxime (10 mg/kg/day once daily) can be used, although there is a small chance of an allergic cross-reaction with these medications in amoxicillin-allergic patients. In cases of serious allergic reactions, clarithromycin (15 mg/kg/day in two divided doses) or azithromycin (10 mg/kg/day on day 1, 5 mg/kg/day ×4 days as a single daily dose) can be used in an effort to select an antimicrobial of an entirely different class. These recommendations are also appropriate in children with CRS, however, the duration of therapy has not been as well defined for chronic infections. Many investigators would recommend treatment for 20–30 days, and in some instances intravenous antibiotics may be appropriate (40).

Fungal infections are unusual in children, with invasive fungal rhinosinusitis most common in immunocompromised children (41). Older children may manifest symptoms of allergic fungal rhinosinusitis in a manner similar to adults with extensive polyposis (42). Systemic antifungal agents are not an option for children.

The fear that steroids, both topical and systemic, could interrupt growth in children is another differentiating factor. Fortunately, it now appears that topical steroids are safe for children, but there is a lingering concern of growth suppression with combined oral steroids and steroid inhalers (43).

Surgical Management
There are substantial differences in the surgical management of children versus adults with CRS.

Adenoidectomy
Adenoid hypertrophy is common in children but rare in adults. An enlarged adenoid pad may present with all the signs and symptoms compatible with CRS. In some cases, the size of the adenoid pad is not a factor. The deep crypts within the adenoid tissue may be in turn associated with increased bacterial overgrowth which may be associated with CRS. There is a good correlation between the core cultures of the crypts of the adenoid tissue and the cause of the rhinosinusitis (44). There is evidence that an adenoidectomy will resolve the rhinosinusitis in approximately 50% of the children (45,46). It is now becoming widely accepted that an adenoidectomy should be performed before intervening with endoscopic sinus surgery (47,48). Adenoidectomy is rarely performed in adults as the adenoid tissue is uniformly resolved by this time. There are no studies correlating the method of performing the adenoidectomy with the effectiveness of clearing the sinus infections.

Irrigation of the Maxillary Sinus
Irrigation of the maxillary sinus was proposed in the past as a primary treatment for CRS. Recently it has been recommended in conjunction with other procedures such as adenoidectomy (40). It does not appear to provide a long-term resolution of CRS and has therefore been dropped as a primary procedure.

Inferior Meatal Windows
Treatment with inferior meatal windows was once commonplace in adults and children. There is a very high rate of closure in children primarily because the window cannot be made large enough (49,50). In addition to the poor patency rates of inferior meatal windows, the ethmoid sinuses, which are involved in 75% of children, are not treated with this procedure. The floor of the maxillary sinus is frequently not low enough, that is, the sinus is not developed well enough, to allow entry into the sinus through the inferior meatus, making the procedure impossible to perform. The bone of the anterior face of the sinus is thick, making a canine fossa tap difficult to perform and requiring a general anesthetic. For these reasons, there is an unacceptably high failure rate (76%) and the procedure has largely been abandoned (50). The procedure may be warranted in children with massive polyps secondary to cystic fibrosis or primary ciliary dyskinesia. However, the problems with window patency still remain.

Endoscopic Sinus Surgery
Endoscopic surgery in children is different from that performed in adults from a number of perspectives. The indications which are not controversial are noted in Table 1. The indications are rare, however. The most common indication, CRS,

TABLE 1 Indications for Endoscopic Sinus Surgery

Complete nasal obstruction in cystic fibrosis due to massive polyposis or closure of the nose by medialization of the lateral nasal wall
Antro-choanal polyp
Intracranial complications
Mucoceles and mucopyoceles
Orbital abscess
Traumatic injury in optic canal (decompression)
Dacryocystorhinitis (infection of the tear/lacrimal sac) due to rhinosinusitis and resistant to appropriate medical treatment
Fungal rhinosinusitis
Some meningo-encephaloceles
Some neoplasms

Source: Ref. 69.

remains controversial and requires judgment in any given patient. There is a trend toward being more conservative with endoscopic sinus surgery in children (48).

The nose and middle meatus are narrower in children and the operative field is therefore smaller than that noted in adults. The middle meatus is not much more than 3 mm in width therefore the use of a 2.7-mm (pediatric) telescope is often required. This takes some getting used to, as the field is smaller and the telescopes are more fragile. Operating off the monitor may be disorienting because of the smaller image. Entire pediatric sets of instruments have been developed which are not only smaller but sharper than their adult counterparts.

MODIFICATIONS IN SURGICAL TECHNIQUE
Pediatric Endoscopic Sinus Surgery

Sinus disease in children is now limited primarily to the anterior ethmoid and maxillary sinuses (48). In general, the surgery has become less aggressive and is now generally limited to an anterior ethmoidectomy and maxillary antrostomy. The more limited surgery has been found to have a success rate similar to more aggressive surgery (51). The frontal sinus is not developed in younger children and there is little need to instrument the frontal sinus recess. Instrumentation of the frontal recess may be associated with scarring and may prevent formation of the frontal sinus. As a general rule, I also am hesitant to perform a sphenoidotomy for isolated sphenoid disease, unless there is a complication of acute or CRS, or there is evidence of persistent headaches or an isolated fungal rhinosinusitis. Opening the maxillary sinus through a Caldwell-Luc procedure is rarely indicated in children. One notable exception is a choanal polyp arising from the roof or anterior wall of the maxillary sinus. Children less than 3 years of age do not respond to surgery as well as children more than 6 years of age (52).

There is controversy regarding how large the maxillary ostium needs to be made (53,54). It appears that surgeons have become more conservative with how much they open the ostium. I personally no longer enlarge the ostium if it can be visualized and noted to be free of obstruction. I will minimally enlarge the ostium if it can only be palpated, is edematous, or has polyps present.

Because the middle meatus is so narrow, extra care must be taken to minimize trauma to the lateral surface of the middle turbinate. If at all possible, mucosa should be left in place over the lamina papyracea. This is best accomplished with sharp through-biting and microdebrider instruments. Leaving the mucosa intact will promote better healing with less scarring. Trauma to the middle turbinate and the lateral wall of the nose will increase the risk of scarring in the middle meatus.

Exposure to the middle meatus is best accomplished with complete removal of the uncinate process up to, but not including, the mucosa at the root of the junction of the middle turbinate to the lateral nasal wall. If this mucosa is traumatized there is increased risk of scarring in the frontal recess and lateralization of the middle turbinate which in turn can result in chronic frontal rhinosinusitis.

Stenting Material
It has long been felt that a stent placed in the middle meatus will help prevent scarring, (55). Initially, silastic and Gelfilm (USP, Pharmacia, Puurs, Belgium) were used; however, there was excessive granulation tissue and subsequent scarring in the middle meatus. The silastic and granulation tissue had to be removed with a second surgical procedure. Because of this, the practice was called into question (56) and other materials were investigated. MeroGel (Medtronics Xomed, Jacksonville, Florida) has been found to be more effective in reducing synechia and forms less granulation tissue than Gelfilm (57,58). Other studies have found equivocal results (59). I have found MeroGel to be superior to other products in children. It is important that the MeroGel is injected with 2–3 ml of saline after it has been placed into the ethmoid cavity. If the stent is not injected, the MeroGel will not be absorbed in the desired two weeks. I also attempt to place it above the maxillary ostium in an effort not to obstruct the sinus. Young children do not have frontal sinuses; therefore, there is less concern about obstructing the region of the frontal recess. Acute infection or obstruction does not appear to be a problem in children with a small frontal sinus.

Second Look
A second look was recommended by many surgeons who used silastic and Gelfilm because of the granulation tissue and because, at the time, this was the practice being recommended in adults. This practice was called into question by Mitchell et al., who found no difference in outcomes in the children who did not undergo a second-look procedure (60). Intraoperative steroids were found to decrease scarring and inflammation of the ethmoid cavity and decrease the need for a second look (61). Fakhri et al. (62) also found that the second look was of no benefit in routine FESS. It appears that the majority of surgeons are now performing pediatric endoscopic sinus surgery with use of MeroGel or no stents and are not performing a second look (48). If MeroGel is used as a stenting material, it is important to remember to inject it with saline.

Postoperative Management
Postoperative antibiotics are used to minimize the inflammatory response and reduce the chance of postoperative infections. I personally will keep the patient on antibiotics until the MeroGel has cleared from the middle meatus, usually for two weeks. Most children will not tolerate suctioning of the nose postoperatively. Older children will tolerate irrigation which can be helpful in removing the MeroGel and crusting from the cavity. An important part of the postoperative management is reinforcement to the parents that children will continue to have recurrent viral infections and this does not necessarily mean the procedure has been a failure.

Complications

The incidence of complications in children (4.1%) is less than that noted in adults (10.5%) (63). Most of the complications are secondary to scarring rather than major complications associated with the eye or brain. There has been a long-standing concern that endoscopic sinus surgery in young children could be associated with interruption of facial growth. This concern was based on experiments performed in piglets that revealed abnormal growth of the snout on CT scans after endoscopic sinus surgery (64,65). Bothwell et al. (66) compared children who had endoscopic ethmoidectomies and maxillary antrostomies at a young age, mean of 3.1 years, with children who had CRS during the same period but had not undergone surgery and with normal facial growth standards. Quantitative anthropomorphic analysis was performed using 12 standard facial measurements for all three groups, and a facial plastic expert performed qualitative facial analysis. Both analyses showed no statistical differences in facial growth between children in the two groups or with normal children of the same age. They concluded that there was no evidence that endoscopic surgery affected facial growth in children.

OUTCOMES

Outcomes of endoscopic sinus surgery have been studied in children and adults. The results are fairly similar, as noted in the meta-analysis performed by Herbert and Bent (67). The rate of improvement is consistently between 80 and 90%. Concerns over facial growth abnormalities after pediatric endoscopic sinus surgery have been used as a justification for long-term intravenous therapy to treat CRS in children. However, the long-term success of this therapy remains to be established (68, 69).

REFERENCES

1. Sobol SE, Fukakusa M, Christodoulopoulos P, et al. Inflammation and remodeling of the sinus mucosa in children and adults with chronic sinusitis. Laryngoscope 2003; 113:410–4.
2. Chan KH, Abzug MJ, Coffinet L, Simoes EA, Cool C, Liu AH. Chronic rhinosinusitis in young children differs from adults: a histopathology study. J Pediatr 2004; 144:206–12.
3. Zadeh MH, Banthia V, Anand VK, Huang C. Significance of eosinophilia in chronic rhinosinusitis. Am J Rhinol 2002; 16:313–7.
4. Cunningham JM, Chiu EJ, Landgraf JM, Gliklich RE. The health impact of chronic recurrent rhinosinusitis in children. Arch Otolaryngol Head Neck Surg 2000; 126:1363–8.
5. Oehling A, Antepara I, Baena CaCE. The viral factor in the etiology of acute asthma attacks in children. Allergol Immunopathol (Madr) 1981; 9:29–36.
6. Lee D, Rosenfeld RM. Adenoid bacteriology and sinonasal symptoms in children. Otolaryngol Head Neck Surg 1997; 116:301–7.
7. Muntz HR, Lusk RP. Bacteriology of the ethmoid bullae in children with chronic sinusitis. Arch Otolaryngol Head Neck Surg 1991; 117:179–81.
8. Brook I, Yocum P. Antimicrobial management of chronic sinusitis in children. J Laryngol Otol 1995; 109:1159–62.
9. Ramadan HH, Mathers PH, Schwartzbauer H. Role of anaerobes in chronic sinusitis: will polymerase chain reaction solve the debate. Otolaryngol Head Neck Surg 2002; 127:384–6.
10. Nguyen KL, Corbett ML, Garcia DP et al. Chronic sinusitis among pediatric patients with chronic respiratory complaints. J Allergy Clin Immunol 1993; 92:824–30.
11. Iwens P, Clement PA. Sinusitis in allergic patients. Rhinology 1994; 32:65–7.
12. Wald ER, Guerra N, Byers C. Upper respiratory tract infections in young children: duration of and frequency of complications. Pediatrics 1991; 87:129–33.

13. Holzmann D, Willi U, Nadal D. Allergic rhinitis as a risk factor for orbital complication of acute rhinosinusitis in children. Am J Rhinol 2001; 15:387–90.
14. Huang SW, Giannoni C. The risk of adenoid hypertrophy in children with allergic rhinitis. Ann Allergy Asthma Immunol 2001; 87:350–5.
15. Monteil MA, Joseph G, Chang KC, Wheeler G, Antoine RM. Smoking at home is strongly associated with symptoms of asthma and rhinitis in children of primary school age in Trinidad and Tobago. Rev Panam Salud Publica 2004; 16:193–8.
16. Kakish KS, Mahafza T, Batieha A, Ekteish F, Daoud A. Clinical sinusitis in children attending primary care centers. Pediatr Infect Dis J 2000; 19:1071–4.
17. Ramadan HH, Hinerman RA. Smoke exposure and outcome of endoscopic sinus surgery in children. Otolaryngol Head Neck Surg 2002; 127:546–8.
18. Kitchens GG. Relationship of environmental tobacco smoke to otitis media in young children (Review). Laryngoscope 1995; 105(5 Pt 2; Suppl. 69):1–13.
19. Calhoun KH, Waggenspack GA, Simpson CB, Hokanson JA, Bailey BJ. CT evaluation of the paranasal sinuses in symptomatic and asymptomatic populations. Otolaryngol Head Neck Surg 1991; 104:480–3.
20. Harar RP, Chadha NK, Rogers G. The role of septal deviation in adult chronic rhinosinusitis: a study of 500 patients. Rhinology 2004; 42:126–30.
21. Stallman JS, Lobo JN, Som PM. The incidence of concha bullosa and its relationship to nasal septal deviation and paranasal sinus disease. AJNR Am J Neuroradiol 2004; 25:1613–8.
22. Aktas D, Kalcioglu MT, Kutlu R, Ozturan O, Oncel S. The relationship between the concha bullosa, nasal septal deviation and sinusitis. Rhinology 2003; 41:103–6.
23. Hamdan AL, Bizri AR, Jaber M, Hammoud D, Baino T, Fuleihan N. Nasoseptal variation in relation to sinusitis. A computerized tomographic evaluation. J Med Liban 2001; 49:2–5.
24. Collet S, Bertrand B, Cornu S, Eloy P, Rombaux P. Is septal deviation a risk factor for chronic sinusitis? Review of literature. Acta Otorhinolaryngol Belg 2001; 55:299–304.
25. Sivasli E, Sirikci A, Bayazyt YA, et al. Anatomic variations of the paranasal sinus area in pediatric patients with chronic sinusitis. Surg Radiol Anat 2003; 24:400–5.
26. Carr MM, Nguyen A, Poje C, Pizzuto M, Nagy M, Brodsky L. Correlation of findings on direct laryngoscopy and bronchoscopy with presence of extraesophageal reflux disease. Laryngoscope 2000; 110:1560–2.
27. Ludemann JP, Hughes CA, Noah Z, Holinger LD. Complications of pediatric laryngotracheal reconstruction: prevention strategies. Ann Otol Rhinol Laryngol 1999; 108(11 Pt 1):1019–26.
28. Burton DM, Pransky SM, Katz RM, Kearns DB, Seid AB. Pediatric airway manifestations of gastroesophageal reflux. Ann Otol Rhinol Laryngol 1992; 101:742–9.
29. Bothwell MR, Parsons DS, Talbot A, Barbero GJ, Wilder B. Outcome of reflux therapy on pediatric chronic sinusitis. Otolaryngol Head Neck Surg 1999; 121:255–62.
30. Phipps CD, Wood WE, Gibson WS, Cochran WJ. Gastroesophageal reflux contributing to chronic sinus disease in children: a prospective analysis. Arch Otolaryngol Head Neck Surg 2000; 126:831–6.
31. El-Serag HB, Gilger M, Kuebeler M, Rabeneck L. Extraesophageal associations of gastroesophageal reflux disease in children without neurologic defects. Gastroenterology 2001; 121:1294–9.
32. Barbero GJ. Gastroesophageal reflux and upper airway disease. Otolaryngol Clin North Am 1996;29:27–38.
33. Yellon RF, Coticchia J, Dixit S. Esophageal biopsy for the diagnosis of gastroesophageal reflux-associated otolaryngologic problems in children. Am J Med 2000 March 6;108 (Suppl. 4a):131S–8S.
34. Suskind DL, Zeringue GP III, Kluka EA, Udall J, Liu DC. Gastroesophageal reflux and pediatric otolaryngologic disease: the role of antireflux surgery. Arch Otolaryngol Head Neck Surg 2001; 127:511–4.
35. Clinical practice guideline: management of sinusitis. Pediatrics 2001; 108:797–808
36. Orlandi RR, Kennedy DW. Surgical management of rhinosinusitis (Review, 26 refs). Am J Med Sci 1998; 316:29–38.

37. Gwaltney JM, Jr., Phillips CD, Miller RD, Riker DK. Computed tomographic study of the common cold. N Eng J Med 1994; 330:25–30.
38. Papsin B, McTavish A. Saline nasal irrigation: Its role as an adjunct treatment. Can Fam Physician 2003; 49:167–73.
39. Chalumeau M, Tonnelier S, D'Athis P, et al. Fluoroquinolone safety in pediatric patients: a prospective, multicenter, comparative cohort study in France. Pediatrics 2003; 111(6 Pt 1):e714–e9.
40. Don DM, Yellon RF, Casselbrant ML, Bluestone CD. Efficacy of a stepwise protocol that includes intravenous antibiotic therapy for the management of chronic sinusitis in children and adolescents. Arch Otolaryngol Head Neck Surg 2001; 127:1093–8.
41. McCarty ML, Wilson MW, Fleming JC, et al. Manifestations of fungal cellulitis of the orbit in children with neutropenia and fever. Ophthal Plast Reconstr Surg 2004; 20:217–23.
42. Manning SC, Vuitch F, Weinberg AG, Brown OE. Allergic aspergillosis: a newly recognized form of sinusitis in the pediatric population. Laryngoscope 1989; 99 (7 Pt 1):681–5.
43. Wolthers OD, Pedersen S. Growth of asthmatic children during treatment with budesonide: a double blind trial. BMJ 1991; 303:163–5.
44. Lee D, Rosenfeld RM. Adenoid bacteriology and sinonasal symptoms in children. Otolaryngol Head Neck Surg 1997; 116:301–7.
45. Ramadan HH. Adenoidectomy vs endoscopic sinus surgery for the treatment of pediatric sinusitis. Arch Otolaryngol Head Neck Surg 1999; 125:1207–11.
46. Vandenberg SJ, Heatley DG. Efficacy of adenoidectomy in relieving symptoms of chronic sinusitis in children. Arch Otolaryngol Head Neck Surg 1997; 123:675–8.
47. Lieser JD, Derkay CS. Pediatric sinusitis: when do we operate? Curr Opin Otolaryngol Head Neck Surg 2005; 13:60–6.
48. Sobol SE, Samadi DS, Kazahaya K, Tom LW. Trends in the management of pediatric chronic sinusitis: survey of the American Society of Pediatric Otolaryngology. Laryngoscope 2005; 115:77–80.
49. Lund VJ. Inferior meatal antrostomy. Fundamental considerations of design and function. J Laryngol Otol Suppl 1988; 15:1–18.
50. Muntz HR, Lusk RP. Nasal antral windows in children: a retrospective study. Laryngoscope 1990; 100:643–6.
51. Chang PH, Lee LA, Huang CC, Lai CH, Lee TJ. Functional endoscopic sinus surgery in children using a limited approach. Arch Otolaryngol Head Neck Surg 2004; 130:1033–6.
52. Ramadan HH. Relation of age to outcome after endoscopic sinus surgery in children. Arch Otolaryngol Head Neck Surg 2003; 129:175–7.
53. Wadwongtham W, Aeumjaturapat S. Large middle meatal antrostomy vs undisturbed maxillary ostium in the endoscopic sinus surgery of nasal polyposis. J Med Assoc Thai 2003; 86(Suppl. 2):S373–S8.
54. Setliff RC. The small-hole technique in endoscopic sinus surgery. Otolaryngol Clin North Am 1997; 30:341–54.
55. Lusk RP, Muntz HR. Endoscopic sinus surgery in children with chronic sinusitis—a pilot study. Laryngoscope 1990; 100:654–8.
56. Tom LW, Palasti S, Potsic WP, Handler SD, Wetmore RF. The effects of gelatin film stents in the middle meatus. Am J Rhinol 1997; 11:229–32.
57. Catalano PJ, Roffman EJ. Evaluation of middle meatal stenting after minimally invasive sinus techniques (MIST). Otolaryngol Head Neck Surg 2003; 128:875–81.
58. Xu G, Chen HX, Wen WP, Shi JB, Li Y. Clinical evaluation of local application of Merogel after endoscopic sinus surgery. Zhonghua Er Bi Yan Hou Ke Za Zhi 2003; 38:95–7.
59. Miller RS, Steward DL, Tami TA, et al. The clinical effects of hyaluronic acid ester nasal dressing (Merogel) on intranasal wound healing after functional endoscopic sinus surgery. Otolaryngol Head Neck Surg 2003; 128:862–9.
60. Mitchell RB, Pereira KD, Younis RT, Lazar RH. Pediatric functional endoscopic sinus surgery: is a second look necessary? Laryngoscope 1997; 107:1267–9.
61. Ramadan HH. Corticosteroid therapy during endoscopic sinus surgery in children: is there a need for a second look? Arch Otolaryngol Head Neck Surg 2001; 127:187–92.

62. Fakhri S, Manoukian JJ, Souaid JP. Functional endoscopic sinus surgery in the paediatric population: outcome of a conservative approach to postoperative care. J Otolaryngol 2001; 30:15–8.
63. Jiang RS, Hsu CY. Functional endoscopic sinus surgery in children and adults. Ann Otol Rhinol Laryngol 2000; 109(12 Pt 1):1113–6.
64. Carpenter KM, Graham SM, Smith RJ. Facial skeletal growth after endoscopic sinus surgery in the piglet model. Am J Rhinol 1997; 11:211–7.
65. Mair EA, Bolger WE, Breisch EA. Sinus and facial growth after pediatric endoscopic sinus surgery. Arch Otolaryngol Head Neck Surg 1995; 121:547–52.
66. Bothwell MR, Piccirillo JF, Lusk RP, Ridenour BD. Long-term outcome of facial growth after functional endoscopic sinus surgery. Otolaryngol Head Neck Surg 2002; 126:627–34.
67. Hebert RL, Bent JP III. Meta-analysis of outcomes of pediatric functional endoscopic sinus surgery. Laryngoscope 1998; 108:796–9.
68. Buchman CA, Yellon RF, Bluestone CD. Alternative to endoscopic sinus surgery in the management of pediatric chronic rhinosinusitis refractory to oral antimicrobial therapy. Otolaryngol Head Neck Surg 1999; 120:219–24.
69. Clement PA, Bluestone CD, Gordts F, et al. Management of rhinosinusitis in children: consensus meeting, Brussels, Belgium, September 13, 1996. (Review, 41 refs). Arch Otolaryngol Head Neck Surg 1998; 124:31–4.

19 Approach to the Evaluation and Medical Management of Chronic Rhinosinusitis

Daniel L. Hamilos
Division of Rheumatology, Allergy, and Immunology, Massachusetts General Hospital, Harvard Medical School, Boston, Massachusetts, U.S.A.

INTRODUCTION

Most experts in rhinosinusitis now subscribe to the concept that "chronic rhinosinusitis is a medical disease." That is simply to underscore the importance of identifying and treating the underlying medical aspects of the disease. The first 18 chapters provide the reader with a foundation for this management. In this chapter, the published literature on medical management is briefly reviewed and a comprehensive medical evaluation and management program is outlined being mindful of the recent consensus definitions of chronic rhinosinusitis (CRS) (1).

CURRENT RHINOSINUSITIS TREATMENTS BASED ON LEVEL OF EVIDENCE

In 2005, the European Academy of Allergology and Clinical Immunology (EAACI) published a consensus document summarizing the level of evidence for published treatments of intermittent (acute) or persistent (chronic) rhinosinusitis (2). With the exception of antibiotics and corticosteroids [and antihistamines for nasal polyp (NP) patients with allergies] none of the other medical therapies achieved a level I for evidence. This was especially true for CRS where none of the other therapies achieved greater than a level III for evidence. As a result, many of the recommendations outlined here for medical management of CRS have not been substantiated by high-level clinical evidence. It is encouraging, however, that over the past two years three important consensus documents have been published that serve to better define CRS, both Chronic rhinosinussitis with and without nasal polyps (CRS with NP and CRS without NP), as well as allergic fungal rhinosinusitis (AFRS) (1–3).

As summarized in the EAACI document, there is level Ia evidence for use of antibiotics for acute/intermittent rhinosinusitis. There is also level Ib evidence for use of topical corticosteroids either as an adjunct to antibiotics or as monotherapy. No other therapies have level I of evidence. Based on this, the EAACI document gave a grade A recommendation for use of antibiotics and use of topical corticosteroids as an adjunct to antibiotics.

For therapy of CRS, there is level Ib evidence only for topical corticosteroids and topical antifungal agents (specifically topical amphotericin B). Based on this information, the EAACI document gave a grade A recommendation for use of topical corticosteroids. However, because the studies of topical amphotericin B have yielded conflicting results, this treatment was given a grade D recommendation. It is worth pointing out, however, that the study by Ponikau et al. (4) found that amphotericin B nasal irrigations provided a modest statistically significant benefit; the study by (5) found that amphotericin B as a nasal spray was ineffective.

In my opinion, it is unfair to lump these studies together and conclude that topical antifungal therapy is ineffective. Subsequent to the EAACI publication, a double-blind, placebo-controlled trial was reported that would also constitute level Ib evidence using the oral antifungal terbinafine (6). This study failed to show benefit for CRS. Clearly, more studies are needed in this area.

For therapy of established nasal polyposis, there is level Ib evidence for use of topical corticosteroids based on several studies, and this treatment was given a grade A recommendation in the EAACI publication. In general, treatment for 12 weeks or longer was required to show a reduction in nasal polyp size, and not all studies demonstrated this effect. There is also level Ib evidence for use of oral antihistamines in nasal polyposis with associated allergies, and this treatment was given a grade B recommendation.

For prevention of nasal polyposis following polypectomy, there is level Ib evidence for the use of topical corticosteroids, and this treatment received a grade A recommendation in the EACCI document. Surprisingly, one study of topical corticosteroids for prevention of polyp recurrence following functional endoscopic sinus surgery (FESS) failed to show efficacy in terms of prevention of polyp recurrence, and therefore this treatment was given a grade D recommendation (7).

Two recent studies using an identical study design and treatment with intranasal mometasone 200 μg daily, or 200 μg bid yielded further evidence for the beneficial effects of topical corticosteroids for established nasal polyps (8,9). Treatment with intranasal mometasone for four months produced a regression in nasal polyp size relative to placebo nasal spray. Both studies also showed symptomatic improvement, and one study showed improvement in hyposmia. The studies formed the basis for FDA approval of mometasone furoate nasal spray (MFNS) as a treatment for nasal polyps in 2004.

Although systemic steroids are often used clinically for the treatment of CRS with NP, no good evidence was available until recently. Hissaria et al. treated subjects with endoscopically documented nasal polyposis with oral prednisolone or placebo for 14 days. They showed a significant improvement in nasal symptoms, as well as significant reduction in polyp size as assessed by endoscopy and magnetic resonance imaging (MRI), in the patients receiving active treatment (10). Similar results were also seen in another study where oral prednisone was administered in a placebo-controlled fashion to patients with CRS with NP (11).

Intranasal Instillation of Topical Corticosteroids with Head Maneuvering

Another recent study demonstrated the benefit of using topical corticosteroid nasal drops for treatment of established nasal polyps (12). In this 12-week, double-blind, placebo-controlled study, subjects were instructed to lie on their back in a bed with their heads hanging down in an inverted vertical position over the edge of the bed while fluticasone propionate drops were administrated (at) 200 μg per nostril once daily. They had to remain in this position for 2 minutes. The primary efficacy endpoint was based on a complicated scoring method that took into consideration patients' symptoms, sinus computed tomography (CT) score, and the physician's impression of the patient's need for sinus surgery. Using this method, fluticasone nasal drops were found to reduce the need for sinus surgery relative to the placebo drops. Fluticasone nasal drops also improved hyposmia and decreased nasal polyp volume as found using a visual analog scale.

I have employed a treatment similar to the fluticasone nasal drops using "off-label" intranasal instillation of budesonide (available in the United States as

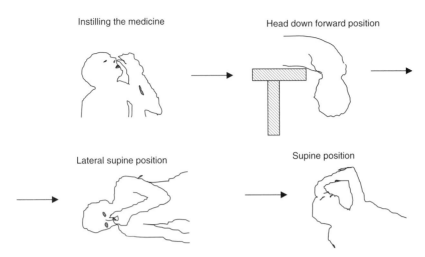

Instilling the medicine

Head down forward position

Lateral supine position

Supine position

FIGURE 1 Intranasal instillation of aqueous corticosteroid mixture. A 0.5 mg Pulmicort Respule® is mixed with 1 teaspoon of saline, and this mixture is instilled in the right nostril once daily first in the head down forward, then right lateral supine position, and finally in the supine position each for 1–2 minutes, following which the remaining nasal solution is expelled from the nose. The procedure is then repeated in the left nostril. A controlled clinical trial of this treatment has not been performed, and the long-term safety of this procedure has not been established. The head-down-forward position can also be accomplished by kneeling and having the top of the head touch the floor.

aqueous Pulmicort Respules®, Astra-Zeneca). The success of this treatment depends on delivery of the topical steroid to the polyp and polypoid tissue near the sinus ostia and in the sinus cavities. Usually a 0.5-mg Respule is mixed with one teaspoon of saline, and this mixture is instilled in the right nostril once daily, first in the head down forward position, then right lateral supine position, and finally in the supine position, each for 1–2 minutes, following which the remaining nasal solution is expelled from the nose. The procedure is then repeated in the left nostril (see Fig. 1). Many patients have responded very well to this treatment. However, a controlled clinical trial has not been performed, and the long-term safety of this procedure has not been established. Therefore, the clinician should be mindful to periodically evaluate the patient for possible systemic effects of the budesonide, including an increase in intraocular pressure.

Antibiotic Treatment for CRS

Whenever possible, the choice of antibiotics for CRS should be guided by appropriately obtained sinus cultures (28). However, when seeing the patient for the first time, an empiric decision about antibiotics is often the most practical approach. Chapter 9 summarizes the bacteriology of CRS and provides recommendations for antibiotic selection. As indicated therein, utilization of a broad-spectrum antibiotic that is beta-lactamase stable, effective against penicillin-resistant *Streptcoccus pneumoniae*, and possessing anti-anaerobic coverage may be optimal for the treatment of CRS. Such agents include: (1) the combination of a penicillin (e.g., amoxicillin) and a beta-lactamase inhibitor (e.g., clavulanic acid), or (2) the combination of a macrolide, a ketolide (e.g., telithromycin), and a fluoroquinolone (only in adults) (e.g., levofloxacin, moxifloxacin, gatifloxacin) or a third-generation cefalosporine along with either metronidazole (e.g., 250 mg tid) or clindamycin (300 mg qid). The regimens differ primarily in their coverage of aerobic gram-negative bacteria. The usual approach is to treat patients for 21–28 days in combination with a short course of systemic prednisone (see "Intensive Medical Treatment for CRS" below).

Empiric antibiotic treatment is not recommended under the following circumstances: (a) if the patient has recently failed antibiotic treatment with a similar regimen; (b) if the patient has a history of infection with gram-negative bacteria (e.g., *Pseudomonas*, *Stenotrophomonas*, etc.) or oxacillin-resistant *Staphylococcus* or another highly drug-resistant bacteria; (c) if the clinical suspicion is that the patient has allergic fungal rhinosinusitis; (d) if the patient shows signs of extrasinus involvement or appears otherwise toxic (i.e., high fever, flushing, hypotensity); or (e) if the patient is highly immunosuppressed and therefore at risk for invasive fungal rhinosinusitis. The exception to this statement may apply to a patient who appears toxic in whom empiric intravenous antibiotics may be started, preferably while awaiting results of sinus cultures.

Antifungal Treatment for CRS

Optimal use of antifungal drugs for AFRS and fungally-driven Th2 chronic inflammation remain to be defined. In the absence of an evidence-based approach, I have used antifungal agents with some success. Unlike culture-directed antibiotic treatment, it is difficult to predict patients' responses owing largely to the limited information available from fungal cultures. As a result, careful follow-up assessment with endoscopic evaluation is essential to assess patients' response to treatment.

In cases where AFRS has been documented or is suspected, treatment is begun with prednisone (see AFRS treatment below). I have also treated patients with oral itraconazole 200 mg bid for 1–3 months in an attempt to reduce the need for prednisone. Liver function tests are monitored on a monthly basis. Caution should be used to avoid use of itraconazole with other potentially hepatotoxic drugs, such as lipid-lowering agents, and the patient should avoid excessive consumption of alcohol or use of acetaminophen. Improvement usually occurs gradually over several months. Patients are reassessed by endoscopic examination in 2–3 months. In the absence of evidence to support their use in the treatment of CRS, systemic antifungals are generally only used if moderate doses of systemic steroids have failed to keep the disease under control.

Topical antifungal sinus irrigation with either amphotericin-B or itraconazole is also recommended, although as stated above the evidence in support of this treatment remains conflicting. The drugs are usually mixed in sterile water at 100 mg/l. I advise patients to administer the antifungal irrigation using the head-down forward, lateral supine and supine positions exactly as recommended for the topical budesonide instillation program (see Fig. 1). Treatments are given either once or twice daily.

Intensive Medical Treatment for CRS

Our group defined "intensive medical treatment" for CRS as therapy that combines a prolonged course of oral antibiotics with a brief course of systemic steroids (13). The typical regimen combines one of the antibiotic regimens outlined above with oral Prednisone 20 mg bid for five days, followed by 20 mg daily for five days. In a retrospective review, we summarized the treatment of 40 patients with CRS with this "intensive" regimen, and reported that 90% of patients improved either symptomatically, radiographically, or both, and that 65% had sustained (>8 week) symptomatic benefit (13). Adjunctive medical treatment, consisting of some combination of intranasal saline irrigations, intranasal corticosteroids, corticosteroid nasal instillations, and leukotriene blocker agents, was also given with this treatment and continued thereafter (discussed further in Chapter 15).

FINDINGS IN PATIENTS WITH DISEASE RECURRENCE FOLLOWING MEDICAL OR SURGICAL TREATMENT
Recurrence Following Intensive Medical Treatment
The study employing "intensive medical treatment" found that a past history or current evidence of nasal polyps and a past history of sinus surgery were associated with early relapses (13). It was further found that these factors were highly related, such that in a multivariate analysis the predominant predictor of early relapse was nasal polyposis. In contrast, atopy, asthma, and persistent obstruction of the ostiomeatal unit were not predictive of relapse. This study identified "uncontrolled" mucosal inflammation as the predominant reason for medical failure. This study did not investigate anatomic factors associated with failure of medical treatment (discussed further below). In a subsequent review of cases seen at Massachusetts General Hospital (MGH), other factors found to contribute to medical failures included: the presence of a gram-negative or drug-resistant bacterial infection in approximately 9% of cases and "suspected AFRS" in 12% of cases. An accurate estimate of the prevalence of fungal Th2 sensitization as a contributor to persistent sinus inflammation is not yet available; however, Ponikau et al. (4) have claimed that this process is responsible for the majority of cases of CRS, both without and with nasal polyposis (14).

Recurrence Following Endoscopic Sinus Surgery
Richtsmeier reported the "top ten" reasons for maxillary sinus surgical failure (15). This study focused on typical patients who had undergone surgery for primarily maxillary sinus disease but excluded patients with pansinusitis, fungal sinusitis, or underlying malignancy. Therefore, the series was not fully representative of all surgical cases; however, it highlighted several important issues in patients who had failed "functional" endoscopic sinus surgery. The most common reason for failure was obstruction of the maxillary sinus ostium, typically caused by a retained uncinate process or a missed maxillary sinus ostium. This accounted for roughly 33.6% of the cases. The second most common reason for failure was disease in the ethmoid or frontal sinus, accounting for 24.2% of the cases. The third reason (13.3%) was the presence of a resistant bacterial infection caused by methicillin-resistant *Staphylococcus aureus*, penicillin-resistant *S. pneumoniae*, or Gram-negative bacterial infection with *Serratia* or *Pseudomonas*. Primary mucosal disease accounted for 7% of cases. The presence of a foreign body, such as a bony chip, dental amalgam, or surgical clip, accounted for 5.5% of cases. This study underestimated the importance of mucosal inflammation as a cause of surgical failure due to the selection criteria which excluded patients with pansinusitis or fungal sinusitis.

Persistence of disease in the narrow clefts of the anterior ethmoid with subsequent spread locally to involve the adjacent sinuses was recognized by Stammberger as a common cause for CRS (16). Similarly, Richtsmeier (15) observed that in some cases an anterior ethmoid air cell had been surgically crushed against the lamina papyracea creating a non-aerated focus of infection and drainage that contaminated the superior aspect of the maxillary sinus ostium. This nidus of infection was often only identified by endoscopic examination due to obliteration of the air cell.

In another study, Musy and Kountakis (17) reviewed anatomic findings in patients undergoing revision endoscopic sinus surgery. All patients had recurrence of disease despite previous sinus surgery and prolonged attempts at medical treatment. The most common findings were: lateralization of the middle turbinate (78%), incomplete anterior ethmoidectomy (64%), frontal recess scarring (50%), retained agger nasi (49%), incomplete posterior ethmoidectomy (41%), middle meatal antrostomy stenosis (39%), retained uncinate process (37%), and recurrent polyposis (37%). They concluded that failure of endoscopic sinus surgery was most often associated with anatomic obstruction in the vicinity of the ostiomeatal complex.

Although these studies did not compare findings to those in control patients who had undergone endoscopic sinus surgery with good outcome, they nonetheless provide important insights into anatomic factors that may be associated with surgical or medical failure. On the other hand, acknowledging that anatomic reasons for failure occur, Stankiewicz (18) emphasized the importance of polypoid CRS as the principal cause of endoscopic sinus surgical failure. Similarly, in the case series reported by Kennedy (19), patients with grade IV mucosal disease (which included patients with nasal polyposis) had a poorer outcome following endoscopic sinus surgery. The bottom line is that there is compelling evidence that both mucosal inflammation and anatomic factors contribute to the persistence of CRS, and these factors deserve careful consideration, especially in the most refractory cases.

SPECIAL CONSIDERATIONS IN THE MANAGEMENT OF CRS WITHOUT NP, CRS WITH NP, AND CLASSIC AFRS

Some of the more common problems encountered in managing patients with CRS are summarized below.

1. Facial pain/pressure may or may not represent rhinosinusitis. The sinus CT scan and rhinoscopic examination can be very helpful in such cases. Often, a "sinus" cause may not be found, but at least the physician is on more solid ground if these procedures have been done. Rhinogenic considerations for localized pain include: oroantral fistula, odontogenic sinusitis, and facial or sinus bone osteomyelitis (also referred to as "osteiitis"). Nonrhinogenic causes were discussed in Chapter 1. The investigation of rhinogenic causes may require special radiographic studies and the assistance of specialists in otolaryngology, oral surgery, or neurosurgery.
2. Fungal stains of sinus mucus are usually inadequate, owing to problems in specimen collection and insensitive staining techniques. Newer staining techniques, such as the use of a fungal-specific chitinase immunostain (20), may eventually improve the utility of this procedure.
3. Intranasal corticosteroids are useful for nasal polyposis but are often inadequate for controlling CRS symptoms. Aqueous corticosteroid formulations applied with topical instillation and head maneuvering improve delivery to the sinus cavities and give superior results.

4. Topical medications, including topical corticosteroids, topical antibiotics, and topical antifungal drugs, are the mainstay of treatment in most cases.
5. The clinical value of antihistamines, antihistamine/decongestant combination, nasal ipratropium, and oral leukotriene blockers in CRS has not been proven, and their use should be individualized based on every patient's symptom profile and the role of allergy in the patient's symptoms.
6. Environmental control measures and immunotherapy are important adjuncts in treatment of CRS.
7. Aspirin desensitization is a useful adjunct for treatment of CRS with NP patients with aspirin sensitivity.
8. Sinus opacification has different significance in CRS without NP, CRS with NP, and AFRS (discussed below).

EVALUATION OF SINUS OPACIFICATION

Sinus opacification in a patient with CRS without NP may represent an infectious process or polypoid degeneration of the mucosa, and these two possibilities cannot be distinguished clinically. In contrast, sinus opacification in CRS with NP most often represents polypoid mucosal thickening in the absence of infection. Sinus opacification in AFRS may simply represent polypoid mucosal disease but may also represent mucus impaction with allergic mucin laden with fungal hyphae.

STEP-WISE EVALUATION OF PATIENTS WITH CRS

The following step-wise approach, which is summarized in Figure 2, is recommended for the evaluation and treatment of patients with CRS.

Step 1: Comprehensive Evaluation of a Patient with CRS
Each patient should undergo a complete history and physical examination. The history should include questions about potential exposure to indoor allergens at home, school, or work. Potential sources of mold exposure include: water seepage or dampness in the basement, leaks in the foundation, walls, or roof; mold growth in the bathroom shower stall, curtain, ceiling, or window sills. Every patient should be evaluated for allergies, particularly indoor allergies, including those to dust mite, cockroach, animal dander, and fungi. Considering that many patients have had previous antibiotic treatment and/or surgery, it is difficult to outline a rational initial treatment plan without having up-to-date information, including a recent sinus CT scan. A rhinoscopic evaluation may be a part of the baseline evaluation, although it may be performed at a second visit, perhaps after an initial empiric course of medical therapy. Three "special considerations" should be kept in mind, as outlined in Figure 2, namely whether the patient warrants an evaluation for hypogammaglobulinemia, gram-negative or drug-resistant bacterial infection, or AFRS. Other contributive factors, such as cigarette smoke, occupational exposures, and comorbid conditions should also be noted.

Step 2: Clinical Classification of CRS
Based on the comprehensive evaluation, a preliminary categorization of the patient is made, and a list of contributive factors is outlined. Precise categorization

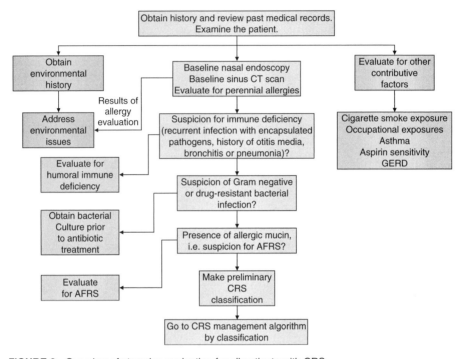

FIGURE 2 Overview of stepwise evaluation for all patients with CRS.

requires rhinoscopic assessment. In the author's experience, longitudinal observation has shown that the vast majority of patients retain the same phenotype of CRS over prolonged periods of time (i.e. years). Furthermore, CRS without NP and CRS with NP likely have different underlying pathogenic mechanisms and tend to respond differently to medical and surgical treatment.

The categories include: CRS without NP, CRS with NP, polypoid CRS, and classic AFRS. In addition, it is useful to examine the temporal pattern of illness. The most common pattern is persistent symptoms with periodic exacerbations. Recurrent acute symptoms (also known as "chronic recurrent rhinosinusitis") are less common and are usually associated with CRS without NP. Patients with this pattern may have asymptomatic periods between episodes (21,22) and are more likely to have underlying hypogammaglobulinemia and a better response to antibiotic treatment (see Chapter 1).

Step 3: Enumeration of Contributive Factors to CRS

The distinguishing clinical features and contributive factors associated with CRS without NP and CRS with NP were discussed in Chapter 1. An awareness of the different clinical subcategories can help the clinician uncover contributive factors to the disease. Certain generalities are noteworthy:

1. CRS without NP is more heterogeneous in underlying cause than CRS with NP. In the former, it is important to rule out chronic sinus infection, anatomic sinus abnormalities, defects in mucociliary function, and immune deficiency.

2. Allergy is common (prevalence ≥50%) and about equally prevalent in CRS without NP and CRS with NP. All patients with CRS deserve an evaluation for underlying allergy.
3. Immune deficiency is more common in CRS without NP and rare in patients with CRS with NP. It is most common in patients with "chronic recurrent rhinosinusitis" (synonymous with "recurrent acute rhinosinusitis").
4. The diagnosis of classic AFRS is difficult to make without surgery unless the patient has had prior surgery and now has a recurrence of disease at the site of the previous surgery.
5. Nearly all patients with classic AFRS have nasal polyps.
6. Asthma and aspirin sensitivity are more common in patients with CRS with NP.

Step 4: Establishing an Infectious Cause of Disease
Empiric Choice of Antibiotics
The microbiology of CRS is changing over time. Traditionally, *S. pneumoniae*, *Haemophilus influenza* and *Branhamella catarrhalis*, and *S. aureus* have been the most common organisms found in the sinus mucus. However, more recent series have found that gram-negative rods and drug-resistant organisms, including methicillin-resistant staphylococci and penicillin-resistant *S. pneumoniae*, are becoming more prevalent. As a corollary, the clinical index of suspicion for a drug-resistant organism should increase if the patient has persistent symptoms and/or sinus abnormalities despite having received antibiotics recently. Repeated use of one class of antibiotics, such as beta-lactams or macrolides, promotes the emergence of resistant organisms, such as penicillin- or macrolide-resistant *S. pneumoniae*. In patients with frequent evidence of mucosal purulence, it is essential to obtain bacterial and fungal cultures to establish the nature of the infection.

Most antibiotics are prescribed empirically for CRS. However, controversies over the role of bacteria versus fungi in the pathogenesis of CRS and the lack of pathogenic bacteria found in most cases provide strong arguments for obtaining bacterial cultures whenever possible, especially in refractory cases.

There is less controversy regarding chronic recurrent rhinosinusitis. Here, the bacteriology parallels that of acute bacterial rhinosinusitis, and it is usually reasonable to prescribe empiric antibiotics in this setting, provided the patient has not received repeated courses of the same antibiotic over several months or years (e.g. amoxicillin or azithromycin). In the latter cases, the likelihood of an antibiotic-resistant organism, such as a penicillin-resistant strain of *S. pneumoniae*, is much higher.

Persistent Infection Despite Multiple Courses of Antibiotics
A history of persistent purulent infection despite treatment with multiple courses of antibiotics may indicate the presence of a gram-negative or drug-resistant bacterial infection or fungal colonization/infection. In such cases, it is essential to obtain mucus samples from one or more sinus ostia for bacterial and fungal culture. This is usually accomplished rhinoscopically, although in some cases it is necessary to perform a maxillary sinus puncture. Representative cultures can only be obtained with proper techniques, appropriate collection vessels and transport media, and timely delivery to the laboratory. Culturing for anaerobic bacteria requires special techniques and handling and is not recommended in the outpatient

setting unless a sinus puncture is performed. In general, obtaining cultures during antibiotic treatment is discouraged. Preferably, the antibiotic should be discontinued for 48 hours.

Cultures should be taken from appropriate areas, especially from the middle meatus (23) or directly from a patent sinus ostium. Care must be taken to avoid contaminating the specimen. Unlike cultures taken from the nose, endoscopically guided cultures from the ostiomeatal unit using Dacron urethral swabs have been found to accurately reproduce cultures taken from within the sinuses, either at the time of surgery or via sinus puncture (23–25). Generally, the most reliable cultures can be expected when the mucus sample is visibly purulent.

Special devices, such as the Xomed Sinus Secretion Collector, are very helpful in obtaining cultures (Medtronic/Xomed). The device consists of a 2-mm plastic malleable catheter inside a protective sheath that is attached to a suction device. The protective sheath minimizes but does not completely eliminate contamination from the anterior nares. After introduction into the middle meatus or sinuses, the outer sheath is retracted, suction applied, and a sample taken. The cultured material is retained within a collection trap. Once collected, the sample can be divided into aliquots that can be transferred to special bacterial or fungal transport media before being sent to the laboratory.

For fungal cultures, a special transport medium is highly recommended as this may help to prevent bacterial overgrowth of the culture and a false-negative result. Whenever fungi may be present, pathogenic bacteria may be present simultaneously, and it is worthwhile sending the sample for both a fungal and bacterial culture. Fungal stains such as Gomor's methamine silver stain (GMS) or PAS are most commonly used, but they lack sensitivity. As a result, a more sensitive fluorescein-labeled chitinase that stains the chitin layer of the fungal organism (e.g. Fungalase, Anomerics, Baton Rouge, FL, USA) has been described but is not yet in general use (20).

Sensitization to Colonizing Fungi vs. Classic AFRS

A high percentage of CRS cases have been found to have evidence of fungal Th2-sensitization whereby their T lymphocytes respond in vitro to certain fungal antigens by producing eosinophil-promoting cytokines, including IL-5 and IL-13 (14) (see Chapter 11). The effect of this sensitization may be to promote eosinophil-predominant, inflammatory mucous exudate devoid of pathogenic bacteria. This is an attractive explanation to account for many refractory cases of CRS. The distinction between a patient with fungal sensitization and one with classic AFRS is that the former may or may not have gross allergic mucin, the mucus is negative on fungal stains and cultures, and there may be no evidence of IgE-mediated fungal allergy. Although such patients do not fit the "classic" definition of AFRS, their underlying pathologic process may be similar to AFRS, and there may be a role for antifungal treatment to reduce fungal colonization of mucus. However, the extent to which the mucus is typically colonized by fungus and the efficacy of antifungal treatment remains controversial.

By contrast, the diagnosis of classic AFRS requires that more strict criteria are met for (a) the presence of gross allergic mucin, (b) the presence of fungi in the mucin, and (c) the presence of IgE-mediated fungal allergy. This definition clearly restricts AFRS to a much smaller percentage of CRS cases, typically only 5–7% of cases. A suspicion of classic AFRS is raised when thick, inspissated "allergic mucin" is identified in a sinus cavity at the time of surgery. Given the insensitivity of fungal stains, the fungal stain of allergic mucin may be reported as negative. It may be worthwhile to repeat the stain and fungal culture to confirm the diagnosis. Classic AFRS may also be suspected based on radiographic evidence of high-attenuation signaling or expansion of a sinus cavity on sinus CT scan or low-attenuation signaling on T1- or T2-weighted images on sinus MRI scan (see Chapter 12). In all cases of "classic AFRS," skin or in vitro testing for IgE-mediated fungal allergy should be positive.

Steps 5 and 6: Initiation of Treatment and Reevaluation

For all types of CRS, it is essential to evaluate an allergic component to the disease and, if present, treat it. Treatment includes institution of environmental control measures to minimize exposure to indoor dust mites, animal danders, and fungi, treatment with medications, and possibly institution of allergen immunotherapy. Special considerations regarding exposure to indoor fungi have been recently reviewed (26). There have been limited studies of the efficacy of environmental control or immunotherapy for any type of CRS.

All CRS patients should also be advised regarding general health measures, such as avoiding exposures to cigarette smoke, noxious chemicals or occupational dusts or fumes and avoiding sick contacts. A yearly influenza vaccine is also recommended. Aside from their role treating allergies, there is no evidence from clinical studies that any other treatment, such as saline nasal washes, decongestants, or intranasal steroids, are helpful in CRS (discussed further in Chapter 15).

CHRONIC RECURRENT RHINOSINUSITIS
Initial

The key clinical features of acute episodes are: purulent anterior or posterior nasal drainage, facial pain/pressure or headache, increase in nasal congestion, and upper tooth pain. These episodes should be distinguished from viral upper respiratory infection (URI) by adhering to the recommendation that they should require symptoms to be present for 7–10 days or symptom worsening after 5–7 days (Fig. 3).

A history of recurrent episodes of purulent infection should prompt evaluation for hypogammaglobulinemia or, less commonly, other types of immune deficiency. This is especially true when a previous infection with an encapsulated organism, such as *S. pneumoniae*, *H. influenza*, and *M. catarrhalis*, has been documented. The evaluation should include checking quantitative immunoglobulins (IgG, IgA, IgM, and IgG subclasses) and specific antibody responses to vaccination with pneumococcal polysaccharide vaccine (Pneumovax®).

Assuming that the patient is not having a recurrent episode, the purpose of the initial sinus CT scan is to rule out a persistent nidus of infection. If sinus mucosal thickening or opacification is present, a course of intensive medical treatment is recommended (see CRS without NP). If the sinus cavities are clear, antibiotics are not indicated. In these cases, the rhinoscopic examination is also typically normal. Certain occupations predispose to recurrent sinus infections, such as working in a day-care center or a nursing home. There is no evidence that any other treatment, such as saline nasal washes, decongestants, or intranasal steroid sprays, help prevent recurrent episodes. Some patients are given prophylactic antibiotics especially during the winter viral season. I avoid this due to concerns about promoting antibiotic resistance.

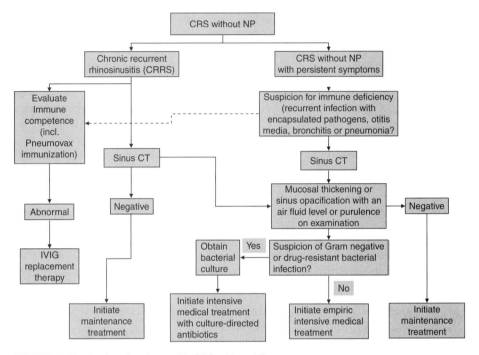

FIGURE 3   Evaluation of patients with CRS without NP.

Follow Up

The status of treatment of allergies and environmental concerns should always be reviewed. If intensive medical treatment was given, the response to this treatment should be assessed. The rhinoscopic examination is used to assess the response to this treatment rather than repeating the sinus CT scan. If the patient has persistent symptoms, management reverts to the algorithm for CRS without NP.

Treatment of Acute Exacerbations

In general, these are treated the same as acute episodes of bacterial rhinosinusitis. It is recommended to avoid using the same antibiotic repeatedly in such patients.

CRS WITHOUT NP
Initial

If the initial sinus CT scan is clear, antibiotics are not indicated (Fig. 3). The rhinoscopic examination is additionally helpful in ruling out focal evidence of inflammation, infection, or polypoid changes. If the sinus CT shows sinus mucosal thickening, opacification with an air fluid level, or there is purulence on physical examination a chronic bacterial sinus infection is presumed. If history raises a suspicion of gram-negative or drug-resistant bacterial infection, a bacterial culture should be obtained so that culture-directed antibiotics can be prescribed. Otherwise, an empiric antibiotic regimen may be selected and "intensive medical treatment" given as discussed above. If the initial sinus CT scan is negative, antibiotics are not recommended.

"Maintenance treatment" is also recommended although there are no published studies to support it. This treatment is guided by the patient's symptoms and by the presence or absence of allergies. Saline nasal washes and intranasal steroids are useful for all CRS symptoms and are recommended for maintenance treatment. Antihistamines are most useful in patients with associated allergies or symptoms of sneezing and rhinorrhea. Oral leukotriene blockers may be of benefit in patients with refractory nasal congestion and postnasal drainage, although the benefit is often marginal. Oral decongestants are generally avoided for maintenance treatment.

Follow-Up Visit

The status of treatment of allergies and environmental concerns should always be reviewed. If the patient has experienced dramatic improvement, a nasal endoscopy is performed to assess the response to intensive medical treatment rather than repeating the sinus CT scan. Assuming there are no signs of persistent infection, the patient is advised to continue with "maintenance treatment".

In patients who fail empiric antibiotic treatment and who have persistent evidence of sinus purulence, sinus cultures for bacteria and fungi are strongly recommended. Infection with a gram-negative bacteria generally requires the use of a quinolone antibiotic, provided the organism is sensitive to this class of antibiotics. In these cases, topical gentamycin or tobramycin sinus irrigation (100 mg/l in normal saline, using 10 cc per nostril once daily in the head-down forward and lateral supine positions only) may also help eradicate the infection. This approach is used mostly in patients who have had previous surgery. Treatment should be guided by appropriate bacterial sensitivities to ensure that the correct antibiotic is used. Electrolytes, blood urea nitrogen (BUN), and creatinine should be monitored, and the possibility of drug-induced sensorineural hearing loss should be considered if this treatment is continued beyond a few months.

Overall, about 15–20% of cases fail intensive medical treatment. Many of these prefer one additional trial of medical treatment before agreeing to undergo surgery. Mindful of the most common reasons for failure of medical treatment, my usual approach is to treat with a different combination of antibiotics, usually including: ciprofloxacin 750 mg bid (to treat possible gram-negative infection) and clindamycin 300 mg qid (to treat anaerobic bacteria), plus prednisone 20 mg bid for five days, followed by 20 mg daily for five days. However, the success rate of this regimen is no better than 50%.

If the patient fails intensive medical treatment and has evidence of persistent sinus disease either rhinoscopically or on repeat sinus CT scan despite these attempts at treatment, sinus surgery is recommended.

Treatment of Acute Exacerbations

In patients who have never had a gram-negative or drug-resistant bacterial infection, acute exacerbations are treated the same as acute episodes of bacterial rhinosinusitis. It is recommended to avoid using the same antibiotic repeatedly in such patients. In patients with a history of gram-negative or drug-resistant bacterial infection, an endoscopic bacterial culture should be obtained before initiating antibiotic treatment.

CRS WITH NP
Initial

It is important to review previous sinus CT scans, and surgical and pathological reports. These may confirm the typical radiographic and pathologic findings (Fig. 4). Special attention should be paid to information that would suggest the presence of AFRS.

The typical patient is bothered mostly by nasal congestion, vague facial or sinus fullness, postnasal drainage, anosmia or hyposmia, and lacks features of acute or chronic infection. Assuming bacterial infection or AFRS is not considered likely, initial treatment focuses on establishing a regimen that reduces mucosal inflammation and regresses nasal polyps. The mainstay of treatment is topical corticosteroids by either the intranasal route or intranasal instillation (see Fig. 1). Leukotriene blocker drugs may be used as an adjunct to topical corticosteroids, but there are no controlled clinical trials to support their use. It is unclear whether 5-lipoxygenase inhibitors (e.g. zileuton 600 mg qid) are any more effective than LTD4 receptor blockers (e.g. montelukast 10 mg qHS or zafirlukast 20 mg bid), but the former occasionally provide superior results. If the patient has extreme nasal blockage, a brief course of oral prednisone may be given to accelerate the regression of nasal polyps.

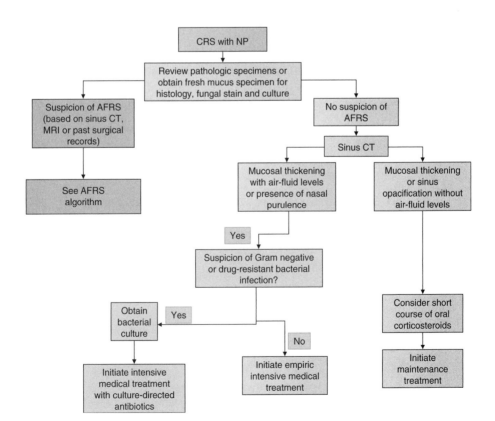

FIGURE 4 Evaluation of patients with CRS with NP.

The presence of mucosal thickening with an air-fluid level on the sinus CT scan or nasal purulence, facial pain, or headache on examination raises the suspicion of superimposed bacterial infection. If there is a clinical suspicion of a gram-negative or drug-resistant bacterial infection, a sinus culture should be performed.

The general recommendations outlined above for CRS should be employed, and coexistent asthma should be addressed. A circulating eosinophil count can be helpful in the evaluation, since a subset of patients will have unusually high levels (e.g., >1000/μl) that require oral prednisone to suppress.

Follow Up

A follow-up visit with nasal endoscopy is usually scheduled for 2–3 months after initiation of treatment, as it may take this long to see significant effects of intranasal corticosteroids. Attention should be focused on whether the cardinal symptoms of CRS are being adequately controlled and whether polyps and polypoid tissues are showing signs of regression. The technique for topical corticosteroid instillations should be reviewed and optimized. Coexisting asthma should be monitored. In patients with eosinophilia, periodic reassessment of the circulating eosinophil count is helpful.

Treatment of Acute Exacerbations

Acute exacerbations can be caused by a recrudescence of the underlying eosinophilic inflammatory process. Alternatively, patients may experience acute infections that may be either viral or bacterial. Acute bacterial infections are generally treated similarly to acute bacterial rhinosinusitis.

CLASSIC AFRS
Initial

Classic AFRS should be suspected when: (a) the patient has thick, inspissated allergic mucin identified from a sinus cavity at the time of sinus surgery, (b) the patient has radiographic features characteristic of AFRS, such as an opacified sinus with characteristic CT hyperdensities or MRI hypointensities, or (c) the patient has persistent symptoms and one or more opacified sinus cavities despite extensive medical therapy, including use of both antibiotics and oral steroids. The latter scenario is the least specific for AFRS. It is also true that the vast majority of AFRS patients have nasal polyposis, but there are exceptions to this rule (Fig. 5).

The evaluation and treatment algorithm for AFRS (Fig. 5) hinges on: (1) establishing the presence of allergic mucin, (2) confirming the presence of fungi in the mucin by fungal stain or culture, and (3) confirming the presence of IgE-mediated allergy to one or more fungi. Furthermore, the sinus tissue pathology should show no evidence of fungal invasion. Only if these criteria are met can the diagnosis of classic AFRS be made, and only 5–7% of all CRS cases meet these criteria. A much higher percentage of CRS cases have allergic mucin but lack the other features of AFRS. These have been labeled "eosinophilic mucin rhinosinusitis" (or EMRS) by some authors (27). When the patient has allergic mucin and evidence of fungal allergy but no fungi by staining or culture, the patient can be considered to be an "AFRS candidate" (see Chapter 16).

The initial evaluation and treatment recommendations for classic AFRS are outlined in Figure 5. Establishing sinus ventilation and drainage is essential and

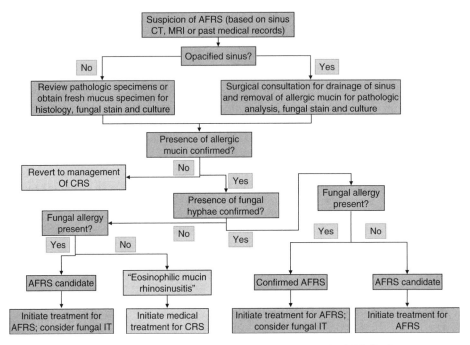

FIGURE 5 Evaluation of patients with allergic fungal rhinosinusitis (AFRS). See comments regarding fungal-specific IgE in Chapter 16.

most often requires initial surgical intervention. Allergy skin testing to fungi, dust mites, and indoor animals is essential. If fungal cultures identify a specific fungal species, evidence of fungal-specific IgE against this organism should be sought. Oral prednisone is the mainstay of initial medical treatment. It is usually started at 0.5 mg/kg daily and tapered over a few weeks to approximately 10 mg daily. Once a dose of 10 mg/day has been reached, the dose is usually tapered by 1 mg/week to the lowest possible dose necessary to maintain control of sinus inflammation. Systemic antifungals are mainly used if moderate doses of systemic steroids have failed to keep the disease under control. Use of an antifungal rinse program with either amphotericin B or itraconazole is recommended, as previously discussed. Fungal immunotherapy is also recommended using a mixture of fungal species based on the results of skin testing and fungal IgE radioallergosorbent test (RAST) tests.

Attention should be paid to the possibility of complications, including mucocele formation, bony erosions, and extrasinus extension of the inflammatory process beyond the bony confines of the sinuses (see Chapter 12).

Follow Up

Follow up is similar to that described for CRS with NP except that in AFRS oral prednisone is typically given for several months at gradually decreasing doses. Oral antifungal treatment may be continued for 1–3 months. Antifungal rinses are recommended as part of the maintenance medication program.

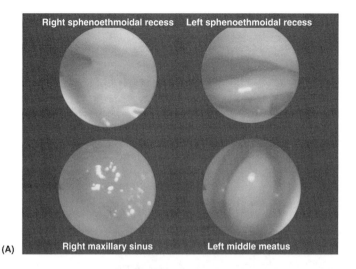

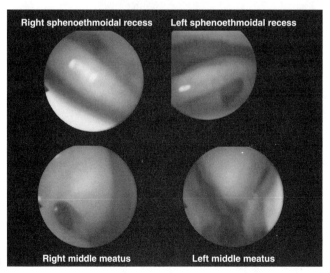

FIGURE 6 (*See color insert.*) Case study no. 1: CRS without NP. The patient is a 36-year-old Caucasian female with a history of recurrent CRS that responded well to antibiotics. Her evaluation revealed no allergies or hypogammaglobulinemia. (**A**) This rhinoscopic examination revealed an acute infection with edema, erythema, and purulence in the right maxillary sinus and in the left middle meatus. A culture of the mucus was positive for *Streptococcus pneumoniae*. The sphenoethmoidal areas, which are illustrated in this photograph, are uninfected. She responded well to antibiotic treatment. (**B**) A second rhinoscopic examination was done at the time of an acute infection. A stream of purulent mucus is seen draining in the left middle meatus from the maxillary sinus. A culture of the mucus was negative suggesting that the infection may have been viral or mycoplasmal.

Case Studies

Figures 6–9 represent illustrative cases of patients with chronic, recurrent CRS, CRS with NP, allergic mucin, and AFRS.

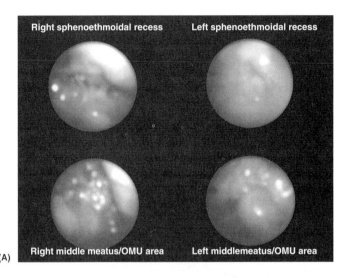

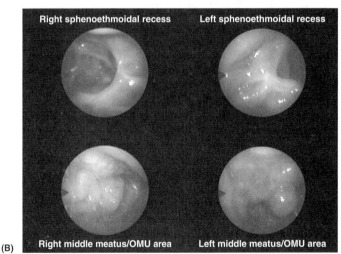

FIGURE 7 *(See color insert.) Case study no. 2: CRS with NP.* The patient is a 65-year-old Caucasian male with CRS with NP. (**A**) On his initial rhinoscopic examination (which is slightly out of focus), extensive polypoid tissue was seen in both sphenoethmoidal recesses and in the middle meatus/ostiomeatal unit (OMU) areas. He was treated with intranasal instillation of budesonide 0.5 mg per nostril once daily along with oral montelukast 10 mg/day. (**B**) A rhinoscopic examination performed 3 months later revealed near-complete resolution of polypoid mucosal thickening in both sphenoethmoidal recesses. In the middle meatus/OMU regions, the polyps have regressed in terms of edema and overlying mucus. The patient had marked improvement in nasal congestion and postnasal drainage and was beginning to have a return in sense of smell.

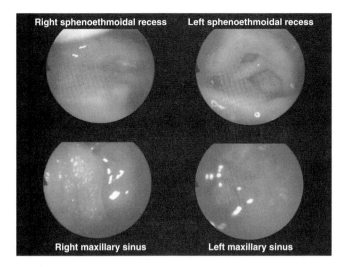

FIGURE 8 (*See color insert.*) *Case study no. 3: Eosinophilic mucin in a patient with AFRS.* The patient is a 52-year-old Caucasian female with a history of AFRS. At the time of this rhinoscopic examination she was feeling well, but a mass of thick greenish mucus was found in the right maxillary sinus that has the typical appearance of "eosinophilic mucin" with associated mild mucosal edema. There is also mild mucosal edema and a small amount of white mucus in the left maxillary sinus cavity.

EVALUATION OF CRS PATIENTS IN THE IMMEDIATE POSTOPERATIVE PERIOD

This topic is covered in Chapters 13 and 20. It is common practice to have the patient return within 1 week of surgery to remove eschar and evaluate the patient for surgical complications and infection. Patients may be seen again in 2–4 weeks and periodically thereafter, depending on their clinical course.

In the postoperative period, it may be difficult to differentiate signs of infection from those of the normal healing process. It is important to inspect for signs of infection during this period, as infection may have a detrimental effect on surgical outcome. The same principles outlined above for obtaining sinus cultures should be applied to the postoperative patient in order to establish the type of infection present.

SUMMARY

Despite the many frustrations involved in the care of CRS, there are many "successes," and most patients experience at least moderate benefit from medical treatment. I cannot emphasize enough the importance of breaking down the evaluation into component parts and addressing each one. Often, successful treatment is only achieved after all elements of the treatment program are in place. Patients are typically desperate for improvement and understand that several different strategies may need to be tried before a successful program is found. Given the high impact of CRS on patients' quality of life, it is not surprising that some of the most grateful patients are the ones in whom a successful medical program has been discovered.

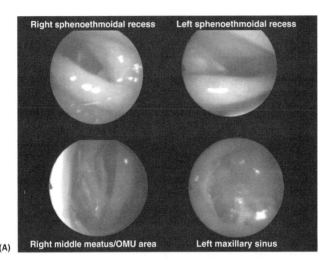

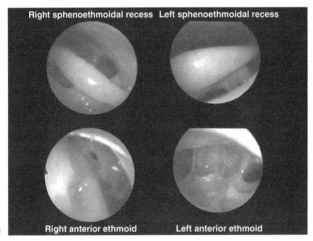

FIGURE 9 *(See color insert.) Case study no. 4: AFRS.* A 42-year-old African American male had a 1-year history of CRS with NP and repeated "infections" for which antibiotics were given. His symptoms included occasional thick green mucus, heavy postnasal drainage, nasal congestion, fullness in cheeks and forehead, and decreased sense of smell. The allergy evaluation revealed positive skin test to several fungi, dust mites, and pollens. Moderate asthma developed coincident with his CRS. His immune evaluation was normal. A preoperative sinus CT showed extensive mucosal thickening and sinus opacification. He underwent sinus surgery. Pathologic examination showed "allergic mucin" with a positive stain for fungal hyphae. (**A**) His postoperative rhinoscopic appearance showed purulent mucus in multiple sinus areas that was positive on culture for *Staphylococcus aureus*. Polypoid mucosal edema is also seen in the left maxillary sinus. He was treated with amoxicillin/clavulanate, topical amphotericin, and prednisone initially at a dosage of 0.5 mg/kg/day for 2 weeks with gradual tapering. Fungal immunotherapy was also started. (**B**) Three months later his prednisone dose was 12.5 mg/day, and he continued to receive topical amphotericin B and fungal immunotherapy. He was symptom-free. The rhinoscopic examination now shows complete resolution of purulent mucus and polypoid mucosal edema. The postoperative appearance of the anterior ethmoid areas is now easily seen. The left nasofrontal duct is also visualized at 3 O'clock in the lower right panel. Over the ensuing months the patient was able to taper his prednisone dose to 5 mg/day without any worsening of the rhinoscopic appearance.

REFERENCES

1. Meltzer EO, Hamilos DL, Hadley JA, et al. Rhinosinusitis: establishing definitions for clinical research and patient care. J Allergy Clin Immunol 2004; 114(Suppl. 6):155–212; and Otolaryngol Head Neck Surg 2004; 131(Suppl. 6):S1–62.
2. Fokkens W, Lund V, et al. EAACI position paper on rhinosinusitis and nasal polyps: executive summary. Allergy 2005; 60:583–601.
3. Benninger MS, Ferguson BJ, Hadley JA, et al. Adult chronic rhinosinusitis: definitions, diagnosis, epidemiology, and pathophysiology. Otolaryngol Head Neck Surg 2003; 129(Suppl. 3):S1–32.
4. Ponikau JU, Sherris DA, et al. Treatment of chronic rhinosinusitis with intranasal amphotericin B: a randomized, placebo-controlled, double-blind pilot trial. J Allergy Clin Immunol 2005; 115:125–31.
5. Weschta M, Rimek D, Formanek M, Polzehl D, Podbielski A, Riechelmann H. Topical antifungal treatment of chronic rhinosinusitis with nasal polyps: a randomized, double-blind clinical trial. J Allergy Clin Immunol 2004; 113:1122–8.
6. Kennedy DW, Kuhn FA, Hamilos DL, et al. Treatment of chronic rhinosinusitis with high-dose oral terbinafine: a double blind, placebo-controlled study. Laryngoscope 2005; 115:1793–9.
7. Dijkstra MD, Ebbens FA, Poublon RM, Fokkens WJ. Fluticasone propionate aqueous nasal spray does not influence the recurrence rate of chronic rhinosinusitis and nasal polyps 1 year after functional endoscopic sinus surgery. Clin Exp Allergy 2004; 34:1395–400.
8. Small CB, Hernandez J, Reyes A, et al. Efficacy and safety of mometasone furoate nasal spray in nasal polyposis. J Allergy Clin Immunol 2005; 116:1275–81.
9. Stjarne P, Mosges R, Jorissen M, et al. A randomized controlled trial of mometasone furoate nasal spray for the treatment of nasal polyposis. Arch Otolaryngol Head Neck Surg 2006; 132:179–85.
10. Hissaria P, Smith W, Wormald PJ, et al. Short course of systemic corticosteroids in sinonasal polyposis: a double blind, randomized, placebo-controlled trial with evaluation of outcome measures. J Allergy Clin Immunol 2006; 118:127–33.
11. Benitez P, Alobid I, deHaro J, et al. A short course of oral prednisone followed by intranasal budesonide is an effective treatment of severe nasal polyps. Laryngoscope 2006; 116:770–5.
12. Aukema AA, Mulder PG, Fokkens WJ. Treatment of nasal polyposis and chronic rhinosinusitis with fluticasone propionate nasal drops reduces need for sinus surgery. J Allergy Clin Immunol 2005; 115:1017–23.
13. Subramanian HN, Schechtman KB, Hamilos DL. A retrospective analysis of treatment outcomes and time to relapse after intensive medical treatment for chronic sinusitis. Am J Rhinol 2002; 16:303–12.
14. Shin SH, Ponikau JU, Sherris DA, et al. Chronic rhinosinusitis: an enhanced immune response to ubiquitous airborne fungi. J Allergy Clin Immunol 2004; 114:1369–75.
15. Richtsmeier W. Top 10 reasons for endoscopic maxillary sinus surgery failure. Laryngoscope 2001; 111(11 Pt 1):1952–6.
16. Stammberger H. Functional Endoscopic Sinus Surgery. Philadelphia: B.C. Decker, 1991.
17. Musy PY, Kountakis SE. Anatomic findings in patients undergoing revision endoscopic sinus surgery. Am J Otolaryngol 2004; 25:417–22.
18. Stankiewicz JA. Management of endoscopic sinus surgery failures. Curr Opin Otolaryngol Head Neck Surg 2001; 9:47–52.
19. Kennedy DW. Prognostic factors, outcomes and staging in ethmoid sinus surgery. Laryngoscope 1992; 102:1–18.
20. Taylor MJ, Ponikau JU, Sherris DA, et al. Detection of fungal organisms in eosinophilic mucin using a fluorescein-labeled chitin-specific binding protein. Otolaryngol Head Neck Surg 2002; 127:377–83.
21. Lanza DC, Kennedy DW. Adult rhinosinusitis defined. Otolaryngol Head Neck Surg 1997; 117(3 Pt 2):S1–7.

22. Bhattacharyya N, Lee KH. Chronic recurrent rhinosinusitis: disease severity and clinical characterization. Laryngoscope 2005; 115:306–10.
23. Vogan J, Bolger W, Keyes A. Endoscopically guided sinonasal cultures: a direct comparison with maxillary sinus aspirate cultures. Otolaryngol Head Neck Surg 2000; 122:370–3.
24. Gold S, Tami T. Role of middle meatus aspiration culture in the diagnosis of chronic sinusitis. Laryngoscope 1997; 107(12 Pt 1):1586–9.
25. Benninger MS, Appelbaum PC, Denneny JC, Osguthorpe DJ, Stankiewicz JA. Maxillary sinus puncture and culture in the diagnosis of acute rhinosinusitis: the case for pursuing alternative culture methods. Otolaryngol Head Neck Surg 2002; 127:7–12.
26. Portnoy JM, Kwak K, Dowling P, VanOsdol T, Barnes C. Health effects of indoor fungi. Ann Allergy Asthma Immunol 2005; 94:313–20.
27. Ferguson BJ. Eosinophilic mucin rhinosinusitis: A distinct clinicopathological entity. Laryngoscope 2000; 110:799–813.
28. Tichenor WS, Adinoff A, Smart B, Hamilos D. Practice parameters for nasal and sinus endoscopy and sinusitis, November 2006. http://www.aaaai.org/media/resources/academy_statements/practice_papers/endoscopy.pdf.

20 Interfacing Medical and Surgical Management for Chronic Rhinosinusitis with and Without Nasal Polyps

Fuad M. Baroody
Section of Otolaryngology–Head and Neck Surgery,
Departments of Surgery and Pediatrics, Pritzker School of Medicine,
University of Chicago, Chicago, Illinois, U.S.A.

INTRODUCTION

Chronic rhinosinusitis (CRS) is a common and difficult disease to manage. As has been detailed in the previous chapters, the pathophysiology is multifactorial and so are the co-morbidities. The previous chapter detailed a comprehensive approach to the medical treatment of this disease. When medical treatment fails, surgery is usually considered. In this final chapter, we will concentrate on surgical treatment and its outcomes as well as possible preoperative factors that might be predictive of surgical outcomes.

FUNCTIONAL ENDOSCOPIC SINUS SURGERY

Although external surgical approaches to the paranasal sinuses are still employed, the vast majority of the surgical procedures targeted at CRS are endoscopic. Details of the surgical technique are not the focus of this chapter and are covered in great detail in specialized publications (1,2). However, a brief overview of the technique and related anatomy will be presented.

Messerklinger was among the first to carefully study the anatomy and physiology of the paranasal sinuses, focusing on nasal endoscopy as a tool to visualize the endonasal structures (3). His initial work was later published and is considered the major reference for endoscopic diagnosis (4). As endoscopes and sinus instrumentation were further developed and improved, Stammberger began teaching endoscopic sinus surgery outside of Germany and Austria (5), and with Kennedy the technique was introduced to the United States in the mid-1980s (6,7). Since then, it has become the mainstay of surgical treatment of rhinosinusitis with over 200,000 procedures performed annually in the United States.

The concept of functional endoscopic sinus surgery (FESS) is based on an understanding of the anatomy of the lateral nasal wall and the osteomeatal unit where most drainage from the paranasal sinuses occurs. The procedure is aimed at improving the drainage pathways of the sinuses that have been affected by chronic inflammation in rhinosinusitis to maintain a functional drainage system. The ostiomeatal unit is bordered medially by the anterior middle turbinate and laterally by the lateral nasal wall. The crescent-shaped uncinate process divides this region in an anteroposterior direction. Anteriorly, the uncinate process joins the posteromedial portion of the lacrimal bone by a membranous attachment. Inferiorly and laterally, it fuses with the medial wall of the maxillary sinus to

321

attach to the perpendicular process of the palatine bone and more anteriorly and medially with the superior surface of the inferior turbinate. The ethmoidal infundibulum lies lateral to the uncinate process, and the posterior aspect of both the infundibulum and the uncinate process is the hiatus semilunaris. The ethmoidal bulla is the most anterior ethmoid air cell and constitutes the posterior boundary of the inferior hiatus semilunaris. The natural ostium of the maxillary sinus, in the medial wall of the sinus, is shaped like an inverted funnel and empties into the inferior aspect of the ethmoidal infundibulum. Once the uncinate process is removed, the ostium can usually be found at a level opposite to the inferior free margin of the middle turbinate. It lies lateral to the more inferior portion of the uncinate process.

The frontal sinus empties through the frontal sinus ostium into the frontal recess. The recess typically drains medial to the uncinate process and lateral to the middle turbinate into the anterior superior portion of the middle meatus. The anterior and posterior ethmoids are divided by the basal lamella, which is the attachment of the middle turbinate. The ethmoidal bulla is the largest cell of the ethmoid complex and is often the first cell encountered when entering the anterior ethmoids. Its lateral wall is the medial wall of the orbit and it drains into the suprabullar or retrobullar recess (sinus lateralis). The sphenoid sinus is the most posterior of the paranasal sinuses. Several important structures including the carotid artery, the optic nerve, and the skull base directly surround this sinus. The natural ostium is located within the sphenoethmoidal recess, a space bordered posteriorly by the anterior wall of the sphenoid, and anteriorly by the superior turbinate. It is safest to enter the sphenoid sinus through its ostium to avoid injury to the important structures that surround it.

Endoscopic sphenoethmoidectomy is usually performed for extensive sinus disease that involves all the sinuses. This usually includes exploration of the frontal recess and establishing adequate drainage for the frontal sinus. Disease limited to the osteomeatal complex only does not usually warrant the complete procedure and might be amenable to limited (anterior) ethmoidectomy and opening the maxillary sinus ostium (maxillary antrostomy). Preoperative computerized tomography in addition to nasal endoscopy in the clinic usually guides the decision on the extent of the procedure that needs to be performed. Advances in instrumentation and improved understanding have led to espousing a mucosal sparing procedure that aims to remove diseased mucosa while preserving as much healthy mucosal lining as possible. Often, nasal septal deviations are corrected (septoplasty) at the same time as FESS to both improve nasal obstruction and facilitate access to, and drainage from, the osteomeatal units.

Image-guided FESS was popularized in the early 1990s and many systems are now available that allow accurate determination of intraoperative surgical position to within 2 mm (8,9) (Fig. 1). Having these systems available is no substitute for a thorough understanding of the anatomy, and these tools are most useful in extensive disease or revision cases as they allow more complete removal of disease with added safety. A recent comparison of quality of life outcomes and incidence of complications following image-guided versus non-image-guided FESS was undertaken retrospectively in 239 patients (10). The results suggested similar outcomes and complication rates including major intraoperative complications (lamina papyracea injury, hemorrhage), major postoperative complications (epistaxis, septal hematoma, delayed frontal mucocele, delayed orbital abscess),

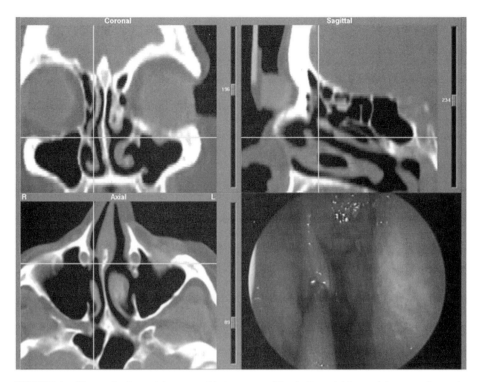

FIGURE 1 (*See color insert.*) Image guided surgery. The bottom right panel is an endoscopic view of a patient's nostril during functional endoscopic sinus surgery with a suction tip that carries the sensor for image guidance. The position of the sensor is seen on the computed tomography scan that was obtained preoperatively and is available in the operating suite. Three views are delineated: coronal, sagittal, and axial.

and number of revision procedures between the two groups. The only difference of note was an observed increase in the number of patients with skull base trauma and cerebrospinal fluid (CSF) leakage, which was experienced in four patients in the non-image-guided group (2.2%), and in none of the patients where image guidance was used. All the leaks were recognized and repaired intraoperatively.

Most surgeons place packing in the middle meatus to prevent adhesions and synecchiae during the healing process. Various packing materials are available and most centers now use absorbable packing such as MeroGel^R (hyaluronic acid; Medtronic, Jacksonville, FL, USA). The postoperative follow up usually includes cleaning of the sinus cavities in the clinic under endoscopic guidance using a 0° or 45° endoscope and local anesthesia. Most surgeons perform these cleanings on a weekly, or every 2-week, basis for the first month or so or until the cavities are healed to the satisfaction of the surgeon as assessed by endoscopic examination. Most patients are placed on antibiotics after surgery until the cavities are healed. Use of adjunct therapies, such as saline irrigation, are at the discretion and the preference of the treating surgeon.

IMPACT OF FESS ON CRS

Many studies have reported on the outcomes of FESS in patients with CRS. Unfortunately, most of these are cohort studies or case series (level III/IV evidence) and very few controlled randomized studies are available. Some reasons why level I/II evidence is lacking are the ethical dilemma of conducting a "placebo"-controlled study when a surgical procedure is involved, and the difficulty of conducting randomized controlled trials for surgical procedures per se. Furthermore, meta-analyses are hard to perform because studies lack a single staging system for the disease, outcome measures are not uniform, and surgical technique might not be comparable across investigators from different centers and is partly determined by the extent of disease at the time of surgery.

Nevertheless, some representative studies which examine both short- and long-term outcome of FESS for CRS will be reviewed. Kennedy evaluated the results of FESS in 120 patients with CRS (age range between 15 and 77 years) with and without polyposis using a mixed prospective and retrospective design with a mean follow up of 18 months (11). He utilized subjective postoperative improvement scales and asked the patients to classify the symptomatic result as no improvement (<25%), mild improvement (25–50%), and marked improvement (>50%). He also performed endoscopic examinations of the postoperative cavities at several time points (6–8 weeks, 4–8 months, and the final follow-up visit). The patients were classified based on the preoperative endoscopic examination or computed tomography (CT) scan into different categories ranging from mild disease to diffuse sinonasal polyposis. Demographic information, as well as the presence or absence of comorbidities such as allergy, asthma, salicylate hypersensitivity, presence of allergic fungal sinusitis, and history of prior surgery were obtained. Overall, 97.5% of the patients reported an improvement in symptoms at the time of the final follow-up examination (85% marked improvement, 12.5% mild improvement, and 2.5% no significant improvement). The degree of symptomatic improvement was comparable in the groups with mild as well as severe preoperative disease. In contrast to the subjective symptomatic outcome, the results of objective endoscopic evaluation of the sinus cavities postoperatively were not as favorable. Cavities were recorded as abnormal if there was any drainage, scarring, inflammation, or mucosal hypertrophy. Using this evaluation, normal cavities were seen in 55.1% of the operated sides and abnormal cavities in 44.9%. Furthermore, the more advanced the extent of preoperative disease, the higher the percentage of abnormal sinus cavities postoperatively. Only 23.5% of the operative sides with diffuse polyps preoperatively were normal postoperatively. Among the other factors considered, the number of abnormal cavities on postoperative examination was higher in patients with previous surgery and in patients with asthma as well as in patients with more sinus disease, as classified by CT scans preoperatively. The persistent abnormalities in asthma patients primarily reflected the increased severity of preoperative disease.

In a follow-up study by the same group, Senior et al. reported on the progress of the 120 patients whose results were reported above (12). Questionnaires were sent to the patients that could be located and responses were received for 72 patients with an average follow up of 7.8 years postoperatively. Subjective improvement was reported by 98.4% of the patients compared to their preoperative status. Thirteen patients (18%) underwent further surgery during the longer follow-up period but the small size of this group precluded any conclusions about predictive factors for subsequent surgery. A trend toward more severe preoperative disease by CT scan was seen in the group that required revision surgery compared to the group that did not. Other studies with similar designs provide similar results. Levine reported his experience in 250 patients with CRS with and without nasal polyps (NP) followed up for a mean of 17 months after FESS (13). Success rate, as determined by subjective criteria, was higher in the subjects with CRS with NP (88.3%) compared to those with CRS without NP (80.2%). There is no mention in this series of the endoscopic status of the sinus cavities postoperatively which might have yielded worse results in the NP group compared to the CRS-only group as reported in Kennedy's series. Similar favorable success rates varying between 91% and 86% were reported 12 and 23 months postoperatively, respectively (14,15). Delank and Stoll evaluated the effect of FESS on olfaction in patients with CRS with and without NP (16). Preoperatively, objective olfactory testing showed 52% of the 115 patients to be hyposmic and 31% anosmic, with the patients with CRS with NP being more likely to have olfactory dysfunction compared to the patients with CRS without NP. Postoperatively, the percentage of patients with anosmia decreased from 31% to 11%, and improvements of either the olfactory thresholds or olfactory discrimination occurred in 70% of the hyposmic or anosmic patients. Similar results were reported by Perry and Kountakis who showed a subjective improvement in olfactory function after FESS (17). Again, patients with polyposis and more severe disease as revealed by CT scan had worse olfactory function preoperatively and greater improvement after FESS. More recent surveys also show an improvement in general and disease-specific quality of life measures in patients with CRS, 2 or more years post-FESS (18,19).

Most recently, Khalil and Nanez performed an analysis of existing publications related to the effects of FESS in CRS (20). Their review focused on reports of randomized controlled trials. Of 2159 abstracts reviewed, nine potential studies were identified, of which only three randomized controlled trials met the inclusion criteria for the review. One of the studies, performed by Fairley and colleagues included 33 patients with CRS and compared endoscopic middle meatal antrostomy with conventional inferior meatal antrostomy (20). They found no difference in the symptom scores after a median follow up of 12 months. Hartog et al. performed a randomized controlled trial of 89 patients comparing medical treatment with sinus irrigation plus loracarbef for 10 days only versus this same treatment followed by FESS in patients with chronic maxillary sinusitis (21). Patients were followed up for a median of 12 months. A significant reduction in symptoms of purulent nasal drainage and hyposmia was seen in the FESS group, but no significant difference in overall cure rates was noted at the end of one year between the groups. In another trial, Ragab et al. compared FESS with medical treatment versus medical treatment alone, consisting of erythromycin and an alkaline nasal douche, followed by a 3-month course of fluticasone propionate nasal spray (22). They randomized 90 patients to the treatments and followed them up for 12 months, at which time only 78 were available for analysis. There was no difference in total symptom scores between the two groups at 12 months. No major complications were reported in either arm of the trial. The authors concluded that maximal medical therapy should be tried initially in patients with CRS and that FESS should be reserved for cases refractory to medical therapy.

Thus, while high-level evidence is not available, there is ample level III and IV evidence supporting the efficacy and safety of FESS in CRS with and without NP. The data suggest less spectacular results in patients with more severe disease and concomitant asthma and aspirin sensitivity and better subjective (symptomatic) than objective (endoscopic) improvement.

EFFECT OF FESS ON ASTHMA IN PATIENTS WITH CRS

Most of the studies that evaluate the effect of FESS on asthma provide level III/IV evidence supporting an improvement in asthma after improvement of sinus-related symptoms after FESS. Ikeda et al. identified 21 adults with asthma and CRS documented by symptoms for at least 3 months and CT evidence of disease (23). Fifteen patients underwent FESS and the other six served as controls and did not undergo any surgical procedure but were maintained on intranasal steroids. Severity of asthma and sinus disease preoperatively was similar between the operated and control groups. Total scores for sinus-related symptoms were decreased at 3 and 6 months postoperatively in the operated patients but did not change in the controls. The average peak expiratory flow following FESS was significantly increased in the patients but did not change over a year of observation in the controls, suggesting a beneficial effect of FESS on asthma in these patients. In another study, Dunlop et al. followed up 50 asthmatic patients with CRS with or without NP who had failed medical management (24). The patients underwent FESS and were followed up for 12 months, and the following parameters were compared pre- and postoperatively: overall asthma control, peak flow measurements, asthma medication requirements including oral corticosteroids, and hospitalizations for asthma. Compared to their preoperative status, in the 12 months after FESS, 40% of patients noted that their asthma was easier to control, 54% stated that there was no difference, and 6% that they got worse. Peak flows were available for 28 of the 50 patients, and, of those 50, 28% improved postoperatively, 6% were worse, 22% remained the same, and 44% did not submit peak flow measurements. There were significant reductions in oral steroid requirements and hospitalizations for asthma after FESS. There were no significant differences in outcome when the groups with and without polyposis were compared. Other studies support an improvement in asthma outcomes as assessed by a variety of measures after FESS (25,26). Dejima et al. examined the outcomes of FESS prospectively in a population with CRS (27). They found that outcomes of FESS were significantly worse in the asthma group, especially when it came to endonasal findings. However, in the patients with asthma, there was significant improvement in asthma symptoms, peak flow, and medication scores after FESS, and the patients with a good FESS result tended to have the greatest improvement in their asthma outcomes.

Not all studies showed uniform improvement in all asthma outcomes or in all patient populations with asthma and CRS after FESS. Batra and colleagues examined asthma outcomes in 17 patients with CRS with NP and steroid-dependent asthma for 1 year after FESS and demonstrated an improvement in CT scores and forced expiratory volume (FEV_1) postoperatively (28). Within this population, the aspirin-sensitive patients did not have a significant improvement in postoperative FEV_1, whereas the aspirin-tolerant group did. In contrast, Nakamura et al. showed a significant improvement in FEV_1 after FESS in patients with CRS and aspirin-induced asthma (29). In yet another such study, significant improvement was seen in diurnal and nocturnal asthma symptoms, as well as asthma medication scores, after FESS in 19 patients with CRS, but no significant change was detected in objective pulmonary function tests (30). In one of the few negative studies reported, Goldstein et al. examined asthma outcomes after first-time FESS in 13 patients with CRS in a retrospective manner (31). They found no improvement in terms of asthma symptoms, medication use, pulmonary function test results, or the number of emergency department visits or hospital admissions. Nothwithstanding that this study was retrospective and observational, and involved only 13 patients, the authors suggested revisiting the common belief that FESS benefits coexisting asthma in patients with CRS.

In summary, the majority of published reports suggest that ameliorating CRS by FESS improves asthma outcomes. Unfortunately, most of the studies are hampered by a myriad of limitations including small sample sizes, limited follow-up duration, retrospective designs, and lack of a control group in most cases.

OUTCOME PREDICTORS AFTER FESS

Many studies have evaluated the predictive value of various parameters on improvement after FESS in CRS. Zadeh et al. performed a retrospective review of patients undergoing FESS for CRS, identified 31 patients with serum eosinophilia $\geq 6\%$, and compared them to 34 randomly selected patients with CRS and serum eosinophilia $<6\%$ (32). When comparing the two groups, a higher proportion of patients with serum eosinophilia had a history of asthma, polyp disease, and allergic fungal sinusitis. Postoperatively, the group with high serum eosinophilia had significantly higher rate compared to controls of recurrent sinus infections and recurrent polyp disease. Although this study suggests that a preoperative high eosinophil count in the serum would be a predictor of worse prognosis after FESS, the study design does not eliminate the bias that the poor outcome is actually a reflection of worse disease preoperatively (more polyposis, allergic fungal sinusitis, and asthma). The serum eosinophilia might just be associated with these diseases which, in and of themselves, carry a worse prognosis for improvement after FESS. Sharp et al. prospectively followed 161 patients with CRS up to 2 years after FESS and analyzed postoperative outcome in relation to preoperative CT score and the presence or absence of any systemic disease that might be related to the pathogenesis of CRS (33). These diseases were asthma, aspirin-sensitive asthma, atopy, bronchiectasis, cystic fibrosis, immunoglobulin deficiency, primary ciliary dyskinesia, sarcoidosis, Young's disease, and diabetes mellitus. There was a significant correlation between the CT score preoperatively and the outcome of FESS at 24 months, with the worse preoperative disease having the poorer outcome. Furthermore, a significant link was found between the presence or absence of predisposing systemic disease and outcome, with the patients with poorer postoperative outcome being more likely to have a systemic disease. Thus, the presence of certain systemic inflammatory diseases and their potential serum markers are probably associated with worse sinus disease and also a higher chance of a poor postoperative outcome.

Along the same lines, some investigators have attempted to identify potential inflammatory changes in sinus tissues that might be useful in predicting postoperative outcome. Lavigne et al. measured several inflammatory cells in the sinus mucosa of patients undergoing FESS for CRS without NP and classified the patients as responders or nonresponders postoperatively by evaluating their symptoms using a visual analog scale (34). Of 15 patients studied, seven were deemed responders at 24 months postoperatively and eight were classified as nonresponders. There were no differences between the number of CD3+, CD4+, major basic protein (MBP+), or tryptase-positive cells between the two groups, and also no difference in cells expressing Interleukin-4 (IL-4) mRNA. The only significant difference between the two groups was a higher number of IL-5 mRNA-bearing cells in the ethmoid biopsy samples of from nonresponders compared to responders, suggesting that the presence of this cytokine is a predictor for worse outcome. In another study, Baudoin et al. studied 100 patients with CRS before and 12 and 24 months after FESS and attempted to correlate symptoms to findings on light microscopy (35). Goblet cells in the sinus tissues were the best predictor, correlating with five postoperative symptoms (patients with higher goblet cell scores might expect better improvement in postoperative itching , but less improvement in congestion, secretion, headache, and cough), followed by subepithelial thickening (a higher subepithelial thickening score may predict better improvement in postnasal secretion but less improvement in congestion, nasal secretion, and cough), mast cell infiltration (higher mast cell scores predicted better improvement in postnasal secretion but less improvement in nasal secretion and cough), and eosinophilic infiltration which correlated with only one symptom (higher esoinophil scores predicted less improvement in nasal secretion after surgery). Thus, some histopathologic characteristics did predict the persistence of certain bothersome symptoms after surgery. In contrast, a small retrospective review of 15 patients with CRS and asthma after FESS did not show a difference in the inflammatory cellular profile of the sinus tissues (B and T lymphocytes, plasma cells, eosinophils, macrophages) between patients who responded to FESS and those who did not respond (36).

Other studies have investigated clinical and radiographic parameters as possible predictors of outcome after FESS. Smith et al. prospectively followed up 119 patients with CRS with and without NP for an average of 1.4 years (37). Multivariate analysis showed that acetyl salicylic acid (ASA) intolerance and depression demonstrated predictive value for outcome. ASA intolerance was a predictor of less improvement in postoperative nasal endoscopy and Rhinosinusitis Disability Index (RSDI), and depression was associated with less improvement of RSDI. In a retrospective review, Dursun et al. followed up 130 patients with CRS after FESS, for a mean of five years (38). Seventy-two of the 130 patients had NP. The preoperative CT scans were staged from 0-III. Regression analysis showed that stage III versus stage I CT, presence of allergy, nasal polyposis, and previous polypectomy were all poor prognostic indicators, whereas age, gender, and anatomic variations were not predictive for surgical outcome in long-term follow up. Watelet et al. prospectively enrolled patients after FESS and followed them up for 6 months postoperatively; 18 patients had CRS without NP and 18 had CRS with NP (39). Preoperative and intraoperative parameters were evaluated by logistic regression analysis to determine whether any of them would be confirmed as independent predictors for the healing outcome. Previous sinus surgery and an initial diagnosis of nasal polyposis showed significantly worse objective outcome of healing 6 months postoperatively. Moreover, the occurrence of intense intraoperative bleeding was significantly predictive for worse postoperative healing, whereas preoperative CT stage had no predictive value. Another study by Bhattacharyya showed that CT scan stage alone did not significantly predict symptom outcomes in 161 patients with CRS followed up for a mean of 19 months post-FESS (40).

Thus, several relatively small studies suggest some predictors for outcomes after FESS in patients with CRS. Most of the studies are in agreement that evidence of systemic diseases such as asthma, aspirin-intolerant asthma, and allergy are predictors of poor outcome after FESS. Worse preoperative disease including nasal polyposis and high-grade disease on preoperative CT scan also seems to be predictive of worse postoperative outcome. These studies help provide treating physicians with information they can use to help give their patients realistic expectations of the results of FESS.

COMPLICATIONS OF FESS

Complications from FESS are major and minor. The major complications include orbital hematoma, blindness, diplopia, epiphora, carotid artery injury, hemorrhage requiring transfusion, cerebrospinal fluid leak, meningitis, brain abscess, pneumocephalus, and focal brain hemorrhage. Minor complications include subcutaneous periorbital emphysema, periorbital ecchymosis, dental or lip pain or numbness, adhesions, epistaxis, and loss of smell. In a large series including 2108 patients undergoing FESS by two surgeons between 1985 and 1992, the overall rate of major complications was 0.85% and that of minor complications 6.9% (41). Most of the minor and major complications were treatable but some were irreversible and permanent. Fortunately these were rare.

POSTOPERATIVE MANAGEMENT

Several modalities are used for the treatment of the nasal and sinus cavities after FESS. Unfortunately, the evidence supporting these treatments is limited. For acute exacerbations of rhinosinusitis, antibiotics are the mainstay of therapy. Topical administration of various agents is common and these include saline, steroids, antifungals, and antibiotics. The reason for topical administration is that the sinus cavities now communicate with the nasal cavity, and it is thought that the topical treatments will have a much higher chance of penetration into the sinus cavities postoperatively than they did preoperatively where virtually no topical intranasal treatment is thought to penetrate the sinus cavities.

Saline

For ongoing treatment of patients with CRS after FESS, saline nasal washes/ irrigations are very popular and are used in the immediate postoperative period and for extended toileting of the now-operated sinus cavities. This modality is described in more detail in Chapter 15. The tonicity of the saline solutions ranges from isotonic to hypertonic, and multiple ways to administer the irrigations are available commercially. It is of note that a recent study comparing hypertonic and isotonic saline spray to no treatment in the first five days after FESS showed that the patients receiving the hypertonic saline did worse with more symptoms and a higher pain score (42). The isotonic saline and no treatment groups had similar outcomes. To be kept in mind is that this was a study where the treatment was only used for five days postoperatively and the administration was in the form of sprays, not irrigation.

Steroids

Another commonly used treatment modality after FESS is intranasal steroids. Two relatively recent studies describe the effect of treatment of the nose with intranasal steroids after FESS on recurrence of disease. Lavigne et al. used a special catheter that they inserted into the postoperative maxillary sinus cavity and secured in the nose to allow irrigation of the sinus cavities on a daily basis (43). They studied 26 patients with perennial allergic rhinitis who had previous FESS for CRS without NP and persistent symptoms of rhinorrhea or pressure-pain resistant to oral antibiotics and intranasal steroids. After securing the maxillary sinus catheter in one of the sinuses, the patients were treated with a 3-week course of placebo or budesonide 256 mg instilled into one sinus cavity. Visual analog scores of symptoms were assessed in the two groups and showed that 11 of 13 patients in the budesonide group improved by more than 50% for a period of 2–12 months. In the placebo group, only four of 13 patients had similar improvements, and the duration of improvement was <2 months. Furthermore, biopsy samples of the sinus mucosa obtained before and after treatment showed a decrease in CD3+ cells and eosinophils as well as cells bearing mRNA for IL-4 and IL-5 after treatment in the group receiving budesonide, suggesting a successful decrease in inflammation coupled with symptomatic improvement. The lack of practicality of securing a permanent catheter in the maxillary sinus has largely limited the use of this modality, but this study provides an important "proof of concept" for topical corticosteroid treatment (discussed further in Chapter 19).

In a longitudinal prospective study, Rowe-Jones and et al. followed up 109 subjects with CRS with and without NP for five years after FESS and also performed a randomized, double-blind, placebo-controlled study to evaluate the effect of fluticasone propionate on disease outcomes over 5 years (44). Seventy-seven of the patients had NP (71%) and the rest had CRS without NP. Overall, FESS was successful in the total group with only 35% of the patients requiring rescue medications during the five year follow-up period. When the placebo and treatment groups were compared, the change in overall visual analog score was significantly better in the fluticasone group at five years. The changes in endoscopic edema and polyp scores and in total nasal volumes were also significantly better in the fluticasone-treated group at four years but not five years. Thus, in this mixed population of CRS patients post-FESS (with/without NP), intranasal fluticasone seems to be beneficial in keeping the disease under control. Many other studies have validated the efficacy of intranasal steroids administered postoperatively in patients with CRS with NP in reducing recurrence of nasal polyps. These studies are described and discussed in Chapter 14.

Antifungals
Antifungal studies have shown small but significant benefit in controlling postoperative disease in patients with CRS and are discussed in detail in Chapter 11. Other studies, however, have shown no benefit (45,46).

Antibiotics
Limited data are available on the use of topical antibiotics in postoperative treatment of patients with CRS after FESS. Vaughan and Carvalho reported their experience with nebulized antibiotics for acute bacterial exacerbations in 42 patients with CRS after FESS (47). The patients had purulent material cultured from the sinus cavities, and nebulized treatment was directed by the culture results. The patients received treatment for three weeks and were followed up for a minimum of three months. The success rate of treatment was around 70% and the

side effects were minimal. This study had many limitations including the absence of randomization or placebo control, and thus the favorable responses must be considered in light of these limitations. In another trial of nebulized antibiotics, Desrosiers and Salas-Prato performed a randomized, double-blind trial of nebulized tobramycin-saline solution or saline-only solution in patients with refractory CRS after FESS (48). The solutions were nebulized three times daily to the nasal cavities by means of a large particle nebulizer apparatus for four weeks. Eighteen subjects successfully completed the trial. Both saline and tobramycin solutions led to clinically significant improvements in quality of life, symptoms, and parameters of sinonasal endoscopy, with the effects first becoming evident only at four weeks and persisting even after cessation of therapy. Comparison of the saline-only and saline-tobramycin solutions showed only minor differences with slightly higher efficacy for symptoms of pain with tobramycin but better nasal congestion scores with saline-only treatment. Thus, nebulized topical antibiotic studies show limited efficacy and, in the absence of more clinical studies, should be used at the discretion and per the personal experience of the treating physician.

COMBINING MEDICAL AND SURGICAL THERAPY FOR CRS

This text provides multiple chapters that address the approach to the treatment of patients with CRS. Chapter 19 synthesizes the maximal medical treatment approach. I will attempt to summarize a rational approach to treatment of the three most common types of CRS encountered with a combination of medical and surgical therapy.

Intraoperative Considerations
At surgery, purulence may be found in one or more sinus cavities. In such cases, mucus and/or tissue samples should be obtained for bacterial cultures and sensitivities as a guide to optimal postoperative management. In cases where gross "allergic mucin" is identified, a sample should be sent for fungal culture and pathologic analysis to confirm the presence of allergic mucin and stain for fungal hyphae.

CRS Without NP
Prior to surgical intervention, medical treatment is the mainstay of therapy for CRS without NP and includes antimicrobials as necessary for exacerbations, topical corticosteroids on an almost continuous basis, and systemic corticosteroids as needed for exacerbations. Maximizing the therapy of concomitant allergies, when existent, is very important. Topical therapies other than corticosteroids probably have very limited proven benefit in this situation, and the drugs have limited capacity to reach the sinus cavities. If all these attempts at medical treatment fail and there is evidence of persistent sinus disease on computed tomography, then FESS should be considered. This invariably leads to a reasonable success rate, but the patients' expectations should be carefully discussed prior to any procedure in the context of CRS. It is rare that a patient's symptoms will be completely "cured" by FESS, and the patient should understand that while surgery is aimed at improving control of their disease, they will continue to require care and follow up after surgery.

After the immediate postoperative endoscopic cleanings and ensuring lack of adhesions and well-ventilated sinus cavities, most patients settle into a maintenance treatment involving intranasal steroids, especially if the patient is allergic. Acute exacerbations can then be treated as necessary with antimicrobials or anti-inflammatories (systemic steroids) as necessary. Nebulized and locally instilled treatments are a little more likely to be effective after FESS than before but supportive data in the literature are still scanty. If the pathology of the tissues obtained at surgery suggests allergic fungal mucin, then topical antifungals might be used. The cumulative evidence in the literature to date does not support treating all subjects with CRS with topical antifungals.

CRS with NP

This entity is reasonably well diagnosed by nasal endoscopy in the office, and usually leads to more significant nasal obstruction than CRS without NP, especially if the polyps are large. There is ample data in the literature to support using topical steroids to attempt to manage nasal polyps and these should be part of any regimen aimed at initial medical therapy and are covered in Chapters 14 and 19. More recently, data have been reported about the efficacy of systemic steroids in reducing polyp size, a fact that has long been known to practicing clinicians (49). Obviously managing concomitant asthma, allergies, and possible acetylsalicylic acid intolerance is essential. If topical and systemic steroids do not result in symptomatic improvement, and if there is significant disease on CT of the paranasal sinuses, then the patient is offered surgery to remove the polyps. Some patients are not bothered by their symptoms and choose not to undergo surgery but many will. FESS in nasal polyposis is useful at removing all disease and draining the sinuses and is usually very successful in improving clinical outcomes. Prior to surgery, many surgeons prescribe oral steroids for approximately one week to shrink nasal polyps, reduce tissue edema, and improve visualization of anatomic landmarks. After the initial postoperative cleaning and healing of the cavities, patients should be restarted on intranasal steroids (see Chapter 14) and followed closely with serial endoscopy. As reported from the many studies above, it seems that the presence of significant NP is a predictor for recurrence of disease postoperatively, and many patients will undergo multiple revision surgeries over their lifetime to eliminate recurrent polyps. Intrasinus instillation of steroids is technically difficult but has shown some promise in preliminary reports. Again, in the absence of obvious eosinophilic fungal mucin suggestive of fungal rhinosinusitis, I would not advocate topical antifungal treatment routinely.

Classic Allergic Fungal Rhinosinusitis

As detailed in Chapter 16, classic allergic fungal rhinosinusitis (AFRS) often presents with specific radiologic features that facilitate making the diagnosis. Unlike the above two conditions, where surgical intervention is reserved for cases that fail maximal medical treatment, AFRS often warrants early surgical intervention to confirm the diagnosis and eliminate all eosinophilic mucin from the sinuses. It is important to send samples of allergic mucin for fungal culture and pathologic analysis as mentioned above. Postoperative management is more aggressive than the above two entities and often includes long-term tapering of oral steroids, possible use of antifungal treatment, and even immunotherapy directed at the offending fungal organisms.

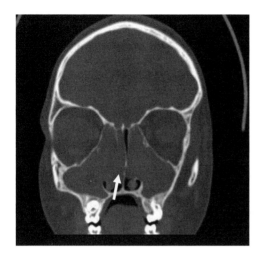

FIGURE 2 Coronal bone windows computed tomography scan of a patient with cystic fibrosis showing pan opacification of ethmoid and maxillary sinuses bilaterally. Notice the obstruction of the nasal passages bilaterally (*arrow*). Very little air is seen in the nasal cavity and most of it is underneath the inferior turbinates. The obstruction is probably a combination of polyps and medial displacement of the medial wall of the maxillary sinuses.

CRS with Cystic Fibrosis

This disease often manifests with intranasal polyposis and a characteristic CT picture which typically demonstrates opacification of all the sinus cavities and mucoceles of the maxillary sinuses with medial displacement of the medial wall of the maxillary sinuses into the nasal cavity (Fig. 2). In fact, we have diagnosed a few patients and referred them for sweat chloride testing based solely on clinical suspicion based on their radiographic picture. Cystic fibrosis is also the most common cause of NP in the pediatric age group. As the life expectancy of patients with cystic fibrosis is steadily improving, it is important to provide appropriate quality of life by controlling sinus disease as well as possible. Medical therapy includes antibiotic treatment aimed at the most common inhabitants of the inspissated mucus, namely *Pseudomonas aeruginosa* and *Staphylococcus aureus*. When the polyps and the maxillary sinus mucoceles become bothersome enough, surgical intervention in the form of FESS is useful in providing a variable disease free interval which has been reported to range as long as 2 years (50). Addition of serial antimicrobial lavages after FESS has also been shown to prolong the disease-free interval and decrease the need for further surgical intervention compared to FESS alone (51). Non-cystic fibrosis patients with CRS have been found to have a higher prevalence of mutations in the cystic fibrosis transmembrane conductance regulator (CFTR) gene (7%) compared to controls (52). However, these patients do not manifest the full phenotype of cystic fibrosis, as they have no other manifestations of the disease and a normal sweat chloride test.

SUMMARY

The development of FESS provided the otolaryngologist with an approach for restoring sinus ostial patency while simultaneously maximizing the restoration of normal mucociliary function. While minor modifications to the basic procedure continue to be discussed, FESS is widely accepted as the standard of care for surgical management of CRS. Image-guided surgery offers further promise of allowing more precise surgery with fewer intraoperative complications. Most patients with CRS who fail medical therapy will benefit from FESS with improved outcomes and possibly improvement in comorbidities, especially asthma. Post-operative medical management and attention to contributive factors for disease, such as the presence of allergies and aspirin intolerance, are key factors toward assuring successful surgical outcomes. The surgical approach and outcomes vary somewhat based on whether the patient has CRS without NP, CRS with NP, or classic AFRS. Furthermore, the goals of surgery depend on whether other under-lying conditions, such as cystic fibrosis, are present. The last section in this chapter provides guidance as to the combined medical and surgical management of various forms of CRS based on existing evidence from the literature.

REFERENCES

1. Hulett KJ, Stankiewicz JA. Primary sinus surgery. In: Cummings CW, Flint PW, Harker LA, Haughey BH, Richardson MA, Robbins KT, Schuller DE, Thomas JR, eds. Cummings Otolaryngology–Head and Neck Surgery. Philadelphia PA: Elsevier Mosby Inc., 2005:1229–54.
2. Lanza DC, Kennedy DW. Endoscopic sinus surgery. In: Bailey BJ, ed. Otolaryngology–Head and Neck Surgery, 3rd edn. Philadelphia, PA: Lippincott Williams & Wilkins, 2001:371–82.
3. Messerklinger W. Endoscopy technique of the middle meatus. Arch Otorhinolaryngol 1978; 221:297–305.
4. Stammberger H. The evolution of functional endoscopic sinus surgery. ENT J 1994; 73:451–5.
5. Stammberger H. Personal endoscopic operative technic for the lateral nasal wall—an endoscopic surgery concept in the treatment of inflammatory diseases of the paranasal sinuses. Laryngol Rhinol Otol (Stuttg) 1985; 64:559–66.
6. Kennedy DW, Zinreich SJ, Rosenbaum AE, Johns ME. Functional endoscopic sinus surgery. Theory and diagnostic evaluation. Arch Otolaryngol 1985; 111:576–82.
7. Kennedy DW. Functional endoscopic sinus surgery. Technique. Arch Otolaryngol 1985; 111:643–9.
8. Anon JB, Lipman SP, Oppenheim D, et al. Computer-assisted endoscopic sinus surgery. Laryngoscope 1994; 104:901–5.
9. Metson R, Gliklich RE, Cosenza J. A comparison of image-guidance systems for sinus surgery. Laryngoscope 1998; 108:1164–70.
10. Tabaee A, Hsu AK, Shrime MG, Rickert S, Close LG. Quality of life and complications following image-guided endoscopic sinus surgery. Otolaryngol Head Neck Surg 2006; 135:76–80.
11. Kennedy DW. Prognostic factors, outcomes and staging in ethmoid sinus surgery. Laryngoscope 1992; 102:1–18.
12. Senior B, Kennedy DW, Tanabodee J, Kroger H, Hassab M, Lanza D. Long-term results of functional endoscopic sinus surgery. Laryngoscope 1998; 108:151–57.
13. Levine HL. Functional endoscopic sinus surgery: evaluation, surgery, and follow-up of 250 patients. Laryngoscope 1990; 100:79–84.
14. Matthews BL, Smith LE, Jones R, Miller C, Brookschmidt JK. Endoscopic sinus surgery: outcome in 155 cases. Otolaryngol Head Neck Surg 1991; 104:244–6.
15. Dursun E, Bayiz U, Korkmaz H, Akmansu H, Uygur K. Follow-up results of 415 patients after endoscopic sinus surgery. Eur Arch Otorhinolaryngol 1998; 255:504–10.
16. Delank KW, Stoll W. Olfactory function after functional endoscopic sinus surgery for chronic sinusitis. Rhinology 1998; 36:15–9.
17. Perry BF, Kountakis SE. Subjective improvement of olfactory function after endoscopic sinus surgery for chronic rhinosinusitis. Am J Otolaryngol 2003; 24:366–69.
18. Damm M, Quante G, Jungehuelsing M, Stennert E. Impact of functional endoscopic sinus surgery on symptoms and quality of life in chronic rhinosinusitis. Laryngoscope 2002; 112:310–5.

19. Khalid AN, Quraishi SA, Kennedy DW. Long-term quality of life measures after functional endoscopic sinus surgery. Am J Rhinol 2004; 18:131–6.
20. Khalil HS, Nunez DA. Functional endoscopic sinus surgery for chronic rhinosinusitis. Cochrane Database Syst Rev 2006; 3:CD004458.
21. Hartog B, Van Benthem PG, Prins LC, Horduk G. Efficacy of sinus irrigation versus sinus irrigation followed by endoscopic sinus surgery. Ann Otol Rhinol Laryngol 1997; 106:759–66.
22. Ragab SM, Lund VJ, Scadding G. Evaluation of the medical and surgical treatment of chronic rhinosinusitis: A prospective, randomized, controlled trial. Laryngoscope 2004; 114:923–30.
23. Ikeda K, Tanno N, Tamura G, et al. Endoscopic sinus surgery improves pulmonary function in patients with asthma associated with chronic sinusitis. Ann Otol Rhinol Laryngol 1999; 108:355–9.
24. Dunlop G, Scadding GK, Lund VJ. The effect of endoscopic sinus surgery on asthma: management of patients with chronic rhinosinusitis, nasal polyposis and asthma. Am J Rhinol 1999; 13:261–5.
25. Palmer JN, Conley DB, Dong RG, Ditto AM, Yarnold PR, Kern RC. Efficacy of endoscopic sinus surgery in the management of patients with asthma and chronic sinusitis. Am J Rhinol 2001; 15:49–53.
26. Senior BA, Kennedy DW, Tanabodee J, Kroger H, Hassab M, Lanza DC. Long-term impact of functional endoscopic sinus surgery on asthma. Otolaryngol Head Neck Surg 1999; 121:66–8.
27. Dejima K, Hama T, Miyazaki M, et al. A clinical study of endoscopic sinus surgery for sinusitis in patients with bronchial asthma. Int Arch Allergy Immunol 2005; 138:97–104.
28. Batra PS, Kern RC, Tripathi A, et al. Outcome analysis of endoscopic sinus surgery in patients with nasal polyps and asthma. Laryngoscope 2003; 113:1703–06.
29. Nakamura H, Kawasaki M, Higushi Y, Takahashi S. Effects of sinus surgery on asthma in aspirin triad patients. Acta Otolaryngol (Stockh) 1999; 119:592–98.
30. Dhong HJ, Jung YS, Chung SK, Choi DC. Effects of endoscopic sinus surgery on asthmatic patients with chronic rhinosinusitis. Otolaryngol Head Neck Surg 2001; 124:99–104.
31. Goldstein MF, Grundfast SK, Dunsky EH, Dvorin DJ, Lesser R. Effect of functional endoscopic sinus surgery on bronchial asthma outcomes. Arch Otolaryngol Head Neck Surg 1999; 125:314–19.
32. Zadeh MH, Banthia V, Anand VK, Huang C. Significance of eosinophilia in chronic rhinosinusitis. Am J Rhinol 2002; 16:313–7.
33. Sharp HR, Rowe-Jones JM, Mackay IS. The outcome of endoscopic sinus surgery: correlation with computerized tomography score and systemic disease. Clin Otolaryngol 1999; 24:39–42.
34. Lavigne F, Nguyen CT, Cameron L, Hamid Q, Renzi PM. Prognosis and prediction of response to surgery in allergic patients with chronic sinusitis. J Allergy Clin Immunol 2000; 105:746–51.
35. Baudoin T, Cupic H, Geber G, Vagic D, Grgic M, Kalogjera L. Histopathologic parameters as predictors of response to endoscopic sinus surgery in nonallergic patients with chronic rhinosinusitis. Otolaryngol Head Neck Surg 2006; 134:761–6.
36. Moran JV, Conley DB, Grammer LC, et al. Specific inflammatory cell types and disease severity as predictors of postsurgical outcomes in patients with chronic sinusitis. Allergy Asthma Proc 2003; 24:431–6.
37. Smith TL, Mendolia-Loffredo S, Loehrl TA, Sparapani R, Laud PW, Nattinger AB. Predictive factors and outcomes in endoscopic sinus surgery for chronic rhinosinusitis. Laryngoscope 2005; 115:2199–205.
38. Dursun E, Korkmaz H, Eryilmaz A, Bayiz U, Sertkaya D, Samim E. Clinical predictors of long-term success after endoscopic sinus surgery. Otolaryngol Head Neck Surg 2003; 129:526–31.
39. Watelet JB, Annicq B, Van Cauwenberge P, Bachert C. Objective outcome after functional endoscopic sinus surgery: prediction factors. Laryngoscope 2004; 114:1092–97.

40. Bhattacharyya N. Radiographic stage fails to predict symptom outcomes after endoscopic sinus surgery for chronic rhinosinusitis. Laryngoscope 2006; 116:17–22.
41. May M, Levine HL, Mester SJ, Schaitkin B. Complications of endoscopic sinus surgery: analysis of 2108 patients-incidence and prevention. Laryngoscope 1994; 104:1080–3.
42. Pinto JM, Elwany S, Baroody FM, Naclerio RM. Effects of saline sprays on symptoms after endoscopic sinus surgery. Am J Rhinol 2006; 20:191–6.
43. Lavigne F, Cameron L, Renzi PM, et al. Intrasinu administration of topical budesonide to allergic patients with chronic rhinosinusitis following surgery. Laryngoscope 2002; 112:857–64.
44. Rowe-Jones J, Medcalf M, Durham S, Richards D, Mackay IS. Functional endoscopic sinus surgery: 5 year follow up and results of a prospective, randomized, stratified, double-blind, placebo-controlled study of postoperative fluticasone propionate aqueous nasal spray. Rhinology 2005; 43:2–10.
45. Kennedy DW, Kuhn FA, Hamilos DL, et al. Treatment of chronic rhinosinusitis with high-dose oral terbinafine: a double blind, placebo-controlled study. Laryngoscope 2005; 115:1793–9.
46. Ebbens FA, Scadding GK, Badia L, et al. Amphotericin B nasal lavages: Not a solution for patients with chronic rhinosinusitis. J Allergy Clin Immunol. 2006; 118:1149–56.
47. Vaughan WC, Carvalho G. Use of nebulized antibiotics for acute infections in chronic sinusitis. Otolaryngology Head Neck Surgery 2002; 127:557–68.
48. Desrosiers MY, Salas-Prato M. Treatment of chronic rhinosinusitis refractory to other treatments with topical antibiotic therapy delivered by means of a large-particle nebulizer: results of a controlled trial. Otolaryngol Head Neck Surg 2001; 125:265–9.
49. Hissaria P, Smith W, Wormald PJ, et al. Short course of systemic corticosteroids in sinonasal polyposis: a double-blind, randomized, placebo-controlled trial with evaluation of outcome measures. J Allergy Clin Immunol 2006; 118:127–33.
50. Rowe-Jones JM, Mackay IS. Endoscopic sinus surgery in the treatment of cystic fibrosis with nasal polyposis. Laryngoscope 1996; 106:1540–4.
51. Moss RB, King VV. Management of sinusitis in cystic fibrosis by endoscopic surgery and serial antimicrobial lavage: reduction in recurrence requiring surgery. Arch Otolaryngol Head Neck Surg 1995; 121:566–72.
52. Wang X, Moylan B, Leopold DA, et al. Mutation in the gene responsible for cystic fibrosis and predisposition to chronic rhinosinusitis in the general population. JAMA 2000; 284:1814–9.

Index

About the Editors

DANIEL L. HAMILOS is Associate Professor of Medicine, Harvard Medical School, and a member of the Division of Rheumatology, Allergy, and Immunology, Massachusetts General Hospital, Boston, Massachusetts, U.S.A. Dr. Hamilos conducts clinical investigations into the immunopathology of chronic rhinosinusitis and nasal polyposis. He is a fellow of the American Academy of Allergy Asthma and Immunology, the American College of Physicians, and the American College of Allergy Asthma and Immunology. Dr. Hamilos received the M.D. degree from Northwestern University in Chicago, Illinois, U.S.A., and his postgraduate training at Washington University School of Medicine in St. Louis, Missouri, U.S.A. He has authored or coauthored more than 50 peer reviewed scientific articles.

FUAD M. BAROODY is Associate Professor of Otolaryngology—Head and Neck Surgery and Pediatrics, and Director of Pediatric Otolaryngology, University of Chicago, Illinois, U.S.A. An expert pediatric head and neck surgeon specializing in allergic rhinitis, sinusitis, and other pediatric disorders, Dr. Baroody conducts research into the pathophysiology and treatment of allergic rhinitis and rhinosinusitis. He is a fellow of the American Academy of Otolaryngology—Head and Neck Surgery, the American Academy of Asthma, Allergy, and Immunology, and the American College of Surgeons, and is a member of the American Society of Pediatric Otolaryngology. Dr. Baroody is the author of more than 80 peer reviewed scientific articles and 19 book chapters on allergic diseases. Dr. Baroody received the M.D. degree from the American University of Beirut, Lebanon, and postgraduate training at the Johns Hopkins University in Baltimore, Maryland, U.S.A.